# The Best Country to Give Birth?

'*The Best Country to Give Birth?* is an extremely good scholarly account of a critical period of change in New Zealand's maternity history. It is thoroughly researched and highly readable. The work is comprehensive, including detailed descriptions of the key events that led to massive changes in the provision of maternity services in this country. As such it is impressive and likely to be a reference for researchers and interested readers alike. Its reception will also be explosive, or at least seen in some quarters as controversial, as it exposes for the first time the political influences at work behind the changes described – but it is factual and totally defendable.'

— Emeritus Professor Peter Stone, Obstetrics and Gynaecology, University of Auckland

'This book examines the changes in midwifery in New Zealand since 1990, relating the unique circumstances that meant there was surprisingly little co-ordinated opposition to the reforms: a subdued obstetric profession, a no-fault medical compensation scheme, an early failure legally to define normal birth, and a rapid change in the nature of midwifery training. Unusual for a study of a profession, the book gives voice to its consumers, and, even more unusual, to their babies. The writing style is clear and accessible and the story is compelling – this will be a thought-provoking addition to midwifery literature.'

— Dr Alison Nuttall, History, University of Edinburgh

'This is a careful, judicious, deeply researched demolition of a retrograde turn in modern attitudes to medicine and science. The story it tells is a scandal where a modern country with an excellent health system allowed itself to be taken over by a self-interested lobby group driven by ideology and science denial. This was an occupational turf war dressed up as liberation of women from male domination, except that mothers and babies died. Readers will detect a clear line from this rejection of biomedicine in childbirth to the anti-vax movement of the Covid pandemic. A quietly spoken book with a shocking story to tell, *The Best Country to Give Birth?* is a crucial step forward in the advancement of reproductive rights, women's health and good medical practice.'

— Emeritus Professor Janet McCalman AC, Population and Global Health, University of Melbourne

'With careful research and meticulous attention to detail, Bryder presents a readable narrative of the intricacies of maternity care in New Zealand over the past several decades. Every statement is well referenced, every argument well put. Bryder demonstrates how, over many years, politics frequently overrode the interests of mothers' and babies' health, often with tragic results for families, and shows how the current situation is still far from perfect. The answer to her question "is New Zealand the best place in the world to give birth?" must still be a resounding "no".'

— Professor Caroline de Costa, Obstetrics and Gynaecology, James Cook University

# The Best Country to Give Birth?

*Midwifery, Homebirth and the Politics of Maternity
in Aotearoa New Zealand, 1970–2022*

LINDA BRYDER

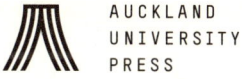

First published 2023
Auckland University Press
University of Auckland
Private Bag 92019
Auckland 1142
New Zealand
www.aucklanduniversitypress.co.nz

© Linda Bryder, 2023

ISBN 978 1 77671 108 6

A catalogue record for this book is available from the National Library of New Zealand

This book is copyright. Apart from fair dealing for the purpose of private study, research, criticism or review, as permitted under the Copyright Act, no part may be reproduced by any process without prior permission of the publisher. The moral rights of the author have been asserted.

Book design by Carolyn Lewis

Cover image: 'Newborn baby with mother', photograph by Cara Dolan, Stocksy

This book was printed on FSC® certified paper

Printed in Singapore by Markono Print Media Pte Ltd

*I dedicate this book to my wonderful sons,
Dennis (born 1992) and Marty (born 1997).*

# CONTENTS

Introduction     1

| | | |
|---|---|---|
| ONE | Homebirth 1970s-style | 7 |
| TWO | 'Everyone should do it': Why choose homebirth? | 30 |
| THREE | Homebirth and maternity services 1970–1990 | 49 |
| FOUR | The meaning of autonomy for homebirth midwives in the 1980s | 70 |
| FIVE | 'A highly focused and effective campaign': Homebirth as a political movement in the 1980s | 89 |
| SIX | The 1990 Nurses Amendment Act and midwife autonomy | 113 |
| SEVEN | Midwifery autonomy and partnership in the 1990s | 137 |
| EIGHT | The politics of maternity services and 'shared care' after 1990 | 157 |
| NINE | The practice of midwifery and the 'midwifery model' in the 1990s | 182 |
| TEN | The new century: 'When things go wrong' | 207 |
| ELEVEN | Maternity system under fire: The Midwifery Council's first decade | 230 |
| TWELVE | Research into maternity outcomes during the 2010s | 251 |

Conclusion: 'NZ – the best place to give birth?'     276

Notes     286

Bibliography     365

Index     380

# INTRODUCTION

IN 2012, FOLLOWING HIS investigation of the deaths of two babies in childbirth at Waikato Hospital, Hamilton coroner Gordon Matenga asked, 'Does New Zealand have the safe, world-leading system the Government says we do, or are we losing babies because the balance has swung too far towards the idea that because childbirth is natural, then the philosophy of "non-intervention" is best?'. 'Babies' deaths reignite maternity row', the *New Zealand Herald* announced.[1]

This 'maternity row' over how mothers and babies should best be cared for during pregnancy and childbirth was a deep and divisive debate in New Zealand. It has a long history and forms the subject of this book.

To understand this row one must go back to the start of the homebirth movement in the 1970s. The tenets of that movement provided the foundational philosophy behind much midwifery practice in this country over the following decades. The 1990 Nurses Amendment Act, which forms the centrepiece of this book, was the moment the direction of childbirth services in New Zealand changed irrevocably. This Act gave midwives the same status in childbirth services as general practitioners (GPs), allowing them to practise independently in the community, and paved the way for new direct-entry midwifery training programmes (meaning prior nurse training was no longer required). The reform was widely acclaimed internationally and by the newly established New Zealand College of Midwives as liberating

New Zealand midwives from the shackles of medicine and nursing, and as recognising midwifery as an independent profession.

The first half of this book is devoted to explaining the genesis of this important reform, the result of a highly orchestrated campaign by a small group of homebirth midwives and homebirth activists led by the self-proclaimed socialist and radical feminist homebirth midwife Joan Donley.[2] In the first two chapters I outline and unpack the values and beliefs underpinning the homebirth movement. The campaign was part of and drew inspiration from an international feminist homebirth movement showcased at the first International Homebirth Conference in London in 1987. In Chapter 3, I examine the responses to the new movement by those overseeing New Zealand's maternity services: the Board of Health's Maternity Services Committee and the New Zealand Nurses' Association. In doing so, I consider their attempts to accommodate homebirth within existing structures and their suggestions for a possible path forward. This did not satisfy the homebirth lobby, which interpreted their actions as an attempt to shut down the homebirth option in the interests of medical control. Chapters 4 and 5 set out the demands of homebirth activists and their extensive and effective lobbying campaign. In Chapter 5, I also explore the social and political climate of the 1980s which allowed the homebirth lobby to gain such traction. The introduction of 'midwifery autonomy', 'midwifed' through Parliament in 1990 by Labour's Minister of Health Helen Clark, forms the subject of Chapter 6.[3]

The 1990 Nurses Amendment Act was designed to give all women the choice of homebirth, with politicians persuaded that this was what women wanted. As it turned out, most didn't, and homebirth never rose above 3% to 4% of all births. Nevertheless, the tenets of the homebirth movement – natural childbirth and women's empowerment through their birthing experience – remained core to the philosophy of the New Zealand College of Midwives, set up in 1989 as the overseeing body of midwifery in New Zealand. In Chapters 7–9 I investigate the immediate aftermath of the 1990 Act as the new system of midwifery autonomy was embedded, with so-called independent or self-employed midwives setting up practice in the community. Chapter 7 explores the College's understanding of midwifery practice as a partnership with birthing mothers, how this was viewed by others within childbirth services and how it played out in practice. The College continued to enjoy government support, and Chapter 8 outlines how a new funding system consolidated independent midwives' primacy in maternity services in the 1990s, ousting GPs, in the face of considerable opposition from GPs themselves as well as some midwives and consumers. In Chapter 9, I turn to other issues arising from what the College labelled the midwifery model of childbirth as opposed to the medical model, with the former underpinning the teaching in the new midwifery programmes. I investigate frictions which adherence to the midwifery model caused when it came to independent midwives' interactions with hospital medicine and with medical technology, including early childhood immunisation. The College and the Ministry of Health in the 1990s celebrated New Zealand's unique woman-centred midwifery-led system, but not everyone saw it as a cause for celebration, believing that safety was being compromised in the interests of an anti-medical or 'natural birth' philosophy.

The final three chapters look to the early twenty-first century to see whether those tensions of the 1990s were resolved once midwifery got its own regulatory body, the Midwifery Council, set up in 2004. I examine growing concerns emanating from a number of quarters, and the responses of midwifery leaders. Chapter 10 considers the findings of coroners and health and disability commissioners tasked with investigating when things went wrong; these attracted considerable public attention. Chapter 11 turns to other platforms of discontent, focusing on systemic issues rather than individual cases. These included qualms about midwifery training and mentoring, and practices in the midwife-run maternity primary-care units. In this chapter, I consider appeals from new consumer groups, primarily formed by parents who had experienced adverse events in childbirth. Chapter 12 investigates significant academic research and the reports of the government's Perinatal and Maternal Mortality Review Committee from 2007 and their findings of inequities across population sectors, including New Zealand's Māori population. Across these three chapters, I look to responses by midwifery leaders and the Ministry of Health to these manifold criticisms.

This book is the first comprehensive study of an important period in the history of New Zealand's childbirth policies and services and the debates underpinning them. In 2008, GP obstetrician Lynda Exton charted policy changes in maternity services from 1990, specifically from the perspective of GP obstetricians who were increasingly excluded as providers of those services.[4] In 2010, two leading midwives, Karen Guilliland and Sally Pairman, examined maternity policy from a midwifery perspective in their in-depth history of the New Zealand College of Midwives.[5] This book sets out policy changes over a longer timeframe than these previous studies, encompassing 50 years from 1970, and draws on evidence from all sectors including midwives, nurses, doctors and above all consumers – the mothers, babies and their whānau (families) for whom the services were constructed.

Maternity care was, and is, a highly politicised area of healthcare, and one in which the stakes are high. This book shows that, while most births proceed without mishap, the results are tragic and life-changing for the entire family when they do not. It is even worse when those adverse outcomes are deemed to be preventable. The repercussions of the changes to the maternity system introduced in 1990 and entrenched in the following decades have been contentious and remain the subject of much debate. This includes two recent commentators who offered evaluations of the current issues facing midwifery in New Zealand. In June 2021 freelance journalist Sally Blundell contributed an article entitled 'NZ – the best place to give birth?' to *Newsroom*, which describes itself as 'an independent, New Zealand-based news and current affairs site [which delivers] . . . in-depth storytelling for thinking audiences'. Her title reflected an upbeat assessment offered by the New Zealand College of Midwives.[6] In contrast to this, Ollie Neas, a Wellington barrister and freelance writer, penned an article titled 'Risky Business' for the investigative magazine *North & South* in May 2022. This article examined issues faced by midwifery services and claimed that birth 'doesn't need to be this risky.'[7] This book explores how and why the nature of these services became so contested and whether Aotearoa New Zealand can rightfully claim to be the best country in which to give birth.

# ONE

## Homebirth 1970s-style

THE HOMEBIRTH MOVEMENT WAS to play a central role in the build-up to the 1990 Nurses Amendment Act which changed the face of maternity services in New Zealand, and it continued to influence those services well beyond 1990, even though homebirth itself remained a minority activity. It is therefore important to investigate the nature of this movement which the government so enthusiastically endorsed in 1990 and in the years that followed. This chapter will do so by profiling its participants, both clients and practitioners, investigating what homebirth meant to them. It will be shown that it was so much more than a decision about where to give birth.

### From home to hospital and back again

By the 1970s, most mothers in New Zealand, as elsewhere in the Western world, gave birth in hospital. This had not always been the case. A century earlier most had birthed at home. The move from home to hospital was driven by two developments. The first was anaesthesia. Chloroform was discovered in the mid-nineteenth century and became widely accepted in childbirth after Queen Victoria famously used it at the birth of her eighth child in 1853. Other methods of pain relief followed, and by the twentieth century women began to demand it as of right. This effectively meant birthing in hospital. The second development, the discovery of bacteriology or the germ theory of disease in the late nineteenth century, led to a safer hospital environment, adding to the attraction of hospital birth. In New Zealand, the Health Department launched a Safe Maternity Campaign in the 1920s, instructing nurses and midwives in the importance of a germ-free environment and separating birthing mothers from surgical patients. This significantly reduced the death rate from the major cause of mortality in childbirth at the time – puerperal sepsis, commonly known as childbed fever.[1]

Women themselves played a prominent role in the move from home to hospital births in New Zealand as elsewhere.[2] By the 1920s about 35% of all births in New Zealand occurred in hospital (including institutions with two or more beds), and this rose to almost 82% by 1937, compared with only 15% to 25% in England and Wales at that time.[3] Women who gave evidence to New Zealand's 1938 Inquiry into Maternity Services suggested that among the reasons women wanted to birth in hospital were the availability of pain relief and a sense of greater safety there. The First Labour Government had come to office in 1935 promising welfare 'from the cradle to the grave', and women lobbied for universal free maternity care in hospital. The maternity benefit introduced in 1939 provided women with 14 days of free care at childbirth, at home or in hospital, and most chose the latter. Fully 92.5% of all births in the first year after the introduction of the benefit occurred in hospital.[4]

It was, however, scientific developments in obstetrics from the 1930s onwards that clinched the hospital as the preferred place of birth for many. Starting with the discovery of the sulphonamides to treat puerperal sepsis in the 1930s, other advances followed. These included the drugs ergometrine and oxytocin (with others known collectively as ecbolics) used in the third stage of labour to prevent or treat postpartum haemorrhage (bleeding after childbirth), along with penicillin and other antibiotics to control infections, improved blood transfusion methods, better antenatal care for eclamptic toxaemia, and less invasive forms of pain relief such as epidural anaesthesia. The post-Second World War period also witnessed improvements in the care of the newborn, with the setting up of neonatal wards, initially called premature units, reflecting prematurity as the major cause of illness and death amongst the newborn. These wards increasingly housed incubators, and offered other forms of treatment such as exchange blood transfusion for Rhesus haemolytic disease from the 1950s and corticosteroids for respiratory distress disorder from the 1970s, significantly enhancing survival rates. Improved diagnostic techniques at childbirth such as ultrasound scans and fetal heart monitoring were also developed from the 1950s onwards.

There was a steep and constant decline in maternal mortality from the 1930s, leading British maternity historian Irvine Loudon to claim that the conquest of maternal mortality from the mid-1930s had been 'one of the most remarkable achievements of modern medicine'.[5] While acknowledging the contribution of broader social factors, New Zealand neonatologist Ross Howie called improvements in the survival rate of babies from the early 1950s 'one of the greatest success stories of public health in this country and arguably the greatest achievement' of New Zealand's National Women's Hospital where he worked.[6]

Most New Zealand women chose to take advantage of this modern technology. There was, for example, widespread celebration at the opening in 1964 of National Women's Hospital, the largest purpose-built maternity hospital in the southern hemisphere, for which women had lobbied. As midwife Dorothy McAleer, who was working there when it opened, later said, 'Everybody wanted to have their baby at National Women's.'[7] In 1960, 93% of all Pākehā women and 90% of all Māori women gave birth in hospital; by the end of that decade, it was almost universal for both.[8]

Hospital training for midwives had begun with the 1904 Midwives Registration Act which provided for the training and registration of midwives in the world's first state maternity hospitals, the St Helen's hospitals set up following the Act. Dr Duncan MacGregor, Inspector-General of Hospitals and Charitable Institutions, declared that with the passing of this Act, 'the day of the dirty, ignorant, careless woman, who has brought death or ill health to many mothers and infants, will soon end'.[9] While this was offensive to many former excellent midwives, it was indicative of the Western professionalisation of nursing and midwifery, based on modern hygienic practices. The 1904 Act allowed practising midwives without formal training to continue working, but regulations were tightened by the 1925 Nurses and Midwives Registration Act which established two routes of entry to midwifery training and registration. One followed general nurse training; the other followed maternity nurse training, which had lower entry requirements. This effectively meant that some midwives did not have a general nursing background, and it remained the case until the 1970s, when all new entrants to midwifery training had to have a nursing degree first and midwifery became a postgraduate course.

The seven St Helen's hospitals set up around the country in the early twentieth century provided subsidised care for the wives of working men either at home or in hospital. Both options continued following the introduction of maternity benefits in 1939. Midwives conducting homebirths were known as district midwives or domiciliary midwives and were contracted to the Department of Health which oversaw the services. St Helen's hospitals stopped offering district services following the Second World War, owing to a lack of demand, but domiciliary midwives could continue to practise independently and be paid by the department.[10] The Board of Health's Maternity Services Committee, which was set up in 1960 to oversee childbirth services, recorded only eight domiciliary midwives working around the country by 1976; a 1980 estimate was just seven.[11]

The 1970s, a time when hospitals were considered by many women and midwives as central to maternity services, saw the kernel of a new social trend: a return to homebirths. While there were only 13 recorded planned homebirths in a population of over three million in 1973, there were 90 in 1975, and 289 in 1979. This latter figure was still only 0.6% of the 52,279 births in New Zealand that year but, commenting on the trend, the Maternity Services Committee noted that this total did not include homebirths where the domiciliary midwife was not contracted to the Department of Health or where the birth was conducted without professional assistance.[12]

A small group of domiciliary midwives led the trend. At their head was Auckland midwife Joan Donley, a Canadian-born nurse who immigrated to New Zealand in 1964, undertook midwifery training at Auckland's St Helen's Hospital in 1972 and conducted her first homebirth in 1974. Donley along with a handful of other domiciliary midwives helped to found associations around the country to promote the movement. The first appeared in Christchurch in 1976, and Auckland followed in 1978, leading to the founding of a national Home Birth Association (HBA) in 1980. Through its newsletter, the HBA publicised the number of homebirths; in 1985 it recorded only 300 (0.6% of total births) and 680 in 1988 (with 12% – or 82 – of the latter transferred to hospital).[13] Auckland led the way, with 45% of all planned homebirths in 1988, although this still amounted to less than 2% of births in Auckland.[14] In 1981, eight homebirth midwives set up their own professional organisation, the Domiciliary Midwives Society. They remained a small group, with just 35 practising midwives in 1987.[15] Despite its size and the fact most mothers still chose hospital birth, the homebirth movement was to have a major impact on New Zealand's maternity services over the following decades.

## The profile of homebirthers in the 1970s and 1980s

Almost all homebirth parents in the 1970s and 1980s were of European descent. A mid-1980s study pointed out that homebirths accounted for almost 1% of Pākehā births but only 0.02% of Māori births.[16] The HBA had its own analyst of homebirth statistics, Stan Gillanders, the Wellington HBA secretary's husband, who noted that Māori were under-represented in the homebirth movement.[17] He classified 'Maori' and 'Other' statistics for the first time in 1989, finding that in 1988 only 35 of 680 recorded homebirths (5%) were Māori, at a time when Māori made up about 12% of the population. These 35 homebirths (of whom three were transferred to hospital, one with postpartum haemorrhage) made up under 0.5% of 6,767 Māori births recorded that year. A 1987 Health Department report also commented that homebirth was an 'almost exclusively pakeha' movement.[18]

Another standout feature of homebirthers was that few smoked cigarettes, in marked contrast to the general population at that time. In 1980 Professor Dennis Bonham, head of the Postgraduate School of Obstetrics and Gynaecology at National Women's Hospital, noted that about 30% of European women and 75% of Māori women smoked in pregnancy; and a 1991 study found 68% of Māori women smoked in pregnancy.[19] This feature alone might have excluded many Māori women from the homebirth option, as Joan Donley stated in 1978: 'The midwives have a rule they won't attend women who smoke.'[20] The link between smoking in pregnancy and premature delivery and low birth weight, with their attendant health problems, was only just being recognised, possibly deterring homebirth midwives from taking on smokers. Nevertheless, a significant number slipped through the net; Gillanders noted in 1988 that 7.2% of its non-Māori and 36.4% of its Māori mothers were smokers.[21]

The homebirth movement rejected smoking not explicitly because of identified risks but in line with its overall health philosophy. Lyn McLean, a Wellington homebirth midwife, explained in 1980 that women who chose homebirth were 'generally highly motivated toward mental and physical health'.[22] Interviewed by the *New Zealand Woman's Weekly* following the first homebirth she attended in 1978, she explained how her clients were drawn to health foods.[23] The HBA commented in 1980 that these women were 'in tip top physical condition . . . They do not smoke, or take harmful drugs. They pay especial attention to their diet and prepare calmly for their labours with the invaluable help of their partners.'[24] Homebirth midwife Sian Burgess later reflected that the women she and other midwives looked after 'seemed to be so extraordinarily knowledgeable. They were knowledgeable about homeopathy and herbs and nutrition . . .'[25]

Others, too, noted this interest in nutrition. In 1982, as part of a Massey University course, Dave West, a member of the Wellington HBA whose wife had just given birth at home, surveyed 37 couples who chose homebirth. He found that many of them were vegetarian or ate little meat, and 'all were keen to avoid processed and packaged foods, preservatives, food additives and chemicals, and chose a diet high in fresh and raw fruit and vegetables, wholefoods and grains'.[26]

Another feature identified by the HBA was that most homebirth parents were in stable relationships (over 90% for Pākehā and 85.7% for Māori in 1988).[27] West too noted this, and also that 'most home birth fathers are actively involved in the antenatal care and preparation of their ladies'.[28] This was consistent with the comment by a father whose involvement in his wife's homebirth was reported in the *New Zealand Woman's Weekly* in 1978: 'I felt totally involved this time,' said Ralph. 'It was my birth as much as it was Nikki's.'[29] The homebirth movement encouraged this; at its 1982 annual conference, the HBA ran a workshop on 'The New Fatherhood – Tenderness in Men'.[30] A 1986 article in the local feminist magazine *Broadsheet* commented: 'Motivation for a homebirth in some cases comes from a partner, willing to accept responsibilities which men would previously have been unhappy about.'[31]

West also found that homebirthers expressed a desire to live cooperatively. He noted their greater involvement in social and political movements such as trade unions and Amnesty International, and that they seemed to have fewer religious affiliations than the general population. Investigating 'occupation and education', he found that both homebirth mothers and fathers tended to be 'more heavily weighted toward the professional group than is the norm'. Half of his respondents were university graduates, and half of these had postgraduate qualifications.[32] Gillanders concurred; in 1988, he found that 58.4% of the non-Māori and 25.3% of the Māori mothers recorded as having homebirths had tertiary education – well above national averages.[33] This profile fits the two women who helped to set up the Auckland HBA, which held its inaugural meeting at the University of Auckland.[34] Derryn Cooper, who had a homebirth in 1978, was a psychology lecturer at the university; her husband Geoff Bridgman was a child psychologist and also involved in the HBA.[35] Barbara Macfarlane, who had had three homebirths by 1989, was a practising lawyer.[36] Joan Donley spoke quite frankly in 1986 of the women coming from 'a higher income bracket'.[37] She reinforced this in a later interview when she said, 'All the women that we look after are middle class and can afford this and that.'[38]

In other words, the profile of those who chose homebirth was: educated (many university graduates), non-smokers, in 'tip top' health, very careful about their diet, predominantly Pākehā, and in stable relationships with partners who also supported homebirth. Homebirth doctor John Grieve called them a 'highly motivated group of women'.[39] A 1990 homebirth survey published in the *Medical Journal of Australia* found homebirthers there were 'older, and wealthier than the average', and that '[v]ery high proportions neither smoke tobacco nor drink, but a significant minority use marijuana'.[40]

## Homebirth and counterculture

Wellington homebirth midwife Lyn McLean commented in 1980 that those opting for homebirth 'may be counter-culture to some degree'.[41] The Auckland HBA described its membership in the 1980s as 'made up predominantly of women and with anti-establishment values and goals'.[42]

The counterculture movement, which emerged across the Western world in the 1960s and 1970s, rejected conventional society and the values of the modern technocratic age. Those embracing the movement were sometimes known as hippies. Some in New Zealand, following the United States, lived collectively in communes where they sought to be self-sufficient, and for a short time gained government support under the Third Labour Government (1972–75). Prime Minister Norman Kirk, a man of strong spiritual convictions, set up a scheme in 1973 to accommodate communities on Crown land, and viewed a kibbutz-type environment as an antidote to the materialism of modern society.[43] The scheme, called Ohu, attracted much interest from alternative lifestylers, but only eight were established before the succeeding

National government dropped the scheme. Many more communes were set up privately or through trusts.

Homebirth was a central part of their rejection of mainstream culture. In 1979, the Maternity Services Committee noted that some medical officers of health and public health nurses had expressed concern that they had no information on births in some of the country's communes, which meant they were unaware of any deaths.[44] The Committee expanded on this concern in a 1982 report on homebirths, under the heading 'Alternative Life Style Deliveries'. It had found individuals who, based on ideological grounds, were not prepared under any circumstances to consider hospital births, regardless of complications or the risk to themselves or to their babies. The Committee commented that the environment in which deliveries took place was often unsuitable, 'with no running water and substandard sanitation and hygiene'.[45]

Some homebirth midwives were also involved with the counterculture movement and lived in communes. For her 2007 PhD thesis, homebirth midwife Maggie Banks interviewed eight of her homebirth colleagues. She found that one, who practised homebirth from 1978, had been exposed to the idea by social contacts in an 'alternative life-style community where home birth was the norm'.[46] Banks also noted that the seed for homebirth practice for midwife Anne Sharplin occurred when a good friend acted as a lay (unregistered) midwife for women in an alternative community in 1976.[47] Two Auckland homebirth midwives, Rhonda Evans (later Jackson) and Yvette Watson, resided at the Centrepoint Community in Albany, north of Auckland, founded in 1979 by self-proclaimed therapist Bert Potter.[48] Christchurch midwife Ursula Helem's first homebirth was in 1974 for a couple at Springbank Christian Community in North Canterbury (which eventually relocated and became Gloriavale Christian Community).[49]

Homebirth midwife Bronwen Pelvin told her how she had hated the regimentation of nurse training in the 1970s, explaining:

> Of course it was the Woodstock era and I was very drawn to peace and love and music and all that. People thought I was a bit weird and [during study] I started dressing in hippie-type clothes, you know, long skirts and tie dyed calico – things that I'd made myself and all that . . .[50]

Following nurse training, Pelvin attended her first homebirth in 1974 at an alternative community near the Whanganui River called Jerusalem (a commune founded by renowned poet James K. Baxter in 1969), and was inspired to become a midwife. She trained at Christchurch Women's Hospital in 1976 and worked at Palmerston North Hospital for 15 months before a friend wanting to birth at home in Canvastown outside Nelson sought a midwife.[51] Pelvin then embarked on her career as a homebirth midwife at the Riverside Community in Lower Moutere, Nelson.[52]

Riverside had originally been set up by a group of Methodist pacifists as a cooperative 'intentional community' in 1941, and by the late 1960s its membership was largely middle aged to elderly. This was to change with an influx of people interested in communal ways of living in the 1970s and after the commune had dropped the requirement that members should be practising members of a Christian church. The period 1970–90 saw 126 people join the community, but only 40 of those stayed beyond a probationary period. It was not a large community; in 1972, there were 22 adult members and 10 children, and in 1990, 33 adult members and 32 children.[53]

Pelvin was a member of Riverside from 1980 to 1990, and a 1991 history of the community explained that since 1980 most Riverside children had been born at home.[54] In 1985 Pelvin recorded that she was 'ever grateful for the support of Riverside Community, without whom I would find it hard to continue'.[55] On her departure in 1991 she wrote them a poem in tribute.[56] The Riverside Community was also the address of the Nelson HBA from 1980, and hosted the 1991 meeting of the Domiciliary Midwives Society prior to the HBA national conference at Bridge Valley Christian Ranch, Nelson.[57]

Nelson district was a hub for communes, housing at least 12 by the 1970s. Pelvin lamented in 1982 that despite the number of alternative-lifestyle people in the region, they tended to be 'conservative about home birth'.[58] Here, as elsewhere, not all alternative lifestylers favoured homebirth, nor were all homebirth midwives drawn to the counterculture. Reflecting on her career, Lynley McFarland commented, 'It was frightening that people classed me as a hippie because I was attending home births.'[59]

Coromandel was another location for those choosing an alternative lifestyle. A midwife who worked in the small Coromandel hospital (with just five maternity beds) from 1966 to 1990 later recalled, '[T]here were quite a few communes up here, 30 years ago and those girls wanted to go without anything, but when it came to the screaming and the shouting they changed their minds, and boy could they shout!'[60]

Dr Christopher Harison, who worked at Thames Hospital, the peninsula's base hospital, was strongly opposed to homebirth and wrote a submission to a Maternity Services Committee inquiry into homebirths in 1980. Drawing on information he received from three or four alternative-lifestyle doctors, he wrote that at one large commune set up around 1970, couples were free, in theory, to make up their own minds about where to birth, and yet group discussions at which horrific tales about hospital delivery were recounted would make it very difficult to choose that option. He also commented on the power of the commune 'father figure'. Harison described numerous occasions when tensions arose over the use of forceps and the handling of breech presentations, for example, when women did end up in hospital. This was, he said, stressful for all concerned. He gave examples of women having to go to hospital postnatally, and described the 'considerable unpleasantness . . . experienced from the accompanying friends'.[61] Harison was not alone. In Nelson in 1982, two obstetricians remarked on the difficulty of treating 'uncooperative and untrusting homebirthers'.[62]

In the wake of the world-famous Woodstock music festival in America in 1969, New Zealand hosted its own Nambassa festivals on farms near Waihī and Waikino from 1978 to 1981. At its peak in 1979, Nambassa attracted over 65,000 attendees.[63] These festivals were premised on concepts of peace and love, and offered not only music but also workshops and displays advocating alternative lifestyles and medicines. One of the 'cultural guests' at the festivals in 1978, 1979 and 1981 was American Stephen Gaskin.[64] In 1978 and 1981, his wife Ina May Gaskin, a lay midwife and author of a homebirth manual *Spiritual Midwifery*, accompanied him, causing much excitement within New Zealand's homebirth circles.

Homebirth midwife Kiet Moonen attended the 1981 five-day event and soaked up the atmosphere, relating how the 15,000 attendees 'lived peacefully together on a beautiful site . . . and shared a wide variety of experiences . . . no-one stopped smiling'. She explained how each day there were well-attended talks, workshops, films and discussions on homebirth; a two-hour homebirth panel attracted 600 people. Members of the panel included Moonen herself, Helen Brew (co-producer of a 1977 film with R. D. Laing, see below), Waimauku homebirth GP John Nealie, and 'consumer' Rukmini Venkataiah. The star of the panel was Ina May Gaskin, whom Moonen described as a 'tremendously good midwife . . . she's totally untrained officially, all her training is through reading and practical experience'.[65]

Gaskin had helped her husband Stephen found The Farm, a self-sustaining community in Tennessee, where they settled in 1971 after Stephen had toured America with more than 200 followers in a convoy of school buses to promote his spiritual and social revolution. Wendy Kline explained in her history of the homebirth movement in America that up to 750,000 Americans lived in around 10,000 communes in the early 1970s, although few survived as long as The Farm.[66] Kline related how, for Gaskin and his company, childbirth became a 'community event, a source of spiritual awakening and transcendence, and even a psychedelic experience'. She described how, on his pilgrimage, what 'started as an experiment in alternative birthing became an established profession, a blending of spiritual theories, trial and error, and medical advice'.[67] It was at The Farm that Ina May Gaskin launched her career in midwifery, set up a birthing centre and published *Spiritual Midwifery*. Kline noted that many stories featured in *Spiritual Midwifery* referred to communal out-of-body experiences. In this context, she wrote, 'birth was truly a communal experience – not just witnessed by others, but felt by others as well', which made it transformative.[68] In her history of the alternative birthing technique known as Lamaze, Paula Michaels also referred to The Farm. Lamaze is a system of childbirth without medication promoted by French obstetrician Ferdinand Lamaze from the 1950s, and it became popular with American parents in the 1970s. Michaels wrote that the use of Lamaze in homebirth, attended by a midwife and 'imbued with mysticism, marked a new turn in childbirth experience', and she pointed to The Farm as 'a particularly vivid and prominent example' of this kind of 'social birth'.[69]

Gaskin made it clear to midwives that they should be 'avid students of physiology and medicine', consult doctors and take their client to hospital if necessary. Nevertheless, as her book's title makes clear, her philosophy was infused with spiritual and religious overtones. She described The Farm as a church. She told midwives they should 'take spiritual vows just the same as a yogi or a monk or a nun', and that 'love and compassion and spiritual vision' were the most important tools of their trade. The spiritual midwife was not to charge for her service, as this would undermine its spirituality.[70]

New Zealand midwives were well aware of Gaskin and her book, whether or not they encountered her at Nambassa. Years later, in 2004, midwifery lecturer Jean Patterson wrote in the *New Zealand College of Midwives Journal*, 'Who can forget the impact of Ina May's "Spiritual Midwifery" published in 1975? Every midwife I knew had at least heard of it, read it or owned it. Many well thumbed and tea stained copies remain on bookshelves as testament to its popularity and appeal.'[71] Jane Stojanovic, a midwife who started attending homebirths in 1988, explained in her PhD thesis that *Spiritual Midwifery* was influential in the re-emergence of the homebirth movement in New Zealand in the late 1970s and 1980s.[72] Maggie Banks related how one of the homebirth midwives she interviewed said that a friend had given her a copy of Gaskin's book to ensure she became 'the right sort of midwife'. Another told Banks that she had been exposed to homebirth 'in her everyday reading of books such as *Spiritual Midwifery*'. Bronwen Pelvin recalled taking *Spiritual Midwifery* to work with her when she was a midwife at Palmerston North Hospital in the late 1970s.[73] Homebirth mothers knew of it too; in his 1980 submission to the Maternity Services Committee, Harison appended a letter written by a homebirth mother in a Coromandel commune – top of her reading list was Gaskin's book.[74] The book was number two of 10 recommended readings for mothers at Centrepoint Community in 1982.[75] Gaskin's popularity persisted into the next century. Pelvin contributed a chapter on 'Life skills for midwifery practice' to a 2006 midwifery textbook, and one of the four items on her recommended reading list was Gaskin's book. It also appeared in the reference list for a chapter in the same textbook by two New Zealand midwifery lecturers, Sally Pairman and Judith McAra-Couper.[76] Personal connections persisted too. New Zealand homebirth midwives kept in touch with Gaskin, with Rhonda Jackson, who lived at Centrepoint, visiting The Farm in 1986, and Christchurch's Maria Ware visiting in 1989.[77]

Also present at Nambassa in 1981 was Helen Brew, a founder of New Zealand's natural childbirth association, Parents Centre, in 1952. Brew abhorred hospital birth. In a talk she gave in 1958 she said of homebirths that 'the maternal and fetal death rates were high but were not probably also the satisfactions of motherhood?'. By contrast, in hospital, she declared, the woman 'often feels like a body or pregnant uterus on a conveyor belt'.[78] Parents Centre itself did not reject hospital birth and the use of modern technology, but sought to make childbirth a more pleasant experience for women. Brew found a more receptive audience in the 1970s. In 1977 she collaborated with Scottish psychiatrist and well-known critic of modern psychiatry, Dr R. D. Laing on a 57-minute documentary filmed in hospitals around Wellington and the Hutt Valley. Brew and Laing had met at a conference in London several years before, and made the film whilst Laing was visiting New Zealand as the Vice-Chancellor's Lecturer at Victoria University of Wellington. Entitled *Birth with R D Laing*, the film included footage of more than 12 births and interviews with young parents. Brew was producer and Laing provided the commentary, telling his audience that hospital childbirth was 'one of the disaster areas of our culture'.[79] Screened on TV1 on 24 October 1977, it won the Feltex award for best documentary for 1977 and the Best TV Film at a 1978 Melbourne Festival. One review explained that the film 'caused a row about delivery methods . . . and created interest in home birth'.[80] Brew, like Gaskin, received a warm reception at Nambassa.

## The 'homebirth package'

One of the requirements when opting for homebirth was self-responsibility. As Brenda Hinton, editor of the HBA's newsletter and herself a childbirth educator, explained, 'Women who choose to give birth at home must take responsibility for their own health during pregnancy and prepare themselves physically and emotionally for labour and birth.'[81] In this advocacy, the movement gained endorsement from the renowned Jesuit philosopher Ivan Illich. In his influential 1975 book *Medical Nemesis*, Illich railed against the evils of modern medical technology and exhorted people to take responsibility for their own health.[82] He visited New Zealand in 1978 as the University of Auckland Douglas Robb Memorial Lecturer. Joan Donley approvingly reported him as saying, 'Hospitalisation of birth is among the most powerful ways people are deprived of their own health care.'[83]

While mothers were exhorted to take charge, they were nevertheless given an explicit set of instructions to follow. This is evident in an account from 1975 in the feminist magazine *Broadsheet* by Kitty Wishart, homebirth mother and member of the Auckland Women's Liberation Group formed at the University of Auckland in 1970. Wishart outlined her experiences of giving birth at home under Donley's watch. She described how, during the last three months of pregnancy, she 'knocked back substantial quantities of Vitamin E, Yeast and Raspberry Leaf tea, followed Adelle Davis's "Let's have healthy children" as far as I was able, and hoped that combination would keep me fit'. Donley had also provided her with 'a source of free Black Strap molasses for iron requirements'. At a check-up a week before the due date, she had an elevated blood pressure, and Donley suggested certain herbs and exercises, and booked her to see an acupuncturist. Wishart occupied herself during early labour 'reading my Lamaze method book, practising my breathing at each contraction, sipping the herbal tonic provided by the acupuncturist'. She did have a mild analgesic (unspecified) and had to have one stitch following the birth. Donley's midwifery partner, Carolyn Young, also attended the birth. During the two weeks after the birth, Wishart took 'brandy, yeast and cashew nuts to keep up the breast milk'.[84] Her supplements and treatments were typical of the homebirth package or toolkit.

First, a careful diet was crucial for a homebirthing mother. As midwife Lyn McLean explained in 1980:

> I think I speak for all domiciliary midwives in New Zealand when I say, for example, that we don't accept any patients who smoke but a lot of emphasis is put on good nutrition, and I don't mean just eating lots of meat, cheese, eggs and that sort of thing, it is a much more in-depth education on nutrition.[85]

McLean recommended a health-food diet based on American nutrition expert Adelle Davis's *Let's Have Healthy Children*.[86] Davis warned that women who did not eat well during pregnancy were more likely to suffer from medical problems and their infants could carry 'emotional scars' through life, such as 'hearing defects, eye abnormalities, rickets and anaemia' and even perform badly at school.[87] Flora Davidson, the New Zealand Health Department's nutrition officer from 1950 to 1985, dismissed Davis's advice following publication of the 1959 edition of *Let's Have Healthy Children*, claiming that the book which advocated 'wondrous concoctions of skim milk, brewer's yeast, and blackstrap molasses . . . should be consigned to a corner of the bookshelf plainly labelled Q for Quackery'. Davis's books nevertheless remained popular with homebirth midwives and their clients.[88]

The HBA's advice on home remedies extended into postnatal care as well. For instance, a 1984 article gave instructions for the treatment of whooping cough:

> Press 2 cloves of garlic to a pulp, add 2 tablespoons of olive oil and sufficient flour to make a paste. Divide into two portions and smear it onto the soles of your child's feet. Cover with cotton wool or a cotton cloth and wrap the feet in thick bandages. Allow to remain on all night. Remove the poultices in the morning and smear the feet with olive oil.[89]

One of the herbal concoctions favoured by homebirth midwives was raspberry leaf tea. Donley had advised Kitty Wishart to take it in pregnancy as a muscle relaxant. McLean prescribed it as an alternative source of iron for pregnant mothers, along with blackstrap molasses for calcium and vitamin B. Donley had argued that iron tablets could lead to congenital abnormalities in the baby, and favoured blackstrap molasses.[90] A much later study of raspberry leaf tea in pregnancy found only one published clinical trial, in 1941, and the researcher, a midwife, wrote that, while it was widely used, she discouraged its use until further studies could demonstrate its safety and efficacy.[91] But raspberry leaf tea was so popular in 1980s New Zealand that Donley later recalled that the *Broadsheet* collective called those involved in the homebirth movement the 'raspberry tea brigade'.[92] It was used by 90% of homebirth mothers in 1982, according to statistician Stan Gillanders who was instructed to record its usage. Gillanders did not often comment on the statistics, but he did note that the increased use of raspberry leaf tea that year had not led to a decrease in the number of episiotomies or lacerations.[93]

Other preparations for a homebirth included alternative or complementary medicines. One was yoga. A 1987 Health Department inventory of alternative or complementary medicines, constructed in recognition of their growing popularity, explained that yoga, originating in India, was based on a principle of unity or harmony of mind, soul and body, and incorporated a variety of techniques including meditation, breathing exercises, and mental and emotional attitudes.[94] McLean referred to yoga's inclusion in private classes for couples planning a homebirth, and the HBA ran workshops on yoga for pregnant women.[95]

Another was homeopathy. This had been introduced to the Western world by German physician Samuel Hahnemann in 1820 but had fallen out of favour by the early twentieth century. It subsequently made a comeback amongst certain groups, and was fully embraced by the homebirth movement in the 1980s. In New Zealand, the HBA ran workshops on it.[96] In 1987 the *HBA Newsletter* published an article by a homeopathic consultant who explained how meningitis could be effectively treated with homeopathic remedies. The newsletter also cited a woman planning a homebirth who said she was 'reading many books (homeopathy, homebirth etc)', indicating how closely the two were linked.[97]

Homeopathy, the 1987 inventory explained, is based on a set of rules of similars ('like cures like'). It aims to promote the body's self-healing qualities by prescribing one infinitesimal dose of a remedy that in gross amounts would create medical reactions like those the patient is suffering from. The inventory noted that there were more than 2,000 known homeopathic remedies.[98] Midwives learnt the techniques through the Domiciliary Midwives Society. In its 1985 newsletter, Donley provided readers with the address to purchase three 'inexpensive books from the N.Z. Homeopathy Society'.[99] Veronica Muller, who explained that she had been practising homebirth since 1981 and had attended a naturopath college (presumably the Naturopathic College of New Zealand which taught mainly by correspondence), gave detailed instructions in 1987 on how to deal with problems of pregnancy using homeopathy and naturopathy.[100] Muller continued to practise what she preached for many years. In 2014, a student midwife applauded Muller as a 'wise woman', referring specifically to her teachings on naturopathy.[101]

In 1989 two Northland homebirth mothers explained that they preferred lay (unregistered) midwives because they used homeopathic and other remedies rather than drugs; they subsequently became lay midwives themselves.[102] In a 1990 article on homebirth, the *New Zealand Listener* reported on lay midwives in Northland who dealt with 'breech births . . . and difficult posterior presentation deliveries with homeopathic remedies as their only emergency equipment'.[103] We have no record of how these mothers fared. The article also referred to lay midwife Carly Judd, who had attended 11 births in the Northland town of Hokianga over four years. One of the women experienced a postpartum haemorrhage for which, she explained, 'We used ipecac, a homeopathic preparation and the bleeding stopped.'[104] Ipecac, a syrup to induce vomiting, used particularly for children who ingested poison, is now considered harmful by toxicologists.

When Canterbury homebirth midwife Maria Ware visited The Farm in Tennessee in 1989, she also went to England to learn about homeopathy, where it was equally part of the homebirth package.[105] Indeed, homeopathy became so closely associated with the homebirth movement that the full report from Dunedin in the 1990 *HBA Newsletter* simply read: 'There have been nine home births in Dunedin Nov-Jan. Homeopathic kits are being supplied to the DMs [domiciliary midwives] for use in labour.'[106] A visiting British midwife told her New Zealand audience in the early 1990s that her practice included herbs and homeopathy, and that she referred mothers to alternative practitioners, such as acupuncturists, homeopaths or cranial osteopaths, as appropriate.[107]

Acupuncture, too, was part of the mix, as Wishart had found. A part of traditional Chinese medicine, it is often used alongside herbal medicines, exercise, massage and dietary advice. As the 1987 inventory explained, practitioners use fine needles to stimulate channels of energy running beneath the surface of the skin to effect a change in the energy balance of the body and restore health.[108] Donley had a long acquaintance with acupuncture, having taught herself the practice following a trip to China in 1975 as secretary of the New Zealand China Friendship Society. She not only referred women to other acupuncturists, as she did for Wishart, but also used it with her own clients to induce labour, as pain relief during labour, and for turning breech babies and those with posterior presentation. In the 1985 *Domiciliary Midwives Society Newsletter*, Donley told readers, 'Except on the full moon acupuncture is very effective in establishing labour when membranes have ruptured.'[109] In 1990 another midwife advocated induction via acupuncture, along with 'lamb curry with ginger and garlic, and kumara and pumpkin soup'.[110]

Data on acupuncture in homebirths collected by the HBA shows that it was used in almost a third of all homebirths in the early 1980s.[111] Dr John Hilton, who like Donley worked in West Auckland, explained in 1979 that he had started using acupuncture after seeing midwives practise it, employing it for pain relief, to bring on labour and to turn breech babies. Although he admitted it was not scientifically proven, he thought it appeared to work.[112] This was not always the case; in 1982 a University of Auckland School of Community Health project on homebirth found that two homebirth mothers treated with acupuncture for high blood pressure in pregnancy had ended up in hospital with convulsions.[113]

It is difficult to know how much training domiciliary midwives and homebirth doctors received for acupuncture. It most certainly would not have met the requirements of the New Zealand Register of Acupuncturists, which specified in the 1980s at least three years' study at an approved college and no less than 1,000 hours' clinical training.[114] While registered acupuncturists trained for three years or more, in the 1980s the *New Zealand Medical Journal* advertised courses in acupuncture for medical practitioners which were one week long.[115] Hilton explained that because of his knowledge of anatomy he was able to learn the acupuncture points from a book.[116] It is unclear how midwives trained; as noted, Donley taught herself.

Thus, mothers had a clear path to follow in preparing for a homebirth, but how was the birth itself to pan out? One woman who resided in a Coromandel commune expressed great confidence that she would be able to birth naturally, as in pregnancy she followed a regime of 'a predominantly raw diet, daily yoga [and] perineal massage', and was planning to use Frederick Leboyer's method of childbirth.[117]

Frederick Leboyer was a French obstetrician whose book *Birth Without Violence* was published in 1975. In 1977 the *New Zealand Listener* ran a feature article on his birthing methods 'based on love and happiness', and described him as the father of 'voluptuous birth'. The authors of this article had experienced his methods when their son was born in a Paris clinic run by Leboyer's disciple, obstetrician Michel Odent.[118] In 1983, a documentary about Odent's birthing centre in Pithiviers was screened on New Zealand television, with the *Listener* explaining that the only equivalent in this country was homebirth; the story was accompanied by a photograph of a homebirth at Centrepoint. The article described birth at Odent's centre as a 'mystical, spiritual event', and cited Odent's view that birth was a sexual experience.[119] The documentary was scheduled for 10pm, well after family-friendly viewing hours.

The scheduling time would not have worried Centrepoint residents; children of all ages were encouraged to attend births. The first baby born there, Phoebe Rose, entered the world in 1983 with about 80 people present. This was the norm; as one resident explained, 'when there is a birth here, everybody is involved'.[120] Bert Potter, the commune leader who was later convicted of child sex and drug offences in the 1970s and 1980s, was intimately involved in all births and their preparation. As resident midwife Rhonda Evans explained, the birthing mothers had 'an incredibly close relationship with their support people and particularly with Bert'. She believed this was 'really effective, but now and again I've had to battle through Bert to get in touch with "my ladies"'. She spoke of women being in a state of trance. This was a reference to hypnotism, which Potter provided women before and during labour: it 'seemed to work', according to the resident childbirth educator. Leboyer's *Birth Without Violence* was on the recommended reading list for mothers at Centrepoint.[121]

There were other methods of pain management in labour in the 1980s that did not involve the use of drugs. Wellington midwife Barbara Hasslacher, who had trained in Britain and attended homebirths in New Zealand from 1987, explained how she managed pain through the use of 'homeopathy, acupuncture/pressure, massage, verbalisation, visualisation, hot/cold compresses, diversion, change of position or movement – all dosed with much reassurance and encouragement'.[122] She attributed her methods to British childbirth educator Janet Balaskas, who had trained at Britain's National Childbirth Trust, helped found the London Birth Centre in the early 1980s, and was the author of *Active Birth* (1983).[123] New Zealand midwife Sally Pairman recalled how impressed she was by a seminar on active birth that Balaskas gave at Otago Medical School in 1984. The seminar was, Pairman said, 'packed with women and midwives'.[124] 'Active birth' was included in the Health Department's 1987 inventory of complementary therapies.[125]

Water birth was also part of the homebirth package. One practitioner was an Australian dolphin researcher, Estelle Myers, who set up the Tutukaka Dolphin Centre for water births north of Auckland in the early 1980s. While she was not a midwife herself, Myers employed midwives, and the first birth there in March 1982 was said to be the first water birth in the southern hemisphere. Later that year the *HBA Newsletter* reported that Myers was facing legal action after a mother having a water birth at the centre ended up in hospital 'due to the midwife not having the necessary suturing material'.[126]

The HBA sought to distance itself from Myers and water birth. Following a 'calamitous bathtub birth' in Auckland, HBA publicity spokesperson Henriette Kemp told Radio New Zealand that it was not the sort of homebirth they promoted.[127] Donley told the *Listener*, 'Quite frankly, if you want a water birth, find yourself a friendly dolphin as a midwife.'[128] Donley's catch phrase, 'Whose body is it? Whose baby is it?', insisting that women should be able to decide on their own childbirth experience, did not apply in this instance.[129] The 1984 national HBA conference denied Myers a place as a speaker but allowed her to put information on display and to show a film by Russian water-birth advocate and swimming instructor Igor Charkovsky.[130]

Water births continued to feature in the homebirth movement. The 1986 *Domiciliary Midwives Society Newsletter* reported on a lay midwife in Kaitāia who travelled around doing underwater births.[131] In 1989 Christchurch midwife Celeste McCoy reported positively on a water-birth conference she had attended in London, with speakers including Odent, Balaskas and Charkovsky. In fact, water birth had become Odent's 'trademark' at Pithiviers.[132] McCoy also visited Dr Roger Leachy in Cornwall, whom she described as a well-known homeopathic GP specialising in water birth.[133] Balaskas later became the authority on water birth, and her book *The Water Birth Book* was recommended reading in New Zealand's 2006 textbook for midwives.[134]

## Rejecting modern technology

The range of instructions for ensuring a 'natural' pregnancy, birth and postnatal experience was accompanied by a forceful rejection of interventions associated with hospitals and modern medicine. One specific intervention which attracted the attention of the homebirth movement in the 1980s was ultrasound scans to view the fetus. Developed in the 1950s as an alternative to x-rays, which by then were understood to be dangerous in pregnancy, ultrasound scans became commonplace in pregnancy from the 1970s as the technology improved, and particularly with the introduction of real-time scanning rather than static scanners.[135] Donley advised her readers in 1984, 'If you are not prepared to accept the unknown risk of this procedure you can refuse.'[136] In 1985 she penned a critical submission to the Health Department in relation to its newly released educational booklet *Your Pregnancy*, writing of the section on ultrasound that the department had a responsibility to inform women that it was 'an experimental procedure about which many prestigious professionals were expressing second thoughts'.[137]

Donley herself said that she 'only very very occasionally' sent a woman for a scan, whilst not explaining what would prompt that decision.[138] Others took a similar position. In 1989, *HBA Newsletter* editor Brenda Hinton wrote that, whilst ultrasound scans were becoming routine for most women, information was starting to filter through that they could be dangerous to the fetus. Women were starting to question the procedure, she said, but they were not given full and unbiased information about the risks and benefits, or offered the opportunity to decline.[139] Homebirth advocate Lynda Williams also claimed that many pregnant women reported increased fetal movements after the scan, felt their baby 'didn't like it', and were increasingly declining ultrasound scans.[140] This was wishful thinking, given that women's demands were one of the drivers for the increased use of ultrasound in the 1980s. Routine ultrasounds were also endorsed by medical researchers, including a working party of the Royal College of Obstetricians and Gynaecologists in Britain in 1984.[141]

The 1982 University of Auckland Community Health Project found that homebirth advocates rejected two other interventions – vitamin K for the baby and ergometrine for the mother. Giving a single dose of vitamin K to prevent a rare but very serious and potentially life-threatening bleeding disorder in newborns had been common since the 1940s. Ergometrine was a medication developed in the 1930s to facilitate delivery of the placenta and to prevent postpartum haemorrhage, the main cause of maternal death after puerperal infection had been brought under control from the 1930s. One obstetrician told the 1982 researchers that not giving these drugs was like 'going out into the country and driving around the corners on the wrong side of the road. Just because you can get away with it 99.9% of the time, this does not mean that this practice is desirable.'[142]

Immunisation was another intervention which attracted the attention of the homebirth movement. Immunisation for early childhood diseases had steadily increased in the twentieth century so that by 1970 Professor Dennis Bonham could point to available immunisations for a wide range of infectious diseases including tetanus, diphtheria, whooping cough, poliomyelitis, smallpox, measles and rubella. He believed that 'wise parents' saw the need for protection, whilst others still needed to be educated.[143] The Royal New Zealand Plunket Society, a voluntary organisation which had provided free postnatal nursing services since 1907, encouraged parents to immunise their babies against what had once been killer diseases.[144] But those in the homebirth movement had a different view.

Homebirth campaigner Hilary Butler was prominent in debates around immunisation, forming the Immunisation Awareness Society in 1988. The Auckland HBA advertised Butler's publications in its newsletters and sold them from its Auckland post office box address, paying Butler a royalty. The HBA newsletters also indicate how Butler resonated with its members. A 1986 newsletter reported on a day-long regional conference in Hamilton hosted by the Waikato HBA at which she presented a 'thoroughly researched paper' on immunisation. Another newsletter that year announced that Butler was to give a talk on 'Scans and Immunisation', linking the two technologies. Butler frequently spoke at local homebirth meetings; for instance, in 1990 the Whangarei Homebirth Support Group organised an Immunisation Awareness session led by Butler which was apparently well attended.[145]

In 1987, Butler was invited to speak at the annual HBA conference, leading to an in-depth article in the women's magazine *More*. Founded in 1983, *More* claimed to be more modern in outlook than the *New Zealand Woman's Weekly*, and reached an audience of 60,000 by the mid-1980s.[146] The article informed readers that Butler was not opposed to immunisation but was pro-choice. She urged mothers to question doctors on all their advice. However, it is also clear that she was anti-immunisation. She explained that vaccination was a poor substitute for a healthy lifestyle, and argued that women who had their children vaccinated would then allow them to eat what they wanted – in her words, 'Coke, chips, biscuits' – without any concern for their health. She claimed to have evidence that vaccination caused cancer and other diseases such as AIDS (acquired immunodeficiency syndrome), as it destroyed immunity. She was convinced the polio vaccine could cause brain tumours, and, when asked whether she could live with herself if her unvaccinated child caught polio, she responded she could, since treatments were available and polio was not always fatal or disabling in any case.[147] Those who had lived through polio epidemics prior to the introduction of immunisation in the late 1950s and early 1960s would have been appalled.

The HBA sought information on anti-vaccination more broadly. Its 1988 newsletter reprinted an article from the Whangārei branch newsletter by osteopath Dr Max Belcher on the adverse effects of immunisation against hepatitis B.[148] New Zealand had introduced universal infant hepatitis B immunisation just that year, one of the first countries to do so. In 1989, the *HBA Newsletter* reported on its members' attendance at an immunisation seminar facilitated by the College of Natural Medicine in Christchurch.[149] It noted that almost 80% to 90% of the attendees were women, and that the Department of Health had declined to send a representative. Butler opened proceedings with a talk on 'What doctors don't tell you'. She claimed that it was not in the interests of pharmaceutical companies to present consumers with the full story, as they would lose money if people chose not to be immunised. For that reason, she said, they concentrated on people's fears and emotions rather than presenting the case for immunisation on its merits. She exhorted mothers not only to demand information from doctors but also to take responsibility for their own and their children's health.

Another speaker at the seminar was Viera Scheibner. Czechoslovakian-born geologist Scheibner had immigrated to Australia in 1968. Following her retirement in 1987, she became an anti-vaccination activist, claiming links between vaccination and sudden infant death syndrome (SIDS), also known as cot death. Christchurch GP and homeopathist David Ritchie spoke about measles, maintaining that people got a lifelong immunity from having the disease and not from the vaccine. He advised people to look after the health of their bodies and minds 'over and above the nastiness of the bugs about us'. Ritchie was a member of the International Medical Council on Vaccination, which sought to counter the messages of pharmaceutical companies and others that vaccines were safe and effective.[150] The final speaker was University of Otago Professor of General Practice Campbell Murdoch. A *Metro* article expanded on Murdoch's arguments against immunisation. Murdoch referred to recent diseases such as AIDS, asthma, cervical cancer, SIDS and chronic fatigue syndrome, all (he said) related to the human immune system, and pondered on what had changed in the ecology of the population over that period. He pointed to immunisation as a notable change, and sought to shift the focus from immunisation to health education.[151] As the *Metro* article, which summarised his views, declared, 'Scepticism about vaccination is another aspect of society's current disaffection with the medical establishment.'[152] The HBA was at the core of this disaffection.

## Conclusion

Homebirth in the 1970s and 1980s was part of a cultural movement that embraced a lifestyle philosophy closely tied to the anti-establishment movement, and its adherents were predominantly white and middle class. Choosing to birth at home came with a whole set of worldviews about health and a distrust of modern medicine. Chapter 2 will address how the movement sought to extend its influence beyond those with anti-establishment values to all modern mothers, investigating the arguments it put forward to do so, and revealing it as part of a powerful international movement.

# TWO

## *'Everyone should do it'： Why choose homebirth?*

THOSE ATTRACTED TO THE 1970S counterculture were the first to reject hospital childbirth and all it stood for. But the homebirth movement sought to extend its influence and attract people beyond the small minority who opted out of mainstream society by gravitating to communes, for example. It urged all women to consider birthing at home, arguing that it was in their own interests, as well as those of their infants, their families and the wider community. The first aim of the Auckland Home Birth Association, formed in 1978, was to 'educate the community about the benefits of home births'.[1]

Since the 1940s, proponents of 'natural' or drug-free birth like British obstetrician Grantly Dick-Read had argued that the resultant bonding between the mother and baby had a profound impact on the child's psychological wellbeing and his or her future development.[2] This view persisted, but by the 1970s the spotlight was pivoting from the infant to the mother. Proponents of homebirth argued that the experience empowered her, making her a better mother and a better person, and in this way benefited the whole community. Moreover, they claimed, she had a social responsibility to take this route; by assuming responsibility for her child's birth, she contributed to the emancipation of women from patriarchal control. Their campaign had the support of an international community of homebirth advocates with similar views. This chapter explores how the homebirth movement sought to persuade everyone that homebirth was the right choice.

## Psychology and birth

Psychology was integral to homebirth. When homebirth midwife Lyn McLean was interviewed by the *New Zealand Woman's Weekly* in 1978, she complained that she had received little support from 'conventional medical workers' but had received a grant of $500 from the Mental Health Foundation which clearly valued her work.[3] Another *Woman's Weekly* reporter interviewed Dr Victor McGeorge, an Auckland GP, psychotherapist and one-time president of the New Zealand Association of Psychotherapists, who had delivered babies at home since 1942. McGeorge stressed the importance of bonding for the baby, explaining that if it failed to establish itself in the first 24 hours after birth, 'a vicious interaction may occur instead, with crime, depression, drug dependency and delinquency as its results'. He said those who chose homebirth were not protesters but concerned and responsible parents.[4]

The HBA invited McGeorge to speak at its 1982 annual conference. In his talk, called 'Birthing, Bonding and Mental Health', he claimed that the current zeal for physical survival was at the expense of psychological aspects.[5] That same year he spoke to University of Auckland community health researchers about the dire consequences for the child if bonding did not occur immediately; the researchers reported these without comment. They included a 'flattening of and diminishing of all the desirable qualities of confidence, creativity and warmth', 'aggressive acting out symptoms', neuroses and ultimately 'depressive illness and psychoses'.[6] He added that homebirth enabled the husband to participate fully and 'not feel left out', helping him to bond to the child as well.[7] In 1984 Joan Donley cited an Australian doctor who claimed that even potentially irresponsible parents would become more responsible if the birth occurred at home. Like McGeorge, this doctor claimed the psychological benefits of family bonding were equally if not more important than the physical 'benefits' of advanced technology.[8] Placing 'benefits' in inverted commas indicated his doubt that there were any.

Scottish psychiatrist R. D. Laing, who strongly opposed hospital birth, also focused on infant psychology. He argued that the conditions under which babies were born often led to the presentation of insanity later in life. He spoke of umbilical shock, the moment of cord-cutting when 'a few seconds can make a profound difference for the rest of one's life'. He claimed to remember his own birth as 'a body blow, a searing pain'. According to his biographer, Laing became preoccupied in the 1980s with not only the process of medical birth but also the therapeutic process of rebirthing.[9] The Health Department's 1987 inventory of complementary therapies explained: 'Some rebirthers believe that birth trauma influences an individual's behaviour drastically unless he or she can re-experience the birth and release its memory. Rebirthing occurs when the person feels safe enough to relive the moment of first breath.' An American psychotherapist, Leonard Orr, had developed the technique in the 1970s.[10]

Frederick Leboyer, author of *Birth Without Violence*, believed that the emotional environment of birth had a profound impact and lifelong effects. He drew comparisons between sexual experiences and being born, claiming, 'To make love is to return to paradise, it is to plunge again into the world before birth, before the great separation.'[11] Amongst the outcomes he claimed for his method of natural childbirth was 'a calm, relaxed, often smiling baby and a superior IQ by school age'.[12] By 'superior', he presumably meant superior to those born in hospital.

At the HBA's first national conference in 1980, Dr Geoff Bridgman, research officer for the Auckland HBA, was part of a panel discussion on homebirth. He was a homebirth father (his wife Derryn Cooper had had two homebirths), but he chose to speak in his capacity as a child psychologist working for the Intellectually Handicapped Society. He explained how in this role he saw homebirth as a 'very high priority area because I see some of the effects of botched-up hospital births'.[13]

The long-term negative psychological effect of medical intervention was the subject of lectures by a visiting American speaker in 1984. Joseph Chilton Pearce, a former humanities professor and author of *The Crack in the Cosmic Egg* (1971) and *Magical Child* (1977), asserted that the world was 'set on a path of self-destruction if it continues to assault the newborn'. He explained that induced labour, the use of forceps, the unnatural position of the mother and the premature cutting of the umbilical cord, together with the separation of mother and baby after birth, were all forms of physical and emotional assault. In his view, 'This assault at birth causes stress that limits the child's learning ability later in life' and turned the child to the self-destructive violence that was currently 'all too evident'. Research by the Californian Crime Commission substantiated his claims, he said, with its 1981 report stating that modern childbirth practices were the main causes of crime and violence. He told his audience categorically that 'home born babies could end world violence'.[14]

These ideas about the psychological benefits for infants of a good childbirth experience, which at the very least involved women being conscious at birth so that bonding could commence, went back to the so-called natural childbirth movement of the 1950s. New Zealand's Natural Childbirth Association, promoting drug-free birth, had been set up in 1951 and renamed Parents Centre in 1952. The British equivalent, the National Childbirth Trust, was set up in 1957. The inspiration for both was British obstetrician Grantly Dick-Read, whose concern was primarily the long-term psychological health of the baby. Christchurch psychiatrist Maurice Bevan-Brown, strongly influenced by Dick-Read, helped to found Parents Centre.[15]

At the HBA 1990 annual conference, Australian paediatrician Kerry Callaghan, described in the programme as a psychologist and homebirth father, gave an evening lecture entitled 'Can Birth Affect Our Future?'. Callaghan had specialised in child and family psychiatry and was particularly interested in the effects of early childhood experiences on personality development.[16] Within psychology, birth was viewed as a formative moment. However, while attention to the psychological development of the child continued into the late twentieth century, there was a subtle change within the homebirth movement under the influence of second-wave feminism. The emphasis was shifting from the psychological health of the infant to the psychological health of the mother and her empowerment through the childbirth experience.

## Women's empowerment through childbirth

Researchers for the 1982 University of Auckland Community Health Project on homebirth cited a growing belief that the child could become attached to its parent any time in its first three years, but that the first hours after the birth were crucial for the mother to bond successfully to the child and there was 'no point employing high technology neonatal care to look after a baby only to have it neglected and/or abused later in life due to lack of attachment'.[17] The spotlight was shifting from the infant to the mother.

In 1986 Joan Donley and childbirth educator Lynda Williams were invited to talk to a General Practitioner Continuing Medical Education evening on the future of GP obstetrics. Williams spoke about the negative effects of hospital births for mothers, maintaining that these instilled a lack of confidence to parent effectively. However, she also implicated male doctors' attitudes more broadly, declaring, '[C]onfident, warm parenting is NOT encouraged by beginning with 9 months, or many years, of treating the mother like a puzzled, fragile, dependent creature.' She told them that an unsatisfying birth experience was a contributing factor in maternal depression, mothers' sense of personal inadequacy and poor feelings for the baby. 'IT IS SIMPLY NOT ENOUGH TO GET BABIES BORN SAFELY', she said, written in capitals in the report of her speech for emphasis. She cited British homebirth advocate Sheila Kitzinger's view of birth as part of a woman's psychosexual experience and an event 'intimately connected with her feelings, which can last a life-time, about her body, her relations with others, her role as a woman . . . and her sense of personal identity'. Williams offered the analogy of Sir Edmund Hillary climbing Mt Everest and asked what his sense of achievement would have been had he been taken to the top by helicopter: 'And this is a bit like what happens to women when they are robbed of the experience of giving birth.'[18] She did not draw on her personal experience in this talk, but Williams told the HBA in a keynote address that same year that she had decided to become pregnant with her fourth child in 1984 so that she could experience a homebirth.[19] She later claimed that giving birth at home was 'undoubtedly one of the most empowering experiences of a woman's life'.[20]

Nelson homebirth midwife Bronwen Pelvin went even further in 1990, just as this very subject was being debated in Parliament, when she claimed that giving birth could be 'an empowering experience which will affect a woman for the rest of her life: give her a minute to roll up her sleeves and she'll climb that mountain or become the first woman prime minister'. The converse of this empowering experience, Pelvin continued, was a hospital birth that made a woman feel like a 'victim violated in the worst way'.[21]

Karen Guilliland, the first president of the New Zealand College of Midwives set up in 1989, stressed the importance of allowing a woman's 'genetically transmitted knowledge of birth simply to take over', which it did in a homebirth. She explained that a woman who had just given birth the way she wanted to was 'euphoric, victorious', with Donley adding, 'Nothing she will have to do for that child . . . will be too much trouble.' The implication was that the mother would not love the child unconditionally if she had received medical intervention.[22] After having a homebirth in 1987, Northland woman Mandy Waata explained that she felt 'so wonderful, so strong and powerful' that she passed these emotions on to the baby.[23]

The belief that the birth experience affected a woman's ability to mother was widely canvassed at the time. A 1980 press article, which stated categorically that birth was a normal process requiring a minimum of intervention, advised: 'A woman has to be happy in herself to introduce a child to this society.' Being in control mattered too: 'Having to make decisions about the birth ritual for their child meant having to think positively about their child's whole future.'[24] Homebirth GP Diana Nash warned that a woman who did not have a good birth experience would not mother easily.[25] The draft report of a 1989 Health Department working group on childbirth which included Bronwen Pelvin and Karen Guilliland explained that a woman who felt in control and positive about her birth experience was more likely to have the necessary self-esteem for positive parenting. One of the contributors to the report wrote 'great' in the margin.[26]

A 1983 letter to the *Listener* supporting homebirth declared that research showed a disastrous link between the battered child and his or her mother's experience during and after birth.[27] This claim elicited an angry response from one reader. She described being treated well in hospital, and said that both her children were 'normal, happy and healthy', despite having been separated from her after birth because of problems.[28] The significance of the first few hours for parental bonding was also questioned by a psychology researcher at the University of Auckland in 1981 who analysed 1,100 births at hospital and at home. She found that while bonding could occur soon after birth, for many it might take some weeks to establish, and that either was considered normal.[29] She concluded that place of birth was not strongly associated with 'postpartum maternal attitudes, coping, competence or perception of the baby in the first six postnatal weeks', and that birth itself was merely the start of an ongoing relationship between mother and child.[30] However, there was no national organisation to promote this view of childbirth; nor did it gain wide publicity.

Donley continued to insist that a bad childbirth experience could lead to child neglect and abuse, even when commenting in 1987 on the death of a homebirth mother seven days after giving birth. Diverting attention away from the death itself, she chose instead to focus on possible adverse effects of hospital births, noting that interventions during birth and separation from their babies deprived mothers of their bonding experience, mothering instincts and self-esteem, 'all of which are recognised as a contributing factor in child neglect and abuse'.[31] The implication was that a fatal outcome from a homebirth was better than living with the consequences of a hospital birth.

## Homebirth and feminism

Homebirth implied so much more to its advocates than simply a personal lifestyle choice or even an experience with psychological advantages for the woman and her family. Its advocates suggested women had a responsibility to choose this option to advance the status of women in society. The title of an HBA seminar in 1986 was 'Home Birth – Personal Choice – Political Act'; as Joan Donley explained, having a homebirth was in itself a political act.[32] One commentator later related how three or four days after attending a birth, Donley would talk to the mother to make her aware of the political issues surrounding childbirth.[33] Donley saw her role extending well beyond that of a health professional looking after mothers and babies and attending births; she used the situation as a lobbying opportunity.

Donley's broader political beliefs informed her views on homebirth. In the early 1970s she supported the New Zealand Communist Party, developed an interest in Communist China, and was secretary of the New Zealand China Friendship Society. In this role, she visited China on three occasions, and surveyed the Women's Liberation Movement there. She argued that without socialism, women's liberation could not occur.[34] Turning to homebirth, she explained that when she described it as a feminist and a political act, she meant that it was a 'challenge to the white, male-controlled obstetrics and gynaecology . . . specialty which is trying to gain a complete monopoly of childbirth in New Zealand'.[35] She wrote to the editor of the *Auckland Star* in 1983, 'Let's not kid ourselves and the public on the real issues involved in the debate over home birth. It is a power struggle between obstetricians-hospital boards, with their huge investment in architecture and technology aggravated by a falling birth rate, and women who are trying to regain control over their bodies.'[36] When obstetrician Tony Baird was an invited participant in a panel discussion on homebirth at the first HBA conference in 1980 he pleaded that he and his colleagues in the New Zealand Obstetrical and Gynaecological Society were 'not your enemies, which is what seems to come through from some of the speakers'.[37]

Suspicion of the motives of (male) obstetricians was closely linked to the 1970s second-wave feminist movement and its views on patriarchal capitalist society. Homebirth advocates ignored the arguments of women who opposed homebirth, explaining, in the feminist rubric drawn from the Chinese Cultural Revolution (1966–76), how these women, being unaware of their oppression, suffered from 'false consciousness'. 'The personal is political' was the slogan of the 1970s feminist movement, and health, according to Auckland writer and *Broadsheet* editor from 1972 Sandra Coney, was at 'the cutting edge of sexual politics, the place where women were often at their most powerless'.[38] In her history of the homebirth movement, Donley related how two 'middle class feminist activists', Derryn Cooper and Barbara Macfarlane, had set up the Auckland HBA because of their 'anger at the powerlessness of women being forced into the medical model'. Both, Donley explained, saw homebirth as a focus of women-power.[39] Cooper became spokesperson for the New Zealand HBA on its formation in 1980, and Macfarlane secretary.[40]

The new women's health movement sought to reclaim women's bodies from the medical profession. A major influence in New Zealand, as elsewhere in the West, was the publication in 1971 of the healthcare manual *Our Bodies Ourselves* by the Boston Women's Health Book Collective.[41] In 1980 *Broadsheet* featured an article invoking *Our Bodies Ourselves* entitled 'Knowledge is Power'. The author, Sarah Calvert, was undertaking a PhD on women and mental health at Waikato University, and edited the newsletter of the New Zealand Women's Health Network, set up in 1978. In her 1980 article, she argued that women's bodies formed the focus of the patriarchal goal to control women. Reviewing history, she claimed that at first men had been in awe both of women's powers to produce and nurture life and their talent for healing. However, this soon turned to envy, and men began to control and dominate women, 'colonising' them and leaving them feeling alienated and confused. She explained how the new women's health movement sought to challenge this oppression by uniting women through consciousness-raising groups to understand the commonality of their oppression and provide them with mechanisms to overcome it.[42] Homebirth was one such mechanism. At the 1980 HBA conference, Calvert ran a workshop entitled 'Feminist Point of View on Birth'.[43]

Another participant at the 1980 HBA panel discussion on homebirth was Auckland lawyer Linda Daly-Peoples.[44] She had outlined her views in *Broadsheet* three years earlier, when she claimed that male involvement in childbirth stemmed from their fear of birth because it was beyond their control. This fear had led them 'to substitute "scientific" manipulation for nature's processes, despite incontrovertible evidence that nature has succeeded admirably without them for so long'. As men attempted to assert themselves in childbirth, she wrote, 'propaganda threatening death and damage replace[d] truth'.[45] On a personal level, she explained that the horrible experience of giving birth to her first child in hospital had led to her involvement in the women's movement.[46] Others too found feminism through the birth experience. Mandy Waata had left her husband and was living in a bus when she gave birth, attended there by seven women. She told *Broadsheet* that she became 'so empowered by that birth that I started realising that I was probably a feminist' and subsequently a 'separatist lesbian'.[47]

Sandra Coney proffered a different interpretation from Daly-Peoples about men's involvement in childbirth. She argued that men's involvement stemmed not from fear but from womb envy. She explained that by fostering women's passivity, ignorance and isolation from familiar support systems, and by promoting the view that childbirth is dangerous and unnatural, men 'brainwashed and coerced women into powerlessness' so that they could take over. This gave men the emotional satisfaction of believing that they were giving birth; in her words, 'The inert unconscious woman, hidden behind sterile theatre guards, allows the man to come the nearest he can to really giving birth – he can "take" the baby – symbolically he can birth himself.'[48] Coney's colleague and co-founder of the feminist activist group Maternity Action in 1984, Phillida Bunkle, recounted her experience of total powerlessness at the birth of her first child in 1975. She wrote in 1988, 'As the doctor bullied and yelled and threatened, it became apparent that this was *his* theatre and *his* drama.' She recounted the glee with which he inserted stitches following an episiotomy without anaesthetics, his face 'alive with pleasure . . . My flesh would no longer defy his power.'[49]

When Dr Colin Mantell spoke in favour of hospital births at his 1978 inaugural lecture as Auckland University Professor of Obstetrics and Gynaecology, *Auckland Star* reporter Vanya Hogg contrasted obstetricians with those they served: 'Pacing the carpet square round the lectern in his beautiful imported shoes, Dr Mantell looked every inch a successful professional man. In contrast, his audience of about 100 were a mixed bag of students, pregnant women, grandmothers, lovers of the natural life, and be-suited men who shared the same calling as the professor.'[50] Others were even more forthright in their condemnation of male obstetricians, overlooking the existence of female obstetricians. In 1982, *New Zealand Woman's Weekly* columnist Valerie Davies declared that women's self-determination in childbirth threatened men's jobs: 'No wonder men are resisting and denigrating home births.'[51] Homebirth advocate Judy Larkin agreed. She referred to the 'obstetric empire' which aimed to make money and secure the obstetricians' future by training on women's bodies and by patronising women.[52] Similarly, Christine Bird, founder of The Health Alternatives for Women in Christchurch in 1980, told *Broadsheet* that the health system consisted of 'vested interests and moralistic woman-haters'; only women's health groups, she said, put women ahead of hospital efficiency or profit.[53] Consumer advocate Judi Strid asserted that the medical profession was totally dependent on women's bodies for the clinical material they needed to maintain their high-income obstetrical practices and to train their successors.[54]

Homebirth midwives expressed great confidence in women-power. A group of them sent a submission in 1979 to the Maternity Services Committee's inquiry into homebirths stating that, since women made up the 'clinical material' in childbirth, they would decide whether they wanted 'high technology, actively managed, high risk births which only a specialist can handle, or whether they want[ed] natural childbirth assisted by a midwife!'. The Auckland HBA sent a similar submission signed by 'Barbara Macfarlane, LLB, Secretary HBA, and Geoff Bridgman, PhD, Research Officer'. They warned that whatever the Maternity Services Committee decided, it could be assured that the HBA would 'continue to promote a full and reasoned debate on this issue' and that 'Women will make the final decision, regardless of the law'.[55] Speaking of the homebirth movement in 1985, Joan Donley confidently predicted that as more and more women 'vote[d] with their bums' and opted out of the marketplace, more and more obstetricians would become redundant.[56]

The homebirth movement saw midwives, along with women, as casualties of this capitalist patriarchal structure. In her submission to the 1979–80 inquiry into homebirth, Lyn McLean maintained that as specialists strove for a monopoly over reproduction, midwives were replaced by 'technical institute-trained doctors' assistants under the guise of safety'.[57] Judi Strid asserted that the medical profession's preoccupation with technology was simply a ruse to threaten and further undermine midwives, turning them into doctors' handmaidens.[58]

In 1989 Donley wrote an article for the first issue of the *New Zealand College of Midwives Journal*, in which she claimed that obstetrician Tony Baird had said in a recent speech that the three greatest threats to obstetrics were consumerism, feminism and midwives.[59] In response, Baird wrote to College president Guilliland, explaining that he said no such thing and setting out what he had said, including direct quotes from his speech.[60] The next issue of the journal published part of his letter and his concluding statement that:

> There has been a lot of misinformation about medical involvement in childbirth and it is very destructive. If the current vogue of denigration of specialist obstetricians continues, with the apparent lack of respect for anyone who is not a midwife, the prospect of co-operation between the people who care for women becomes a forlorn hope. The lives of countless women and babies have been saved by medical intervention because even though childbirth is a natural process, it can go badly wrong, like all natural processes.

The editors followed this with a statement apologising for any misrepresentation, accepting Baird's views as expressed in his letter, and offering him their 'unreserved apologies'.[61] At the next meeting of the College of Midwives' national committee, members expressed their 'dismay and concern' at this apology, pointing out that it was contrary to what the committee had agreed and therefore the editor responsible had not acted as an agent of the College. A motion to ask for the editor's resignation was passed unanimously (with one abstention).[62]

In the meantime, Donley's account was repeated in other fora, such as an HBA newsletter and the Health Department's educational magazine in 1989, and in a 2003 PhD thesis entitled 'Midwifery as Feminist Praxis'.[63] Donley herself continued to allude to it, ignoring the apology. Reporting in *Broadsheet* on the first national conference of the College of Midwives some months later, she wrote: 'Each day of the conference was devoted to a specific topic: consumerism, midwifery and feminism – "the three greatest threats to modem obstetrics!"'[64] She repeated the claim that midwives were a threat to obstetrics in articles for the College's journal in 1992 and 1998, and extended it to an international audience in 1995, when one of her concluding remarks was 'to recall the claim of a New Zealand obstetrician that the three greatest threats to modern obstetrics are feminism, consumerism and midwives'.[65] To Donley and others, obstetricians were indeed the enemy.

## An international community

The New Zealand homebirth movement was part of an international network, as was second-wave feminism itself, giving it a significant boost. In a 1981 article for the *HBA Newsletter* entitled 'The International Revolutionary Movement We're Part Of', Joan Donley described how the local movement was aided by an extensive overseas network which provided information on 'the struggle' elsewhere.[66] Both midwives and consumer members fostered the connection, which included attending conferences overseas and reporting back, as well as hosting overseas speakers at local conferences and events.

Through the newsletter, Donley kept readers apprised of what was happening elsewhere. In 1981 she referred to the Association of Radical Midwives in Britain, which, she explained, was fighting to prevent the English midwife from being reduced to the status of a maternity nurse – as had happened in New Zealand. She also referred to the Margaret Marsh Defence Fund Trust in Vancouver, Canada. She explained that Marsh was a Canadian lay midwife who had been charged two years earlier with causing a child's death; while found not guilty, she was convicted for practising midwifery without a licence. Donley concluded, 'The fight for natural normal childbirth is fast becoming an international revolutionary movement' and that only by uniting could women overthrow the vested interests of the medical profession and its increasing mechanisation or 'active management' of childbirth. She cited English social science lecturer Jean Donnison who called this active management the 'latest manifestation of male medical imperialism'.[67] Donnison was the author of a history of women's rights and the professional rivalries between doctors and midwives, published in 1977.[68]

A Canadian by birth, Donley kept in touch with North American midwives. In 1984 she visited Canada and the United States, and excitedly reported back that homebirth was 'proliferating!' there. She explained that lay (unlicensed) midwives, who gained their experience through apprenticeship to other midwives or in birthing centres, attended most homebirths in both countries. She was informed that while nurse-midwives could practise legally in the US, they were not popular with the medical profession; the 350 lay midwives, however, were positively harassed.[69] Historian Wendy Kline later noted that from 1974 to 1980 almost 50 midwives were prosecuted in California for practising without a licence.[70] As a result, American feminist activist Sheryl Ruzek wrote that 'lay midwives and their clients, with all their traditional values, came to be viewed as warriors in the feminist battle for freedom of choice.'[71] After visiting America in 1986, Centrepoint midwife Rhonda Evans reported that homebirth midwives were 'doing quite well' in New Zealand.[72]

The International Childbirth Education Association (ICEA), founded in America in the 1970s, trained women to teach natural childbirth. New Zealander Diony Young, a consumer homebirth activist and educator who was resident in America, became active in the organisation and was editor of ICEA's journal *Birth* from 1990.[73] Young's mother Nancy Sutherland had been a founding member of the New Zealand Parents Centre. Young kept in touch with her home country, visiting in 1984, for example, when she gave public lectures on the 'insidious process of medicalisation of childbirth', declaring, 'While perinatal morbidity and mortality are important, so too is the personal satisfaction of the woman.' Parents Centre traditionally ran antenatal classes, but in 1988 a group of childbirth educators decided that some of the Parents Centre educators were too indoctrinated into the medical model and set up a separate childbirth educators course aligned to ICEA.[74] Donley, herself a consultant for ICEA, claimed that Parents Centre antenatal classes 'jeered' at 'active birth'.[75]

Other New Zealanders also became involved in ICEA. Lynda Williams became a childbirth educator whilst visiting America with her husband in 1979. She continued in this role when she returned to New Zealand in 1980, combining it with activism in women's health and homebirth. She joined the Auckland Childbirth Education Association, and was one of two New Zealand members of ICEA, appointed as its New Zealand coordinator. She maintained contact with the movement in America, attending two conferences there in the late 1980s.[76]

Williams' successor as New Zealand coordinator for ICEA was Dunedin childbirth educator Jenny Drew. In 1990 Drew was appointed to the board of directors of ICEA, which by then boasted 10,000 members in 32 countries and supported the 'philosophy of family centred maternity care and freedom of choice for childbearing families based on knowledge of childbirth alternatives'. Drew had co-founded the Childbirth Education Association of Otago, a group which, she explained, brought the first childbirth educator training course to New Zealand from Australia.[77]

Childbirth educators were an important part of the homebirth movement. Drew expressed concern about the relationship between the homebirth midwives and the childbirth educators. She complained that the former did not regard them as professionals but 'just as active and vocal consumers'.[78] They were, however, very useful allies for homebirth midwives. For instance, Brenda Hinton, a childbirth educator, became editor of the *HBA Newsletter*, and Williams was an outspoken and passionate advocate.

Conferences were an important way to keep in touch across borders. Australian homebirth conferences, the first of which was held in Canberra in 1981, were reported in the New Zealand newsletters and, according to Donley, almost always included a New Zealand delegate.[79] That delegate was usually Donley herself, who took extensive notes and relayed them back home. In 1985, for instance, she submitted to the *Domiciliary Midwives Society Newsletter* an eight-page report on the sixth National Homebirth Australia conference in New South Wales, which she attended on behalf of the Auckland HBA. Among other things, she reported that in her opening address Homebirth Australia's president and founder Henny Ligtermoet claimed that Australian doctors harassed homebirth midwives, and that, as more and more women opted for homebirth and obstetricians' control began to slip, that harassment increased.[80] Such sentiments showed the New Zealand lobbyists were not alone.

There was great excitement within the New Zealand movement when it was announced that the first International Conference on Homebirth was to be held at Wembley Conference Centre, London, in October 1987. The New Zealand HBA elected to send two delegates and fundraised to aid their travel. The delegates were consumer activist Micky Harrower and homebirth midwife Sian Burgess, who were asked by the conference organisers to prepare a 10-minute presentation for delivery at the conference. Harrower was well qualified to speak on homebirth, having had five of her six children at home. She was active in the Kaitaia HBA and the Save the Midwives Direct Entry Midwifery Task Force (see pp. 75–77), and was at the time undertaking a correspondence course in midwifery.[81] She was also described as a 'support person (and sometimes lay midwife) of many births'.[82] Sian Burgess, mother of two and an Auckland homebirth midwife, had trained and practised in the UK before coming to New Zealand. About 10 other New Zealanders also made it to the conference.[83]

This was a grand occasion for the homebirth movement. In her report, Burgess conveyed the excitement of connecting and sharing stories of 'struggles' with delegates, whom she numbered at almost 5,000 from 30 Western countries.

This was clearly an overestimate, as the venue could host only 2,500 people; nevertheless, the mood was electric. Speakers included internationally renowned figures in the natural childbirth movement. Beverley Beech, childbirth activist and president of the British organisation AIMS (the Association for Improvement to Maternity Services), opened the conference. Other speakers included Michel Odent, Sheila Kitzinger, Marjorie Tew, Ann Oakley, Wendy Savage, Janet Balaskas and Marsden Wagner. Burgess described them as 'visionaries with enormous experience who profoundly influenced the people with whom they work'.[84] All would have been well known to the New Zealand contingent.

Speaker Michel Odent had left his maternity hospital at Pithiviers (see pp. 24–25) in 1985 to set up the Primal Health Research Centre in London, where he investigated the impact of birth on health in later life. Reporting on Odent's conference speech, Burgess said she was dismayed to hear that after he left Pithiviers the hospital reverted almost immediately to a 'normal' state hospital – 'no singing group, no water births, no "salle sauvage" [primitive room]'.[85]

Sheila Kitzinger, British social anthropologist, author of many books on childbirth, and so-called 'Earth-Mother-Birth-Mother', was already famous in New Zealand.[86] Two of her books were on the 1982 recommended reading list for intending homebirth mothers at Centrepoint.[87] The 1987 HBA conference cited her belief that every woman was entitled 'to give birth in freedom and in a loving environment', implying that women in hospital were captive and faced hostility.[88] A New Zealand Health Department report on homebirth that same year quoted Kitzinger's view that homebirth was an 'important function of a responsible society'.[89] Burgess enthused that Kitzinger gave the conference 'a dramatic and dynamic presentation as only she can'.[90] Homebirth politicised the mother, Kitzinger said: '[it] represents values . . . which spring from conviction and the courage of the inner power of human beings to resist autocracy and dogma and a political system designed to crush opposition'.[91]

Burgess also explained in her report how Marjorie Tew had become politicised when she stumbled across the surprising fact that statistics did not support the widely accepted claim that hospital birth was safer than homebirth. Tew related how not everyone accepted her findings; the *British Medical Journal* did not publish her work and *The Lancet* accepted just one paper, which she saw as the establishment's attempt to silence her.[92] As neither journal is averse to rigorous debate, this seems unlikely. Tew brought to her analysis an ideological perspective that was also apparent in her 1990 history of maternity.

*Why choose homebirth?*

In this she alleged psychosexual motivations for obstetricians' engagement in childbirth services, and that women and midwives alike were oppressed by the male obstetrical profession.[93] In a 1985 article in the *Journal of the Royal College of General Practitioners*, she argued that homebirth was not a threat to mothers and babies, but to 'the healthy survival of obstetric and medical practitioners'.[94] Burgess reported that Tew received a standing ovation at the 1987 conference.[95] Back in New Zealand, her work was cited in support of homebirth by the Health Department's 1989 working group on safe options for low-risk pregnancy.[96]

In her talk at the conference, Ann Oakley, feminist sociologist and author of *The Captured Womb: A History of the Medical Care of Pregnant Women* (1982), criticised obstetricians for being unscientific in their opinions on homebirth, governed by their own inordinate fear of the birth process.[97] While this followed the usual feminist rubric, Oakley later expressed misgivings about the conference itself, writing an article for *New Society* entitled 'Home Birth: A Class Privilege', in which she criticised the conference for focusing narrowly on the situation for white middle-class women. This elicited an angry letter to the editor accusing Oakley of 'behaving like a reactionary man'.[98]

Another speaker at the conference, Dr Marsden Wagner, an American neonatologist and epidemiologist, had been the World Health Organization's Director of Perinatal Health Care Services European Region since 1978. Wagner held strong feminist views, claiming that the medical profession's attitude to homebirth was part of a much larger issue, which was 'the male struggle to control women'. He argued that, by persuading women they were inadequate to give birth without male assistance, men created a lifelong dependency on them. Homebirth, he argued, was key to overcoming this dependency and empowering women.[99]

'Active birth' advocate Janet Balaskas was one of the conference organisers. In her closing address, Balaskas enthused that women were giving up their posture of helplessness, or the 'stranded beetle position', in childbirth and starting 'to get off the delivery table and to discover how to behave instinctively'.[100] Balaskas, along with Kitzinger, Odent and others, became part of the steering committee for the new organisation formed at the conclusion of the conference – the International Home Birth Movement. In the event, this organisation was to host only one further conference, in Sydney in 1992.[101]

Burgess reported that she and Harrower did not get the opportunity to present to the 1987 conference after all (and received apologies for this) but that they made 'a big impact with people referring to the New Zealand model. We have more independent midwives in Auckland than they do in the UK. There are only six domiciliary midwives in London!'[102] According to one estimate, there were only about 10 midwives practising independently throughout Britain in the mid-1980s, and they were private practitioners who charged for their services.[103] Christchurch homebirth midwife and conference attendee Celeste McCoy boasted that New Zealand was a 'shining example' as one of the few countries where homebirth was free of charge.[104]

In 1987, too, Joan Donley and Judi Strid attended a conference of the International Confederation of Midwives in Amsterdam. There, among other speakers, Australian Carolyn Noble-Spruell urged feminists not to lose sight of the fact that all women were subjected to the powerlessness, control and degradation of current reproductive health practices that continued to use women's bodies as living laboratories.[105] New Zealand feminist midwives and consumers were not alone.

New Zealand also appeared to be an attractive destination as part of the circuit for campaigners, as it had been for Stephen and Ina May Gaskin. In 1986, feminist American author, photographer and filmmaker Suzanne Arms lectured in Auckland.[106] Renowned for her 1975 book called *Immaculate Deception* critiquing American childbirth, Arms had helped found an alternative birth centre in California in 1978.[107] The New Zealand College of Midwives (Otago branch) cited Arms in its 1990 submission in favour of midwifery autonomy in New Zealand.[108] Almost all the dignitaries at the 1987 London homebirth conference visited New Zealand during the 1980s. As well as Arms, they included Janet Balaskas (1984), Sheila Kitzinger (1984 and 1989), Wendy Savage (1988), Michel Odent (1989), Ann Oakley (1989) and Marsden Wagner (1990). In 1988 West German Professor Friedrich Graf, a homeopathic and homebirth GP who had run a workshop at the 1987 conference, visited New Zealand and gave talks on homeopathy in childbirth.[109]

In 1988 the Wellington HBA hosted a public lecture by British obstetrician Wendy Savage, who had worked in New Zealand for a time in the 1970s.[110] Savage had been dismissed from her post at the London Hospital in 1985 following accusations of incompetence, although she was eventually cleared and reinstated following a high-profile inquiry. She had recounted her experiences in a 1986 book, *A Savage Enquiry*.[111] In her 1988 lecture she put in a plea for homebirth midwives, arguing that the only way to return to normal birth was for midwives to move out of the hospitals and become independent practitioners. In Britain, she said, midwives had to obey obstetricians and were resigning because of lack of job satisfaction, so that 'we've lost the strong midwives and those left in the system are often those prepared to go along with it'. This was a clear vote of no confidence in hospital midwives. 'Cheers for Wendy', the HBA write-up of her visit concluded.[112] She also gave a public lecture in Whangārei on 3 January 1989 which Strid transcribed for the *HBA Newsletter*.[113]

Sheila Kitzinger addressed an enthusiastic audience of 400 in Auckland in 1989 on 'Birth, Breasts and the Passage to Motherhood'. She claimed that women's sense of self-worth was attacked by the obstetric profession which had a 'history of violence commencing when they gate-crashed the midwifery field, taking over and bullying women's uteruses into submission'. She reiterated her view that birth in the right environment was a psychosexual experience which was frequently destroyed by the violence of obstetricians, and she even equated hospital birth with rape.[114]

Marsden Wagner was possibly the greatest coup for New Zealand's homebirth movement, arriving just as Parliament was debating the virtues of natural birth under the Nurses Amendment Bill in 1990. As the newly established New Zealand College of Midwives pronounced, he 'sped through NZ challenging the establishment and inspiring midwives'.[115] After he addressed their first annual conference in 1990, his lecture was reproduced in full in the College's journal.[116] Wagner vehemently opposed epidurals, describing them as making women not numb but 'dead' from the waist down, and claimed without providing evidence that they were the second most common cause of women dying during childbirth in Britain. Lumbar epidural anaesthesia had been developed from the late 1950s as less invasive than general anaesthesia, and by the 1980s had been further developed and endorsed by major obstetrical bodies as a safe method of pain relief, generally administered by trained obstetric anaesthetists. The growing popularity of epidurals was driven by women who demanded the right to choose.[117] Such interventions were anathema to natural childbirth advocates such as Wagner, however, who censured all forms of intervention. Combining New Zealand's forceps and caesarean rates (14% and 11% respectively), he condemned the practice of a country where, he stated, 25% of all women were having their babies 'pulled out or cut out'.[118] The homebirth movement had gained some powerful international allies.

## Conclusion

During the 1980s the New Zealand Home Birth Association insisted that everyone should consider homebirth – it was what responsible parents did. It was good for the infant and empowering for the mother, who would then be in a prime position to manage the complex task of motherhood. Moreover, they argued, in adopting homebirth, women were making a stand against the male medical profession who sought to control childbirth in their own interests. This was the message not only from the local homebirth lobby but also from international authorities of high standing.

While homebirth remained a minority activity in New Zealand, those espousing it maintained that more and more women would choose it, if given the opportunity, because of its many advantages. They argued that this was a woman's right, restricted only by the selfishness and misogyny of the medical profession. In 1985 a New Zealand Planning Council report, chaired by sociologist Professor Peggy Koopman-Boyden, commented on the fact that 'while most babies were still born in hospital, there was a growing interest in home birth in recent years'. The report asserted without providing evidence that: 'The limitations appear to be more in the form of organisational barriers than lack of demand, for example, opposition from some sectors of the medical profession, the cost to parents, conditions of work for midwives.' It continued: 'Given greater emphasis on the wishes of mothers and acceptance that choice should be available, it is probable that the number of home births will grow.'[119] They were not the only ones persuaded by the homebirth lobby, but was it truly what women wanted? These assertions would eventually be put to the test.

# THREE

## *Homebirth and maternity services 1970–1990*

BY THE LATE 1970S, medical and nursing professionals, other members of the public, and politicians were cognisant of the new interest in homebirth. Their perspectives were, however, often very different from those within the homebirth movement. They did not accept homebirth advocates' interpretation of hospital birth that it was driven by male obstetricians wishing to control women and make money at their expense. Many saw the homebirth movement itself as self-indulgent and even dangerous, and they believed that health professionals had the welfare of the mother and baby at heart when they favoured the hospital over homebirth. The New Zealand Nurses' Association (NZNA), including its Midwives' and Obstetric Nurses' Special Interest Section, took a leading role in cautioning against, and urging regulation of, the new trend in childbirth.

This chapter explores the debates around the inclusion of homebirth within maternity services in the 1970s and 1980s by reviewing the submissions to and findings of significant government inquiries, and the relevant sections of the Nurses Acts. It argues that the direction taken during this period was very different from that which would emerge in 1990. Those leading the services considered how best to incorporate homebirths within the existing maternity system, with legislation aimed at achieving this. The chapter also challenges the oft-repeated account of this period as one of oppression of midwives and their subsequent liberation in 1990. It does so by revisiting the relevant legislation and examining how it operated in practice, including its effect on the working relationship between doctors and homebirth midwives. It argues that the latter had a level of independence prior to 1990, and that most, although not all, worked collaboratively with doctors. The end of the period, however, saw a growing radicalisation of some homebirth midwives who demanded 'autonomy'. What they precisely meant by autonomy will be further explored in Chapter 4.

## The Maternity Services Committee and homebirth

The Board of Health's Maternity Services Committee (MSC), charged with oversight of maternity since 1960 and composed largely of obstetricians and nurses, published a report in 1982 on services provided in the home at and following birth. The report noted that, while domiciliary (homebirth) midwifery funded by the Department of Health had been part of maternity services since 1939, there had been no overall review of that sector.[1]

This report was preceded by an information paper on domiciliary midwifery written by the MSC in 1979 in light of the 'slight increase' in the number of domiciliary midwives claiming maternity benefits. The paper addressed domiciliary midwifery services in Holland and the UK as reference points. It pointed out that those countries had set criteria for screening homebirths and that no woman lived far from a base hospital. In this latter respect they differed significantly from New Zealand with its scattered population, where outlying hospitals already had staff shortages, and distances militated against rapid transfer to hospital.[2] The MSC also acknowledged the existence of a demand for homebirth. It referred to a 1977 NZNA survey of the Hutt Valley which had found that some women chose to have their babies at home regardless of back-up facilities, and noted that a recent United Women's Convention had advocated homebirth.[3]

The MSC expressed two concerns about domiciliary midwives. The first was whether they complied with the 1971 Nurses Act which required them to notify medical practitioners of a pregnancy so that the latter could assess the suitability of homebirth and provide back-up if necessary. The second related to ongoing professional training to ensure domiciliary midwives kept up to date. The committee claimed that domiciliary midwives were encouraged to attend courses at National Women's Hospital in Auckland or the St Helen's hospitals, 'but to date have shown no interest'.[4]

That same year the MSC published a pamphlet called 'Obstetrics and the Winds of Change'. This, it explained, was written in response to the demands of 'modern women', who included a vocal minority wanting to birth at home even if in a high-risk category. It asked, 'How can we protect the lives and IQs of our future citizens and counter this move away from our hospitals?' The answer was to make hospitals more homely, abandon rigid attitudes, listen to patients' requests and 'make her feel that she is the centre of the universe in her moment of triumph'.[5] Journalist Carole Wall agreed: 'Instead of bowing out of the system altogether and opting for home births in spite of the risks, women must insist that the maternity hospitals gear themselves to the consumers rather than the staff.'[6] Hospitals took this directive seriously, with New Zealand's most high-tech institution, National Women's Hospital, leading the way. As early as 1964, Professor Dennis Bonham had emphasised the importance of humanism in medicine, and in subsequent years measures were introduced such as allowing the husband or other support persons to be present at the birth, relaxed visiting hours and 'rooming in', with the baby kept at the mother's bedside rather than being sent to the nursery.[7]

The Home Birth Association viewed the 1979 pamphlet as a blatant attempt to shut down the homebirth option.[8] Joan Donley thought so too, but also conceded, 'We do not advocate home birth for everyone – only as a viable alternative for those who want it and can meet our conditions, such as no smoking and a good diet.'[9] Elsewhere she confirmed that it was 'up to the girl's doctor to assess if she's a low risk patient. If there is any toxaemia, a heart condition, a breech birth or twins likely the delivery must be in hospital.' She related how she and her midwife partner Carolyn Young had delivered about 200 babies over five years since 1974, with no mortality, although occasionally they had to transfer the mother to hospital.[10] From this account, it appeared to be a safe and carefully controlled option.

The NZNA was not so sure; nor was its special interest group of midwives and obstetric nurses. This group had been set up in 1936 as the National Obstetric Group with a focus on midwifery education.[11] In 1969, the group was formalised as the Midwives' and Obstetric Nurses' Special Interest Section to affiliate with the International Confederation of Midwives. Three years later, the NZNA ratified its constitution to allow this group to speak on maternity issues of national importance.[12] In 1978 those running a midwifery teacher training workshop explained that changing social circumstances during the 1970s had brought increasing public disillusionment with the hospital environment and thus a greater demand for homebirths; like the MSC, they thought this 'unsafe practice' could be countered by making hospitals more family oriented.[13] National Women's Hospital charge nurse Glenda Stimpson, chair of the NZNA Midwives' and Obstetric Nurses' Special Interest Section, who claimed to have had experience of homebirth, spoke against the practice at a 1976 seminar on 'Where to be born?'.[14] Penelope Dunkley, national executive member of the NZNA and chair of the Special Interest Section in 1973, also put the Association's views forward in support of hospital births. If homebirths were to continue, she said in 1979, the NZNA wanted to see domiciliary midwives come under the control of an obstetrician and to have continuing education to keep them up to date.[15] In the same vein the NZNA told the Minister of Health that year that it wished to 'publicly express its extreme concern that domiciliary midwives are not necessarily subject to adequate supervision or control and do not have ongoing educational programmes'.[16]

When the MSC invited submissions relating to homebirths in 1979, the Auckland HBA was quick off the mark. Barbara Macfarlane and Geoff Bridgman wrote the submission, and focused on the NZNA's call for obstetrical control. They declared, 'Since the Branch knows of only one sympathetic obstetrician, we regard this call as nothing less than an attempt at a de facto shutdown of the home-birth option.'[17] The HBA pointed out that during the previous five years the New Zealand perinatal mortality rate for homebirths had been 4 per 1,000, whilst in 1975 the perinatal mortality rate in hospitals was 16.5 per 1,000. Such statistics were misleading, however, since they overlooked hospital transfers and the very small and select group of women who opted – or were accepted – for homebirth.[18]

The HBA's submission to the MSC was not representative of submissions overall, and homebirth midwife Maggie Banks later described the opposition to domiciliary midwifery in the submissions as 'overwhelming'.[19] In their stark rejection of homebirth, many of these submissions had a very different flavour from those sent to the select committee for the 1990 Nurses Amendment Bill just a decade later. Exceptions to that total rejection of homebirth in 1979–80 included the New Zealand Council of the Royal College of Obstetricians and Gynaecologists and the National Council of Women, who instead suggested ways of regulating homebirth to ensure the wellbeing of mother and child, just as they would in 1990.

One of the 1979–80 submissions came from the Hospital Boards' Association, and was written by its chief executive and nursing officer. The latter objected to improving homebirth services on the grounds that this would simply encourage the trend, 'which the nursing service has no desire to do [as] many unsuitable clients would present'.[20] In their submission, staff of St George's Private Hospital in Christchurch worried that even conducting a review could be interpreted as officially supporting homebirth. Recognising that most of the serious complications of pregnancy occurred in labour, they argued that 'nothing said to the contrary can take away from the cold fact that hospitals are best equipped and staffed to deal with such emergencies'. They even opposed the provision of a flying squad (a mobile obstetrical back-up team, one of which had been set up at National Women's Hospital, and commonly used in the UK), as this would simply encourage homebirths. They firmly believed that all women should give birth in hospital.[21] Canterbury Hospital Board also considered it 'regrettable that the Maternity Services Committee should ever seriously consider domiciliary midwifery', maintaining that no one experienced in obstetrics and homebirth would support the idea.[22] Staff from Palmerston North Hospital suggested focusing on 'more friendly and deinstitutionalized' hospital care instead of home deliveries, maintaining that 'emotive factors and an imperfect understanding of the risks' drove the homebirth movement.[23]

In his submission, Dr Christopher Harison from Thames Hospital maintained that establishing an official homebirth service would be a retrograde step and dangerous to mother and child. He calculated that half or more of the patients suffering significant postpartum haemorrhage would be classified as low risk during antenatal screening and that most complications in labour were unpredictable. He described what happened after a homebirth in the Coromandel where the mother lost a considerable amount of blood and went into shock following a retained placenta; it took two and a half hours to transfer her to hospital. There she had to be resuscitated with multiple blood transfusions, the placenta had to be removed manually, and antibiotic therapy administered. Another woman on a commune in the Coromandel ranges had a retained placenta and postpartum haemorrhage, and could not be reached by ambulance; it took nine hours to get her to hospital. 'In both instances,' Harison noted, 'considerable unpleasantness was experienced from the accompanying friends.'[24] Branches of the Obstetrical and Gynaecological Society also opposed homebirth, with Graeme Henderson, president of the Southland Division, telling the MSC that his branch opposed the Health

Department paying midwives for homebirths, adding, 'In fact it is difficult to understand why the Department continues to do this.'[25]

By contrast, the New Zealand Council of the Royal College of Obstetricians and Gynaecologists recognised the need to accommodate the demand for homebirths, and emphasised the importance of adequate medical and social screening, along with assessment of home facilities, a competent and experienced midwife, integrated home/hospital delivery facilities, medical supervision, a flying squad for urgent transfer to hospital if necessary, and support services such as home aides.[26] The New Zealand Medical Association stressed the importance of protecting the mother and 'the one who is more at risk, namely, the child', and recommended that domiciliary midwives have a continuing attachment to a hospital in order to keep up to date.[27] Similarly, in its submission, the National Council of Women, which claimed wide representation and to be a watchdog for issues concerning women and children, did not oppose homebirth, but argued that women considering this option should be carefully vetted for their suitability, with mandatory hospital delivery for cases with known or foreseen complications and for those having their first babies or after their fourth. The Council was also concerned about the level of training homebirth midwives had for independent practice (as opposed to working as a team in hospital), and submitted that this should include 'recognition and acceptance of her limitations'. Above all, they stressed the importance of 'adequate and expert medical aid' being available immediately should intervention be necessary, and the need for good relations between midwives, doctors, and public health and Plunket nurses.[28]

The MSC survey attracted considerable public interest. Journalist Pauline Ray wrote a feature article for the *New Zealand Listener* based on an interview with Joan Donley. Entitled 'Whose body is it? Whose baby is it?', it emphasised a woman's right to choose homebirth.[29] In response, Julia M. Witchalls of Auckland wrote a letter to the editor outlining her own obstetric history, pointing out that even though she would have been in the low-risk category, she and her son would not be alive today had she opted for a homebirth.[30] Another respondent, R. Herrick from Hamilton, defended the hospital experience, advising readers that birthing in a public hospital did not mean the woman had to 'fight every inch of the way to have a choice of alternatives' or had to be separated from her infant and husband.[31] Jess Parker pointed out that homebirth favoured only a limited cohort of women in the community – the better-educated and higher socio-economic group – and that homebirth would only add to the desperate social and economic problems of many other women. She encouraged women to lobby to incorporate all the advantages of homebirth – a friendly and relaxed atmosphere, bonding, freedom of choice – whilst retaining the hospital system's obvious advantages, such as safety measures for emergencies.[32]

Even the alternative community at Centrepoint saw a place for hospitals. Its leader Bert Potter claimed in 1982 to have been very impressed by the cooperative attitude of hospital staff who allowed support people at the birth. He explained that when his twins were born at National Women's Hospital, 'the theatre became a bit like a picnic with people sitting around on the floor waiting for the babies to be born'.[33] Centrepoint's resident homebirth midwife Rhonda Evans declared, 'Hooray for hospitals when you need them'; for labours not progressing, she advised, 'When you've done all you can, it's time to go to hospital.'[34]

Debate about home versus hospital was the subject of a panel discussion at the first HBA annual conference in 1980, attended by 150 people. Three speakers, Sister Patricia Clark from the NZNA, and obstetricians Andrew Mackintosh and Tony Baird, faced a hostile audience. Undeterred, Clark told them that women considering homebirth should have the opportunity for an objective discussion of the pros and cons, and cautioned that problems could and did occur with potentially disastrous speed during labour, even for women categorised as low-risk.[35]

In February 1980, the NZNA Midwives' and Obstetric Nurses' Special Interest Section produced a policy statement on homebirth for the MSC. It began by noting the existence of a relatively small group of 'vociferous' advocates of home confinement. It was correct in seeing this as a small group; whilst the Section itself had 500 members, Donley claimed that she 'never tired of telling all and sundry how EIGHT domiciliary midwives formed [the Domiciliary Midwives Society] to challenge the NZNA speaking for us'.[36] In its statement, the Section considered the reluctance of most midwives and doctors to attend a woman at home 'well-founded', considering how quickly problems could arise, and suggested ways of persuading women to birth in hospital. These once again included making the hospital environment more homelike, and offering early discharge from hospital with domiciliary support.[37] The original 1939 Maternity Benefit had granted women 14 days' free care in hospital following birth. By the 1950s, some hospitals advocated early discharge – after the third or fourth day – provided there were suitable conditions at home for the mother.[38] Mothers no longer valued a lengthy hospital stay following birth, but health and social work professionals continued to express the need to support mothers going home.

The UK was grappling with similar issues to the MSC. The 1980 House of Commons Social Services Committee Report on neonatal and perinatal mortality recommended reducing the number of small maternity units and phasing out homebirths altogether. It recognised a growing lobby of 'mostly very educated ladies . . . who are very pro home confinement'. It attributed this primarily to 'a degree of inhumanity [and] a lack of understanding of the women's needs' in some obstetric units. In light of this and the 'doctor bashing attitude' encouraged by 'trendy' weekly newspapers, the report advised that there must be a 'humanisation' of maternity hospitals, and full explanations given when technological intervention was needed. It concluded, 'We were left with the strong impression that the demand for home delivery and in peripheral units would be reduced if services elsewhere were adequate and of the kind the mothers wanted.'[39]

New Zealand's MSC and others hoped for the same. On the other hand, improving the hospital environment was never going to be enough for some homebirth advocates like Linda Daly-Peoples, who declared in 1980 that she would never have another baby in hospital, no matter how 'homely' hospitals were.[40]

## *Mother and Baby at Home – The Early Days* (1982)

The MSC published its report on domiciliary midwifery and early discharge from hospital in 1982. It was titled *Mother and Baby at Home – The Early Days*. The committee's remit was to consider the provisions for three groups of women: those wishing early discharge following birth in hospital; those who planned a homebirth but were prepared to transfer to hospital if necessary; and those who rejected contact with, or admission to, hospital under any circumstances.[41] The MSC noted that, because there were very few practising domiciliary midwives, it had managed to interview most of them: 11 in total.[42] It named only three of these: Joan Donley (described as the spokesperson for the Auckland midwives), Lyn McLean and Jennifer Sage.[43] The latter had expressed her views forcefully the previous year when she declared that working in hospital 'led to a warped, incorrect concept of childbirth, with an unnecessary emphasis on danger and risk'.[44]

The MSC introduced its report by defining reproduction as a biological process, and that 'like all biological processes, things could go wrong with it'. It reported a World Health Organization statement about the risk of dying at birth: 'Regardless of the level of child mortality the probability of dying is at its peak at the time of birth, including the period immediately before birth, and declines thereafter.'[45] It also referred to the legal requirement for doctors' involvement in homebirths (the 1971 Nurses Act), explaining that the reason Parliament had legislated for this was that *the unborn baby has rights as well as the mother and the father, and society should ensure that adequate care is provided for the baby*.[46] The committee did not believe there would be any substantial increase in the demand for homebirth in New Zealand but thought it probable that a small number of women would continue to choose this option. With that in mind, it wanted to ensure the highest standards of care, with optimal back-up services from a nearby obstetric unit.

The report addressed the training and regulation of homebirth midwives and general practitioners practising childbirth (commonly known as GP obstetricians). It recommended that midwives should be connected to the nearest obstetric unit and contracted to the local hospital board rather than the Department of Health. Hospital boards had already set up review committees to oversee obstetric standards of GPs, and the MSC thought these should include domiciliary midwives. It believed that all midwives practising in the community should have undertaken general nurse training along with their midwifery training, and not simply maternity nurse training which had been the alternative route to a midwifery qualification since 1925. They should also have had 'recent and appropriate experience in a modern obstetric unit'. This experience should include at least two years' post-registration continuous midwifery practice in an approved hospital, with six months in an antenatal clinic, one year in the delivery unit, and six months devoted to postnatal care.[47] For GPs, the MSC recommended ensuring adequate postgraduate and continuing education in obstetrics for those doing homebirths (National Women's Hospital had run obstetric diploma courses for GPs since 1958), and that GPs should hold a current hospital board contract to enable them access to hospital facilities if necessary.[48] It advised that all homebirths should be attended by a midwife and a doctor if possible.[49]

The Netherlands was often held up by the HBA and others as the model for homebirth. *Mother and Baby at Home – The Early Days* repeated the contention that, unlike in New Zealand, all Dutch women lived less than half an hour away from a hospital. Above all, it noted that in the Netherlands there was a 'great emphasis placed on the selection of risk', with no fewer than 100 risk indications leading to free hospital care under a specialist. As a result, about 38% of Dutch women delivered at home, 35% delivered free of charge in hospital because of a specific medical indication, and a further 27% delivered in hospital for social or personal reasons.[50]

*Mother and Baby at Home* was in keeping with the 1980 NZNA Midwives' and Obstetric Nurses' Special Interest Section policy statement.[51] The NZNA and the MSC appeared to be on the same page. However, their suggestions were strenuously resisted by homebirth midwives, who would eventually win governmental support in 1990.

## The Nurses Amendment Act 1983

The 1983 Nurses Amendment Act was the immediate predecessor to the 1990 Nurses Amendment Act, but it could not have been more different. Parliamentary debates on the two pieces of legislation also had a very different flavour. Something very significant was to occur in the seven years between them.

The 1983 Act repeated the clause in the 1971 and 1977 Acts that it was an offence to undertake obstetric nursing without a medical practitioner taking responsibility for the care of pregnant woman (Section 54 (1)). Following the recommendations of the MSC and the NZNA, Section 54 (3) specified that all midwives practising outside a hospital setting had to be trained in both general nursing and midwifery. However, another clause, Section 54 (5), provided an exemption from having to be trained nurses for midwives already in practice. This was added following extensive lobbying by homebirth midwives (and will be further explored in Chapter 4). Another clause in 1983 (Section 58 (2)) authorised a medical officer of health to suspend a midwife from practice 'where such suspension appears to him to be necessary in order to prevent the spread of infection or where he has reasonable grounds to suspect any such nurse to be practising in an unhygienic manner'.[52]

During the parliamentary debates in December 1983, Labour Opposition MP Margaret Shields (later Minister of Women's Affairs 1987–90) explained that 'one of the fountainheads of the Bill was the unfortunate case of the baby that was born in a bathtub'.[53] This was reinforced by National's Health

Minister Aussie Malcolm when he noted some 'pretty peculiar and amateurish attempts' to deliver babies, referring to the same case.[54] While the HBA had sought to distance itself from water births, it too acknowledged that 'Auckland's waterbirth debacle provided the climate for the introduction of the Nurses Amendment Bill', as it had raised concerns about the safety of some homebirth practices.[55]

Homebirth in general did not receive a favourable coverage in these debates. Shields acknowledged that it was 'not a popular choice, but one that should be made available for second births and for low risk patients [sic] who choose that option'.[56] In other words, she was supportive, but only under very specific conditions. National MP Roger McClay argued that the Bill was 'aimed only at ensuring the greatest possible safety to the mother and baby', and stated that:

> I was amazed that those making submissions in support of home births talked about the mother and the father in almost every case, and perhaps about some other members of the family, but I do not recall – although other members may correct me – anybody talking specifically about the health and welfare of the baby. The clause is aimed at ensuring that no possible risk exists that could be avoided.[57]

Labour MP for Eastern Maori, Peter Tapsell, who had graduated in medicine in 1952, also commented on the HBA's submission. He believed women had a responsibility to do their best to ensure their baby's survival and wellbeing. Referring to the claim that birth was a normal physiological function, he said, '[W]e all know that physiological functions run awry from time to time.' When this happened, he said, it was important that the birth took place 'in close proximity to a modern and well equipped operating theatre where instruments are available to clear the baby's tubes, to provide oxygen, and perhaps to supplement the blood supply of the child'. It was 'unacceptable for a woman's medical adviser, whether doctor or nurse, to acquiesce in any arrangement that falls short of those requirements'.[58]

In the lead-up to the 1983 Nurses Amendment Bill, the MSC and legislators received a clear message from health professionals, including doctors, nurses and hospital midwives, that the hospital was the safest place in which to give birth. They accepted that women had the right to choose homebirth, but looked to ways to make this as safe as possible and stressed the rights of the baby as well as the parents. Later, in 1989, when the Health Department launched a review of the 1983 Nurses Amendment Act and invited submissions, the National Council of Women's submission included comments on Sections 54 and 58 of the Act. On Section 54 it stated: 'We consider the restrictions under this section are important for the safety of both women and babies.' And on Section 58: 'The powers conferred here are important for the protection of new-born babies and their mothers.'[59] Despite this assessment, debates on a new Nurses Amendment Bill would take a very different turn just a few months later.

The politics that led to this dramatic shift are the subject of Chapter 5. The following section explores how the 1971 Nurses Act and the subsequent amendments in 1977 and 1983 played out in practice, and specifically in respect of the relationship between homebirth midwives and doctors. The changes and continuities in their relationship during this short period provide an important backdrop to the 1990 Act and the events that followed.

## Homebirth midwives and GPs

The 1971 Nurses Act has been interpreted by some as hugely significant in the history of midwifery. As noted, Section 52 of the Act (Section 54 of the 1977 and 1983 Acts) specified that it was an offence for a person to 'carry out obstetric nursing in any case where a medical practitioner has not undertaken responsibility for the care of the patient', except in emergencies. Donley described the 1971 Act as the death knell for the midwifery profession, because it meant they could no longer practise without doctors' supervision. Yet, she admitted, 'There was not a murmur of protest from midwives!'[60] In a similar vein Karen Guilliland, president of the new College of Midwives in 1989, reflected on this legislation:

> The Nurses Act of 1971 removed the right of midwives to practise autonomously. New Zealand midwifery changed from a community-based profession into a hospital-based workforce ... The midwives became sort of obstetric nurses – the obstetrician looked after the woman and the nurses did as they were told. Medicine ruled.[61]

This chronology is incorrect; in 1971 most midwives worked in hospital, with only a handful in the community. Nor did these hospital midwives simply 'do as they were told'. And there was also a very good reason for the lack of protest that Donley identified. Most midwives did not feel aggrieved by the legislation. History researcher Samantha Skiff, who interviewed eight midwives working in maternity hospitals in New Zealand at that time, concluded, 'The law was not seen to change social or medical practice for many.'[62] Glenda Stimpson, charge nurse in the delivery suite at National Women's Hospital, told Skiff, 'I don't believe it made any difference to my practice, I did what I had to do.'[63] Midwives also continued to run St Helen's hospitals. Gabrielle Bourke, researching Auckland's St Helen's Hospital, wrote of the Act, 'To say that nothing really changed for hospital midwives in 1971 disrupts the story of a repressed profession that rises from the ashes in 1990', yet she found 'not an anguished group of St Helen's midwives, but one happily accepting the legislation'.[64] Life continued as before, as midwives ran delivery suites, calling in medical assistance in the case of emergency.

The legislation potentially had more impact for the small number of midwives working outside hospitals. Introducing Section 52 to Parliament in 1971, Minister of Health Don McKay said, 'Only a small number of people will be affected, since this provision is restricted to obstetric nursing at home.'[65] As there were only 24 recorded births outside the hospital setting in 1971, it was almost a non-issue. The clause was repeated in the 1977 Nurses Act (Section 54), but in 1978 there were still only 15 domiciliary midwives registered with the Health Department, and not all of these were claiming fees.[66] They were a very small minority.

In 1989, amid publicity that women's rights were curtailed by the requirement that a doctor attend all homebirths, Gayle O'Brien from the Health Department's Advisory Committee on Women's Health asked for a legal opinion on medical supervision of birth. She explained, 'I am aware that Section 54 of the Nurses Act states that a medical practitioner must be responsible for each patient. I am unclear whether a doctor must be present, your clarification of this matter would be appreciated.' The response was: 'The short answer to the question is – no, the legislation does not require the presence of a doctor at every birth.'[67] Rather, as a 1979 Health Department information sheet explained, the midwife had to notify the GP of the pregnancy, and the latter then approved domiciliary confinement, as in the Netherlands. The midwife was to maintain contact with the GP through the pregnancy and inform the GP when the patient went into labour.[68] This was a contingency plan in case of emergency; for normal births there was no oversight. Yet the myth that midwives had to be supervised was to become part of the campaign for midwifery autonomy.

While it was not a legal requirement for doctors to attend uncomplicated births, there appears to have been an expectation (and, for many, a preference) during the 1970s and 1980s that a doctor would attend those births. Joan Donley, who in the 1990s made the explosive claim that the 1971 Act spelt the end of midwifery, appeared to work well with doctors in the 1970s, telling the press in 1978: 'Most of our doctors are very interested and they attend the birth, but they usually stay in the background. We notify the doctor about the labour and let him know how advanced it is.'[69]

Homebirth midwives had worked with doctors before the 1971 legislation. For example, Pat Minnell, a domiciliary midwife in the 1950s, said in an interview that she, like her colleagues, would attend a woman in her home only if she had the back-up of a doctor. Similarly, the daughter of a midwife who had graduated from St Helen's in 1930 and attended homebirths in Pukekohe, Auckland, recalled that her mother only ever worked as a domiciliary midwife alongside a doctor.[70] Carolyn Young, a homebirth midwife in Auckland from the 1970s, later explained that she worked alongside 'many dedicated and good GP's who would get up in the middle of the night and walk 2 or 3 km's up a dirt road to get into a place and be there and really bring a positive nurturing attitude to birth'. She recalled 'a very close working relationship with a group of GPs who would support home birth because we still needed them'.[71] Reflecting on her career in 2004, GP obstetrician Helen Rodenburg commented that before 1990 she used to attend home deliveries to 'support the midwives'.[72]

In its submission on homebirth to the MSC in 1979, the Auckland HBA defined a homebirth as one 'where a domiciliary midwife and a doctor are always in attendance', a definition it repeated to a journalist in 1980.[73] In 1981, the HBA listed 105 homebirth GPs around the country who were willing to support the 17 practising homebirth midwives.[74] This number does not support Donley's later claim that, by the 1970s, 'There were still a few GPs who would provide the necessary "medical supervision" despite peer pressure.'[75]

One woman who had two homebirths in the 1970s defined the doctor's role: 'The doctor will come at any hour and though seldom even helps at the delivery he will be in the room relaxed, chatting and friendly but alert for any sign of trouble, providing sedation if necessary.'[76] Ina May Gaskin, the role model for many homebirth midwives, always had the back-up of a doctor for homebirths conducted at The Farm in Tennessee.[77] Auckland-based homebirth doctor John Grieve spoke at the first HBA conference in 1980. Grieve was happy to support midwives in homebirths, but also explained:

> I personally feel it is essential that a doctor be present at all home births, partly because if he is not there and anything goes amiss it brings the home birth movement into disrepute. Having said that, the doctor, while there should keep as low a profile as is humanly possible. Seen as little as possible, and not heard at all.[78]

Wallace Metcalfe, a Wellington GP obstetrician, told the HBA in 1981 how he was often relegated to holding the mirror and taking the photographs during a homebirth.[79] He was happy in that role. Other midwives commented on the doctors' tea-making skills. Midwife Tina Gilbertson, who gave birth at home in 1990 with midwife Sally Pairman in attendance, remembered, 'We had to have a doctor present and he made the cup of tea so that was good.'[80] Nelson GP Bryan Hardie Boys, who had long been involved with home deliveries, told Minister of Health Helen Clark in 1990 that he thought it important for both doctor and midwife to be present at a homebirth, and that the former's presence need not interfere with the midwife's autonomy. He believed that removing either from the delivery would put babies and mothers at risk.[81]

Lynley McFarland explained that in the late 1970s she was paid $25 for attending a birth – six hours of work. She said, 'The doctor came along to make the cup of tea and take the photos, they used to get paid $75. It was the way things were then.'[82] This $25 fee was in fact just part of the $98 midwives earned for each homebirth, including pre- and postnatal visits.[83] The pay imbalance for the birth attendance could be regarded as a pay equity issue, but GPs' presence could equally be seen as a security measure. Metcalfe certainly saw it this way. He held the honour, according to the HBA in 1983, of being the first GP to speak publicly in favour of homebirth when he appeared on Radio NZ's national programme.[84] But he was also very frank about the role of the doctor. He told *Listener* journalist Pamela Stirling in 1990 that about 70% of births were trouble-free but that he did not feel like a fraud for accepting payment for 'basically doing nothing at most deliveries'. He said,

'I'm there as crash fireman.'[85] His 2018 obituary noted, 'Dr Metcalfe, known to friends and patients alike as Wally, will be remembered for his energy and ability to need but little sleep, an essential attribute in someone called out at all hours to attend upon births.'[86]

Some doctors were prepared to support midwives without attending the birth, and this was permitted in law. As homebirth midwife Barbara Hasslacher explained in 1988, 'Although the doctor has the legal responsibility and determines the criteria for acceptance of a home-birth case, it is the midwife who assists the woman during delivery.' She relished the responsibility of conducting homebirths without a doctor looking over her shoulder.[87]

Homebirth midwives prior to 1990 practised relatively independently. In 1987 the Health Department compiled a report based on interviews with homebirth midwives and advocates. It noted that the department's contract for domiciliary midwives had been drawn up in 1938 and had not been amended in the intervening 49 years. The contract was with the district health office, and the function of that office was to ensure that practitioners complied with the legislation and to administer claim forms and benefits, not to monitor the competence of the midwife. In response to a question relating to accountability, the midwives explained they were 'responsible to themselves, their peers, and their clients'. They objected to suggestions that their contracts be moved from health offices to hospital boards, with the report explaining, 'The main reason for rejecting this option was the real concern the midwives had that they might lose their autonomy and the right to use their professional judgement.' Nor did they wish to be contracted to a GP, as this 'could restrict their freedom of practice' and 'result in loss of independence', a clear acknowledgement of how much autonomy or independence they had under the current legislation.[88]

The relationship with GPs appeared to be working. In 1981 the HBA declared: 'The GP must . . . have faith in the competence of the D.M. [domiciliary midwife] to whom he entrusts his patient – for whom he is still ultimately responsible. All in all, it takes a special kind of doctor to back your home birth, and he deserves to be appreciated.'[89] The Auckland HBA reiterated this in 1987, when it thanked these doctors for their commitment to homebirth and for their support.[90] The Domiciliary Midwives Society noted supportive GPs in its newsletters, and Donley reported in the late 1980s that Auckland homebirth midwives met quarterly with homebirth doctors, holding 'frank discussions'.[91]

While Carolyn Young praised doctors who attended births, she also said that 'a lot of them just rubber stamped it', and that '[t]he official requirement of a GP endorsing the said event was fulfilled by an obliging but distant doctor'.[92] Auckland obstetrician Tony Baird and many of his colleagues were concerned by this, with Baird complaining during the 1980 HBA homebirth panel discussion that some doctors accepted nominal responsibility for homebirths without making adequate arrangements either to assist or supervise the delivery.[93] He said the same to the MSC in his submission about homebirths on behalf of the Auckland Division of the Obstetrical and Gynaecological Society.[94]

Another concern was the vetting of women for homebirth by both doctors and midwives. In listing who was not eligible for a homebirth in 1980, the HBA included those who had previous caesarean sections.[95] Yet, two years later, a study noted that some Auckland GPs and midwives accepted women for homebirth who had experienced a caesarean delivery, as well as those who displayed other risk factors such as heroin addiction. However, the researchers commented that concern about the failure of vetting did not account for women who might refuse to go to hospital, and that if women chose to birth at home it was better to have some professional attendance than none, as happened in California.[96]

## Midwives practising alone

There is evidence from the late 1970s that some homebirth midwives were not involving doctors in their practices. The MSC revealed that there had been 55 homebirths in Auckland in 1978, and that many doctors attended at least in the third stage of labour, but added, 'Unfortunately when the doctor was not present there was no indication that the midwife had notified the doctor.'[97] The committee's 1979 survey into homebirths discovered that, in one unidentified health district in 1978, 75% of the homebirths occurred without medical practitioners taking responsibility for the pregnant woman. According to midwife Maggie Banks, this was 'amongst the prompts' for the MSC to set up its review into homebirth.[98] As noted, one of the recommendations of the resultant 1982 report was that both doctor and midwife should attend homebirths if possible.[99]

A case of a midwife not complying with regulations came to official notice in Christchurch in 1981. The local medical officer of health and the principal public health nurse reported to the Health Department that a certain domiciliary midwife continued, despite their 'not inconsiderable efforts', to accept women for home delivery prior to an antenatal visit to the GP, and often without a routine referral note from the GP indicating the woman's suitability for homebirth. They wondered whether they could withhold payment from her.[100] In its response, the Health Department advised that she was indeed open to prosecution.[101] It is unclear what happened in this case, but the department did seem reluctant to prosecute midwives, as Bronwen Pelvin would also find.

In 1985 Pelvin told the Domiciliary Midwives Society that the two local obstetricians in Nelson were 'at least tolerant of home births', and that the younger one was 'most relaxed and commonsensical when dealing with any of our clients'.[102] Yet the following year she reported that the obstetricians, along with the local hospital medical superintendent, had called a meeting of all GPs to outline standards for accepting women for homebirths and reminding them of their 'responsibilities' in decision-making. She claimed this had made the GPs 'somewhat jittery!'[103]

In November 1988 the *Nelson Post* ran a story headlined 'Homebirth midwife breaks the law', declaring, 'Ms Bronwen Pelvin thinks she is the first midwife in New Zealand to admit publicly she has delivered a baby in an illegal birth – when she knew no doctor had agreed to be responsible . . .'[104] Pelvin recorded this episode in the *Domiciliary Midwives Society Newsletter* under the title, 'A New Zealand Midwife's Tale'. She began, 'Well, it has finally happened. I've attended an "illegal" home birth.' She explained how she and the woman 'decided to leave a doctor out of the picture entirely', though she understood that she could be prosecuted or reported to the Nursing Council. Aware that she was not 'covered' by a doctor, she said, '[Y]ou see I don't believe that I need to be covered. I am a professional person. I am responsible for what I do in any situation. I am prepared to stand in a court of law or at a disciplinary hearing and be responsible.' She pointed out that she had discussed the situation with the medical officer of health, the principal public health nurse, a lawyer who was also a homebirth father, and 'even my friendly local obstetrician'. All of them were very sympathetic, she said, but none was willing to provide the necessary legal back-up. The nurse had spoken to the Health Department's nurse advisor, who confirmed that Pelvin should try to find a doctor who was 'prepared to be a backup and safeguard' for her. If she could not do so, she was to explain this to her client and get the latter to 'sign a written, witnessed statement taking full responsibility for her own delivery and any consequences arising from it'.[105] Pelvin wrote that after receiving this letter she thought, 'Stuff it! I'm sick of this.' She went ahead with the homebirth, apparently without mishap, adding, 'It remains to be seen if I get paid!!' She felt 'really good about it' and thought it was 'what any good midwife would do'. If the woman had had to transfer to the hospital, she continued, her GP would have attended her, 'because he had agreed to do that originally. If I'd rung him and told him it was an emergency and that he had to come, then he would have had to come or we could've reported him to the Medical Council.'[106]

The *Nelson Evening Mail* noted that by conducting a homebirth with no doctor involved, Pelvin incurred the wrath of local doctor Graeme Loveridge, who said, 'Deliberately not involving a doctor but assuming one would attend in an emergency was imposing on a doctor's good will.' He fumed, 'There should always be at least liaison with the doctor, who had some skills domiciliary midwives did not have. In an emergency those skills could be crucial.'[107]

Donley reported the following year that, after Pelvin's 'public stand' in undertaking a homebirth 'without medical supervision', 1989 had been her busiest year; she had 'done three more home births without medical supervision' and had been paid for them by the department.[108] It was this wording – 'without medical supervision' – which had led Gayle O'Brien from the Health Department's Advisory Committee on Women's Health to express confusion and seek legal advice as to whether doctors had to be present at births, only to be told the law did not require this presence 'at every birth'.[109] Taking responsibility did not mean supervision for births that proceeded normally. Yet Pelvin for one felt that as a midwife she was a professional who had no need to involve a doctor at all. The 1989 AGM minutes of the Domiciliary Midwives Society, of which Pelvin was secretary, stated under the heading 'Legalities': 'Women without Doctors at all – just attend them, what can anyone do about it.'[110]

High-profile midwives such as Pelvin were not prosecuted for apparently infringing the law, possibly because local health officers feared a public backlash in the likely event of considerable media attention. In early 1990, as midwifery autonomy was being debated in Parliament, the *New Zealand Listener* ran a story strongly endorsing the new Nurses Amendment Bill. The author, Pamela Stirling, quoted Pelvin, who asked, 'Who is the childbirth service in

New Zealand for? Is it for women and their babies or is it a commercial venture for doctors on their own terms and at their own convenience?'[111] Doctors were cast as selfish and pecuniary, and resistant to change regardless of women's interests. Yet Stirling also cited one GP obstetrician expressing concern about midwives attending births alone. Obstetric Standards Review Committee North Shore (Auckland) representative Dr Jonathan Wilcox fumed:

> It is absolutely hazardous . . . for midwives to deliver on their own. We had a recent case up here where the home-birth midwife was the only person at the delivery and the baby was exposed to thick meconium ... and the midwife wasn't able to intubate that baby by passing a tube down into the larynx and lungs to get that meconium out. I mean, that is an absolute disgrace.

He also referred to a case where the midwife had not identified a prolapsed cord, and claimed recently to have been horrified to find a midwife had never heard of a common heart disorder. What GPs wanted, he said, was a team approach.[112]

## Conclusion

The 1971 Nurses Act did not spell the end of midwifery either in hospital or in the home. It set up a system where GPs would vet those women deemed suitable for a homebirth, and be available to attend at least in an emergency, as in the Netherlands. Many homebirth midwives accepted this and worked collaboratively with amenable GPs, many of whom were happy to attend homebirths as back-up. However, there were ongoing concerns about whether both doctors and midwives were carrying out their responsibilities under the Act, and whether there were enough safeguards, such as ongoing professional development, to ensure a good outcome.

Given the concerns about the need for additional safeguards for homebirth expressed by the MSC, as well as by many medical and nursing professionals and others such as the National Council of Women, allowing midwives to act on their own without clear statutory regulations was not a done deal. At the start of the 1980s the NZNA Midwives' and Obstetric Nurses' Special Interest Section itself did not support homebirth without strict controls in place. All indications were that childbirth services from the 1970s were moving in the direction of regulation, monitoring and teamwork. With legislators and others expressing so much caution, how can we explain the about-turn in 1990 allowing homebirth midwives to practise alone in the community?

When Bronwen Pelvin made a public stand against the law and confidently proclaimed, 'Roll on autonomous practice!', hers was not a lone voice but part of an organised campaign that gained considerable traction.[113] That campaign is the subject of Chapter 5, but to better understand what the government was signing up for in 1990 when it granted midwives 'autonomy', the next chapter explores what exactly this meant to the homebirth midwives and their supporters.

# FOUR

## *The meaning of autonomy for homebirth midwives in the 1980s*

IN APRIL 1989, LABOUR'S Health Minister Helen Clark wrote to her departmental officers, 'Please provide me with information about the midwives campaign for "autonomy". I am supportive of it and would like to see how it can be progressed.'[1] But what exactly did 'midwife autonomy' mean? On one level it meant the right of midwives to practise with no interference from other health professionals such as nurses and doctors – an autonomy that some homebirth midwives felt they already had to a large degree. However, for some radical homebirth midwives the concept of autonomy involved much more than this, implying a wholesale rejection of what those other health professions stood for. Firmly rooted in the homebirth movement, advocates of autonomy eschewed contact with hospitals in training and in practice, and in this regard differed significantly from those involved in homebirth services in the Netherlands. Some of this antipathy to hospital medicine was to survive within the new College of Midwives set up in 1989, making that body very different from its counterparts in the UK and Australia. This chapter unpacks the meaning of autonomy in homebirth midwives' pursuit of independence from doctors, nurses and hospitals in the 1980s.

## 'Homebirth midwives are the only real midwives'

The quest for 'midwifery autonomy' was led by homebirth midwives. As Joan Donley later said, it was this cohort who led all midwives out of their 'nursing bondage'.[2] The promotional material for Donley's 1986 book *Save the Midwife* stated that it explored the history of midwifery in New Zealand to show how midwives as independent practitioners had been constantly undermined so that their very survival was now at stake.[3] The editor of the *Domiciliary Midwives Society Newsletter*, Auckland homebirth midwife Heather Waugh, enthused that it should be compulsory reading for all midwives.[4] The book explained that the midwife had been 'refurbished to become a nurse-midwife, a hybrid, a medically oriented handmaiden, while the real midwife is an endangered species'.[5] Nurses along with doctors had contributed to this trend, 'colonising' midwives, according to homebirth midwife Maggie Banks, whose 2007 doctoral thesis examined the influential role nursing and hospital-based midwifery had played in trying to stamp out domiciliary midwifery.[6]

In 1982, the Home Birth Association set out to define the qualities of 'real' midwives compared to hospital or nurse-midwives. The former, they said, were independent-minded and liked to query doctors' decisions, whilst the latter always followed doctors' orders, courting their favour.[7] According to Wellington homebirth midwife Lyn McLean, not only did the 'nurse-midwife' defer to authority, but she also expected everything to go awry during birth and had a 'hearty respect' for modern technology. By contrast, the 'midwife', as the 'protector of the normal', respected the natural process.[8] Homebirth advocate Lynda Williams was another who disparaged hospital midwives for being over-reliant on technology.[9]

Not surprisingly, hospital midwives did not accept this characterisation, as researcher Samantha Skiff found when she interviewed eight midwives who worked in New Zealand hospitals from 1960 to 1990.[10] Hospital midwives valued what they described as teamwork with doctors. As Val Fitzpatrick put it, '[I]t was a good working relationship. I felt they respected me and my knowledge. Especially the older ones. Some of the young doctors sometimes felt they knew it all, but they soon got put back in their little places.'[11] Researching the history of Auckland's St Helen's Hospital, Gabrielle Bourke found that midwives there were proud to be part of team-based maternity care. Her interviews with midwives and with obstetrician Ian Ronayne affirmed the respect and reciprocity between the two groups.[12] Midwife Margaret

Scanlan insisted, '[W]e were never handmaidens.'[13] Ronayne described the midwives as excellent and experienced practitioners, with 'constant circulation of opinions' between them and the doctors.[14] Cooperation was celebrated in a 1971 article on St Helen's entitled 'Team work turns hospital into a model centre'.[15] Others spoke of these midwives as highly skilled and respected practitioners. Homebirth midwife Lynley McFarland who trained at St Helen's commented that it was 'run by very strong women . . . They taught a lot of good practical skills. A lot of them were great role models.'[16]

A classic midwifery textbook, written by internationally renowned Scottish midwife, teacher and author Maggie Myles, encapsulated the hospital midwife's perspective. Myles's textbook was used around the world, including in New Zealand, which she toured to deliver lectures. Trained in 1922, her many years of midwifery embraced what she called the 'bad old days of natural childbirth' when maternal and infant mortality rates were 'appallingly high'. She described childbirth in those days as 'long, painful, exhausting, lethal and with little to commend it'. Her own experience and 'logical reasoning' had convinced her that modern obstetrics, as practised by teams which included and gave responsibility to midwives in a modern, electronically equipped maternity hospital, backed up by experts on the medical conditions that might complicate childbearing, was the 'ideal blue-print for future planning'. She believed that no childbearing woman should be deprived of the monitoring and other scientific devices which had made childbirth 'safer, easier, shorter and more fulfilling'. Referring to modern obstetric advances in bacteriology, endocrinology, biochemistry, radiology, haematology, genetics and ultrasound, she wrote that midwives could not have accomplished this alone, but only as 'competent and co-operative members of the obstetrics team as we know them today'.[17]

She clearly wrote with an eye to those who romanticised the past. Others too questioned the notion of a golden age of midwifery and its subsequent subordination to medicine. In her 2009 PhD thesis on the history of midwifery in Victoria, Australian midwife and historian Madonna Grehan disputed the historical narrative espoused by some midwives which portrayed 'victimisation and oppression by the dual villains of nursing and medicine'. She argued that their desire to return to 'the wisdom of original midwifery devoid of the impediments of nursing' had created a romantic and nostalgic picture of their occupational past, which her research did not support. Rather, she found that midwifery's association with nursing from the late nineteenth century had successfully elevated the work of caring for women in childbirth from quasi-domestic employment into a professional practice, and that the new title of 'obstetrical nurse' was an indication of higher prestige and status, not lower.[18]

The alignment of nursing and midwifery in New Zealand had been formalised with the founding of the Nurses and Midwives Board in 1925, part of the professionalisation of both groups, setting standards and regulations. The New Zealand Nurses' Association (NZNA) included the Midwives' and Obstetric Nurses' Special Interest Section, which wrote a paper on homebirth that was incorporated into the NZNA's 1981 Policy Statement on Maternal and Infant Nursing (see p. 55). Describing those who promoted homebirth as 'fanatical' and 'vociferous', it incurred the wrath of members of the Auckland HBA who called the document 'authoritarian and elitist'.[19] Donley and her colleagues were further riled by the paper's description of a midwife as a nurse who specialised in childbirth, contrary, they said, to the World Health Organization definition of a midwife as a 'person' who provided childbirth services.[20] The NZNA policy statement advocated further training for domiciliary midwives, to which homebirth midwife Lyn McLean retorted that it was not the latter who needed training but rather hospital midwives who had been blinded by their male 'superiors' as to what birth was all about.[21]

Not all homebirth midwives and others in the HBA supported such an antagonistic stance towards the NZNA; the HBA national executive, then divided between Dunedin and Wellington, wished to establish better relations with the NZNA, and apologised for the 'personal antipathy' towards the NZNA displayed by some domiciliary midwives. Different approaches amongst HBA branches led the national organisation to disband in 1985 and to establish separate HBAs instead.[22]

There was further controversy after the 1983 Nurses Amendment Bill proposed that midwives working outside a hospital setting should be trained general nurses as well as midwives, rather than coming to midwifery through the maternity nurse training route. Objecting to this requirement of general nurse training, as the *New Zealand Listener* reported, 'Local midwives . . . have hastily formed a Save the Midwives Association . . . adamant that theirs is a separate profession [from nursing].'[23] Donley said of the 1983 Act that it 'did have one good aspect – it roused midwives from their long slumber and politicised them very quickly!'.[24] By 'midwives' she meant homebirth midwives, and especially those in Auckland where the new Save the Midwives Association was based.

Auckland HBA publicity officer Geoff Bridgman presented his organisation's evidence to the select committee on this Bill. He explained that, because they dealt with illness, nurses were very different from midwives. Another HBA member who attended the hearing, Henriette Kemp, reported that Bridgman's description 'brought strong mumbling reactions' from the Nursing Council (which had replaced the Nurses and Midwives Board in 1971) and the NZNA. The latter responded that nursing encompassed more than the treatment of illness; it included community health and preventative medicine.[25] Part of the rationale for moving nursing education from hospitals to tertiary institutions (following the 1971 Carpenter Report, see below) had been to ensure a broad base for training. A 1972 Health Department report explained that nursing was becoming more involved in the prevention of illness and the promotion of health, and that while hospital training was important, nursing students also required experience in other community health agencies where many of them would ultimately work.[26] Later, in 1989, a Health Department memorandum complained that some midwives failed to understand the extensive emphasis on health promotion in nurse training. Plunket nurses were a good example of this community focus, as were those working in contraception, public health and safety, and health education.[27]

As noted in the previous chapter, the homebirth lobby succeeded in getting a 'grandmother' clause inserted into the 1983 Nurses Amendment Act; this specified that a domiciliary midwife without general nurse training who had a contract with the Department of Health before 1 April 1984 could continue to attend homebirths. The original ban would have applied to those who qualified as a midwife through the maternity nurse training route or under a different system overseas, but in any case the department established that it would have affected only two of the 21 domiciliary midwives then practising in New Zealand, with the rest having a general nursing background.[28] Nevertheless, the achievement was symbolic, effectively acknowledging that midwives did not need nurse training. In 1987, Judy Larkin, a consumer advocate who helped to set up the Save the Midwives Association, made the exaggerated claim that without their successful intervention, the 1983 Act 'would have effectively eradicated midwives and midwifery in this country'.[29]

When the Labour government, elected to office in 1984, set up a Women's Health Committee to replace the Board of Health's Maternity Services Committee in 1985, the Auckland HBA sent the new committee a submission castigating the NZNA. It argued that the latter sought to limit the availability of homebirth, and that its 'denigration of the midwife' meant that 'mothers and babies [were] suffering'.[30] Again, by 'midwife', it meant the homebirth midwife, who was the only 'real' midwife.

## Save the Midwives Direct Entry Midwifery Task Force

Claiming autonomy from medical and nursing control also meant establishing an independent path for midwifery qualification that required no prior nurse training before entry into midwifery training. Valerie Fleming, Professor of Midwifery at Glasgow Caledonian University before coming to New Zealand, where she embarked on further study at Massey University, commented that the Save the Midwives Association sought to develop direct-entry midwifery training programmes 'to emancipate midwifery from domination by the medical and nursing professions'.[31] For this purpose, it set up a Direct Entry Midwifery Task Force, convened by consumer activist Judi Strid.[32] Task force members included midwives Joan Donley, Anne Sharplin and Karen Guilliland, and homebirth activists Brenda Hinton, Lynda Williams and Micky Harrower.[33]

Midwifery training, like general nurse training, had been hospital based since the early twentieth century. This changed following the 1971 government-commissioned report by Dr Helen Carpenter, Dean of the Faculty of Nursing at the University of Toronto and World Health Organization consultant, who had been asked to evaluate nurse education. She recommended that nursing and midwifery training occur in the tertiary sector rather than through apprenticeship in a hospital.[34] From the mid-1970s, nurses who trained at a technical institute became known as 'comprehensive nurses'; after two years' experience as a registered nurse, with at least one year working in their chosen specialty, they could undertake another six months' study leading to an Advanced Diploma. Midwifery education was an option in the Advanced Diploma in Maternal and Infant Nursing. From 1979, the St Helen's hospital midwifery training programmes were discontinued.[35]

The NZNA Midwives' and Obstetric Nurses' Special Interest Section lobbied to extend the postgraduate maternity course from six to 12 months.[36] They also wanted to separate it from the Advanced Diploma. The limited number of places available in the Advanced Diploma, the prerequisites needed to enrol, and the Nursing Council's requirements for midwifery registration led to a huge drop in the number of graduating midwives, from 120 registered in 1980 (which included those still coming from hospital-based programmes) to just 27 in 1985.[37] By 1989, Advanced Diploma maternity courses were still offered in Waikato and Christchurch polytechnics, but new midwifery postgraduate courses were introduced in Auckland, Wellington, and Southland/Otago polytechnics. These were independent from the Advanced Diploma but were still postgraduate courses, following general nurse training.

Carpenter had argued that midwives should be familiar with advances in medical science and technology, and that they should be trained nurses.[38] Some midwives saw value in prior nurse training, as Skiff had found in her interviews. Margaret Brown felt that she used her general training 'almost every day' in midwifery – for instance, if someone came in with a stroke or heart problem.[39] Catherine Young did not agree with the perception that midwives who were trained nurses were 'too medically oriented', but rather saw the broad background as a 'big advantage'.[40] Bourke found the same at St Helen's; Pat Minnell, who worked as a domiciliary midwife for 25 years following her St Helen's training, believed this training stood her in good stead for homebirths.[41] In 1989, Sheryl Smail, chief nursing officer in the Department of Health (1988–92), informed Health Minister Helen Clark of the department's belief that women in childbirth should have access to the combined skills of nursing and midwifery.[42]

In contrast to those views, Joan Donley argued that the time spent by midwives in technological obstetrical wards during their nurse training was enough to make them paranoid about birth and see it as abnormal, and she wondered how they could possibly function as 'guardians of normal birth' when they qualified.[43] The new postgraduate midwifery courses were, under her influence, subtly shifting away from hospital training. Sally Pairman, coordinator of the Southland/Otago course, explained that students would do practical training at several small maternity units and attend a homebirth.[44] Donley also explained the new Auckland midwifery course was 'home birth oriented'.[45]

In its plea for direct-entry midwifery training, the Save the Midwives Association claimed that domiciliary midwives who moved from the hospital to the community had expressed the need to 'unlearn' their nursing background, seeing it as an obstacle to practice. Using a curious analogy, it argued that requiring midwives to train as nurses was 'as sensible as requiring aspiring lawyers to train as policemen first!'.[46] It cited UK homebirth midwife Caroline Flint's view that nurse training preceding midwifery training was 'absurd': 'Undoubtedly useful knowledge is gained during the nursing training, but perhaps Midwives should also train as Chiropodists to help them learn communications skills, or as Florists to ensure a satisfactory standard of floral arrangements in the labour ward.'[47] Homebirth midwife Bronwen Pelvin argued in 1987 that the hospital-trained midwife had to 'unlearn a lot of things to satisfy the consumer' and observed 'how nursing training had to be "unlearnt", to change from nurse to midwife, to domiciliary midwife'.[48] The NZNA Midwives' Section, which appeared to have now dropped 'obstetric nurses' from its title, shared this view, arguing in 1988 that midwives who moved from hospital midwifery to the community often found they had to 'deprogramme' themselves and 'unlearn nursing and medical attitudes that are not appropriate when attending home births'.[49]

This statement was a complete turnaround for the Section, given that domiciliary midwives had not felt represented by it as recently as the early 1980s. The reason for the change appears to have been the increasing involvement of a new generation of feminist midwives such as Sally Pairman and Karen Guilliland; the latter chaired a regional committee and became part of a new national strategy committee set up in 1986.[50] Pairman explained that her passion for homebirth had begun when, on holiday in Auckland, she attended a birth with Donley – 'a magical experience and unlike any birth I had witnessed' – that was reinforced when she attended a lecture by British childbirth educator Janet Balaskas in 1984. Her political involvement began when she joined the Midwives' Section that same year.[51]

These new midwives oversaw the Section's change of focus, including persuading the NZNA in 1985 to adopt the World Health Organization definition of a midwife as a 'person' and not a 'nurse'. In 1987, after Guilliland was elected Section president, she became the Section's representative on the Save the Midwives Direct Entry Midwifery Task Force.[52] Donley's influence was key; Guilliland and Pairman later noted that her 'lucid analysis' had convinced them of the benefits of direct-entry midwifery education.[53]

## Lay midwives

The ultimate form of autonomy from the shackles of hospitals, doctors and nurses was lay midwifery, also sometimes called 'empirical midwifery', carried out by unlicensed practitioners outside the confines of the law. Historian

Wendy Kline estimated that there were at least 2,350 lay midwives in the United States in the mid-1970s.[54] Prominent Australian homebirth midwife Maggie Lecky-Thompson stated in 1995 that there had been a large number of lay midwives in Victoria in the 1970s; she noted admiringly that they were 'not as limited as the registered midwives'.[55] In 1989 homebirth midwife Barbara Hasslacher reported on a 'stimulating paper' presented at a Sydney conference by an American lay midwife working there, but 'unfortunately', she added, 'the New South Wales Nurses Registration Board is able to prosecute any person or persons unauthorised to practice midwifery and attending a woman at birth'.[56]

There were also some lay midwives practising in New Zealand in the 1980s, despite the law banning such activity unless in an emergency, and they were generally very open and candid about it. Northland seems to have had more than its share of lay midwives. The small Northland town of Kaitāia, home to around 5,000 people, had its own HBA, and one of its members, Micky Harrower, represented the New Zealand HBA at the 1987 London homebirth conference. Harrower described herself at New Zealand's 1987 national homebirth conference as a 'support person (and sometimes lay midwife) of many births'.[57]

In Hokianga, Rāwene hospital employed two homebirth midwives to attend births within a 10-kilometre radius of the hospital. Two local women, Mandy Waata and Tracy Dalton, wrote in the local newspaper about their experiences of having these hospital midwives conducting their homebirths.[58] In their view, it had been much the same as having a hospital birth, as the authority still lay with the midwife. Waata subsequently became a lay midwife and assisted in the birth of Dalton's third child, along with lay midwife Carly Judd. The latter attended other births, where the mother did not qualify for a homebirth because they lived too far from Rāwene hospital or did not want a trained midwife. The Domiciliary Midwives Society reported in 1989 that the medical officer had mounted a witch hunt against Judd and threatened to prosecute her but then dropped the case.[59] A 1990 *New Zealand Listener* article on maternity services referred to 'Lay midwife Carly Judd' and the 11 births she had attended in the Hokianga in the previous four years, one of which had ended in a postpartum haemorrhage. It did not report the outcome, but cited local doctor Tony Birch who spoke of a near-disaster when lay midwives attended one difficult birth.[60] Mandy Waata had also engaged in what she called 'traditional' unpaid midwifery for five years by 1990.[61] Waata and Judd believed that until midwives became autonomous and were no longer required to train as nurses, women would continue to use lay midwives.[62] They endorsed Donley's viewpoint that if domiciliary midwives became too medicalised, more women would turn to lay midwives.[63]

Yet, even in Northland, which the local medical officer of health said had the second-highest rate of homebirths after Nelson, only 25 out of the 2,200 births in 1988 were homebirths.[64] It remained a minority activity, and appears to have attracted few Māori, even in an area with a high Māori population. Around 60% of the population of Kaitāia was Māori in the 1980s, but none appear in reports on homebirth. The Hokianga HBA recorded one Māori homebirth for a young couple's first baby in 1986, and wrote, 'We're hoping it's the beginning for many more Maori women.'[65]

From 1988, lay midwives were granted membership of the Domiciliary Midwives Society, effectively legitimising them within the homebirth movement.[66] The following year the Society asserted that it was the only group to support lay midwives, adding, 'Being outside law gives them more freedoms that DMs [domiciliary midwives] don't have.'[67] When the New Zealand College of Midwives was set up, it too was sympathetic to the work of lay midwives. The College's stance on lay midwives was certainly on the agenda for a working party to establish the College in October 1988.[68] The Health Department expressed concern not only about the new College's lobbying to exclude the requirement of nurse training for midwives, but also its sanctioning of no training. Sheryl Smail, the department's chief nursing officer, noted, 'Although there is no documented evidence, it appears that "lay" midwives . . . are developing and offering a service. We understand that the NZCOM [New Zealand College of Midwives] may be including lay midwives in their membership.'[69] The Health Department's 1989 Working Group on Safe Options for Low Risk Pregnancy, of which Donley, Guilliland and Pelvin were members, also wanted New Zealand to consider ways of recognising the training which lay midwives received overseas, presumably referring to those from North America.[70] Guilliland and Pelvin argued that introducing direct-entry midwifery courses would attract those unregistered midwives, and Judd confirmed that she would take such a course if it were available.[71]

Guilliland told *Listener* journalist Pamela Stirling in 1990 that she was reluctant to condemn unqualified birth attendants who had 'a lot of instinctive knowledge' and were responding to what women wanted. She claimed there were lay midwives practising in Auckland, Coromandel, Taranaki, Gisborne and Northland. Pelvin told Stirling of lay midwives attending 'breech births . . . and difficult posterior presentation deliveries with homeopathic remedies as their only emergency equipment'.[72] A group of midwives from the Nelson Hospital birthing unit subsequently wrote to the College of Midwives, concerned about the impression given in Stirling's article that the College supported lay midwifery. The College's national committee responded that they did not feel the College and its leaders had been misrepresented in the article.[73]

## The Netherlands as a model

In their goal for recognition of midwifery as an autonomous profession, homebirth midwives looked to the Netherlands. Donley and Strid, on behalf of the Save the Midwives Direct Entry Task Force, attended a conference there in 1987. Donley's extended report of what they found revealed significant differences from the system that homebirth midwives proposed for New Zealand, as expressed by the Save the Midwives Association and the Domiciliary Midwives Society, although she did not draw attention to the differences. Those differences related first to midwifery training, secondly to monitoring and auditing of homebirth services, and thirdly to the relationship of homebirth services to hospitals broadly. I will address each of these in turn to better explain what New Zealand homebirth midwives envisaged when they sought autonomy.

Donley related that there were about 1,000 midwives in the Netherlands, 80% of whom worked independently. She explained how they were legally a medical and not a nursing profession, taking the Hippocratic Oath on graduation like doctors. There were midwifery training centres in Amsterdam, Heelem and Rotherham, each attached to a large obstetrical-gynaecological unit with a special baby care unit. Training was a three-year course with the curriculum laid down by statute. Candidates had to be at least 19 years of age, and have five years' secondary education with an A-level (equivalent to university Bursary in New Zealand at the time) in chemistry and biology. Of approximately 800 candidates annually, around 60 were selected. Students needed to undertake 40 deliveries to graduate. In their subsequent practice, midwives had to be assisted at the birth by a maternity nurse, who also underwent three years' training.[74] In short, Dutch midwives were admitted to a programme that was highly competitive, with science featuring in admission criteria; they were trained in a hospital environment; and they could not practise alone.

This system differed significantly from the one the New Zealand homebirth midwives envisaged. The first difference was the emphasis on science and academic excellence in admission criteria. By contrast, the Save the Midwives Direct Entry Midwifery Task Force explained in 1989:

> The Taskforce saw the lack of an academic basis to the anticipated midwifery course as a positive advantage over the current system requiring nurse training. They thought this would be particularly suited to Maori and Pacific Island women . . . [who were] often overwhelmed by the theoretical structure of the course and ultimately by having to partake in tests and examinations in a language that is not their own.

This could be seen as disparaging of these women's intellectual capabilities; the existence of a language barrier is also questionable, given that most Māori and Pasifika resided in urban or semi-urban areas and their young people attended English-speaking schools. But above all it is clear that the task force valued experience over science when it explained, 'Rather than academic achievements, it is more desirable to value previous childbearing experience and motherhood, and a positive attitude to health, healing, birth and parenting.'[75]

Not only did they view experience in motherhood as more valuable than academic training, but there was also no suggestion the training would be located in high-tech hospitals, as in the Netherlands. The task force did not set out the specifics of the new programme it envisaged for direct-entry training, but made it clear that it would not be hospital based, and that experience would be gained in homebirths and small maternity units. Resistance to any link with high-tech hospitals in the training programme was a significant difference from the Dutch model. Donley had, as noted, argued in 1982 that training in an obstetric unit would be counterproductive for homebirth midwives with their philosophy to 'guard the normal labour against the abnormal'.[76] She stated this more forcefully in response to the suggestion in 1990 that midwives be required to work for two years in a hospital immediately after qualifying, claiming that it would be 'completely counter-productive!'.[77] Training in base hospitals was, by contrast, in keeping with the recommendations of

New Zealand's 1982 Maternity Services Committee report which had so incensed Donley and homebirth midwives.

That desire to eschew all links with hospital medicine in the training programme also differed from the trend in Britain. In 1987, only one hospital – Derby City Hospital – offered a direct-entry midwifery course, where eight midwives qualified each year. An account of the course explained:

> Their training whilst excluding subjects like geriatrics and orthopaedics, is intended to equip them for every eventuality . . . They learn about diseases affecting childbearing women, they gain medical and surgical experience and go to the gynaecological wards, they study paediatrics and they work in acute admissions to give them the knowledge to recognise conditions like a diabetic crisis, or pulmonary embolism, which might affect pregnant women.[78]

The second way in which the scheme proposed for New Zealand by the Domiciliary Midwives Society and others within the homebirth movement differed from the Dutch model was in the monitoring of the service. The midwives in the Netherlands were, Donley explained, under the control of a Medical Audit Board. In New Zealand, hospital board-run obstetric standards review committees had been set up around the country from 1980; these set out guidelines for contracts for GPs to practise in hospital board facilities.[79] The 1982 Maternity Services Committee report took the view that, with the addition of a midwife, they would be the most appropriate monitoring body of homebirth midwives as well.[80] However, the Domiciliary Midwives Society proposed a peer-review structure for homebirth midwives that eschewed medical involvement. In 1988 the Society set up its own standards review committee in Auckland, consisting of Donley and three consumers, including homebirth advocates Lynda Williams and Brenda Hinton.[81] The committee's structure, it explained, was 'based on birth as a social event, as well as a normal physiological function, and home birth as a safe and viable option which an increasing number of women are demanding as of right'.[82] The committee formulated standards, including that midwives had to 'provide clients with accurate information'. 'Conversely', it continued, 'the responsibilities of the pregnant woman and her family should be honestly stated – her responsibility to maintain good nutrition, to refrain from the use of alcohol, tobacco, marijuana and social or medical drugs, and her responsibility to accept medical intervention if this becomes necessary.'[83] In other words, the client too had to take responsibility. When asked by the Department of Health about indemnity insurance in 1989, homebirth midwives responded, '[T]he idea of it was a waste of time and a bit of a joke. It was not a worry for midwives, they had an equal role, a partnership with the mother/client. They do not want to alter their principles and practises [sic] for fear of being sued – there was no problem here.'[84]

In 1989, Dr Graeme Cable, chair of the Auckland Obstetric Standards Review Committee, congratulated the midwives on setting up their own standards review committee. He assured them of the New Zealand Obstetrical and Gynaecological Society's support, and wondered whether they had considered asking that society to nominate a representative to serve on their committee.[85] Dr Tony Baird, chair of the New Zealand Medical Association, also suggested to Donley that the domiciliary midwives' standards review committees work closely with obstetric committees.[86] Donley responded that this was not possible, and explained why there was no obstetrician on their committees: 'Since domiciliary midwives practice [sic] midwifery outside the parameters acceptable to the majority of obstetricians, it would not be reasonable nor politic for them to be assessed by those supporting the medical model of childbirth.'[87]

The Thames Hospital Board had set up an obstetric advisory committee in 1982, which produced guidelines for homebirths.[88] In 1989, the board suggested to the Waikato Area Health Board (which had replaced the hospital board following a 1989 Act) that it establish formal mechanisms for reviewing the competence and standards of practice of health professionals involved in homebirth, and that it also include domiciliary midwives on its obstetric advisory committee. Donley responded that this was the very thing the domiciliary midwives standards review committees were 'set up to avoid!'.[89] Midwifery standards review committees were subsequently set up around the country, each with eight members – four consumers, two midwives (one community and one hospital), a GP nominated by the HBA, and a medical officer of health representative, usually the principal public health nurse.[90]

Homebirth midwives also resisted the suggestion to transfer their contracts from the Health Department to the hospital boards and the subsequent area health boards. The 1982 MSC report had suggested integrating homebirths with hospital services.[91] The Domiciliary Midwives Society, however, told

Health Minister David Caygill in 1988 that such a transfer would be counterproductive, with the present system allowing midwives to remain 'independent of the constraints of the medical model of childbirth', once again suggesting homebirth midwives had a degree of independence prior to the 1990 Act, as noted in Chapter 3.[92] Even though the new area health boards sought to embrace preventative as well as curative healthcare, midwives resisted any association with them because they were still connected to hospitals. The homebirth midwives' pursuit of autonomy was therefore very different from homebirth in the Netherlands that was overseen by a Medical Audit Board.

The role of hospitals in maternity services in the Netherlands generally, and not just in training and monitoring of services, was a third point of difference. In the Netherlands the screening system for pregnancies was generally accepted. By contrast, Donley described it as of 'concern' when the hospital board service planning guidelines, supported by the Department of Health, stated, 'Every effort should be made to ensure that women with identified risks are delivered in hospital.'[93]

Donley also reacted negatively to the setting up of smaller birthing units attached to hospitals, allowing a more informal setting for childbirth with back-up services. She was very cynical about the motivations behind this trend. When Nelson Hospital set up a new maternity unit, officially opened by Professor Dennis Bonham in 1987, Donley reported: 'THE GRAND OPENING OF THE "HOME-LIKE" MATERNITY UNIT or OBSTETRICIANS ARE NICE GUYS AFTER ALL'. The report claimed that those initiating the project saw it as a 'bulwark against the "rot" of home birth'.[94] Another unit set up in 1987 was Birthcare, a privately run facility located a short distance from National Women's Hospital in Auckland that provided a 'medically safe alternative to hospital'. Risk factors – such as diabetes, heart problems, poor obstetric history, past caesarean section – made some women ineligible for birthing at the centre.[95] A 1985 report for the Health Department had deemed small maternity units just as safe as larger hospitals, but with the important proviso that there was back-up to transport any emergencies to those better-equipped hospitals.[96]

Another late-1980s alternative to homebirth was the so-called Domino service (Domiciliary in-and-out), a scheme also operating in Britain. Under this scheme, domiciliary midwives would accompany their clients to hospital for the birth but would ensure continuity of care. In 1989 the Northland

Area Health Board reached an agreement with two homebirth practitioners, Lynley McFarland and Feliz Barnett, to provide a short-stay hospital birth with continuity of care before, during and after the birth. The board paid the midwives for their hospital attendance, and the Health Department for their work in the home as before. The board's Medical Officer of Health Dr David Sloan welcomed this as 'an important and sensible arrangement'.[97] The Bay of Plenty and Wellington Area Health Boards followed that same year.[98] Donley later made her disdain for the Domino service clear, explaining, '[T]he only place a midwife is an independent practitioner is in the community.' She maintained that Domino services were simply another means of maintaining medical control.[99]

A 1990 press article comparing the Australian and New Zealand homebirth movements remarked on the anti-hospital nature of New Zealand's lobby.[100] The article cited Hilda Bastian, Homebirth Australia co-coordinator from 1986–91 and founding editor of the *Homebirth Australia Newsletter* 1984–89, who argued that the New Zealand movement was more 'dogmatic' than its Australian counterpart. Bastian herself changed her mind about homebirths after participating in a survey which found that the mortality for planned homebirths was double that in hospital.[101] She argued that there should be more collaboration between home and hospital birth services. The article reported, 'Both Hilda Bastian and obstetricians here [in Australia] point to the Dutch system where anti-hospital feeling would be seen as totally out of place', with its clear referral criteria and thorough risk assessments. Bastian commented, 'For some home birth purists the move to greater co-operation with the hospitals is treason' and referred specifically to comments by the New Zealand delegate at a recent Australian homebirth conference.[102] It is unclear whether that delegate was Donley. Others shared her views; for instance, Pelvin said of the much-cited risk assessment in 1990, 'Motorbike riding is far more dangerous than having a baby and yet we don't limit that to hospital grounds under supervision of a doctor.'[103]

## Homebirth and the NZNA Midwives' Section

In their quest for autonomy, homebirth midwives had to strengthen their professional base. With just 31 members in 1987 (and 52 in 1988 when they opened membership to supportive midwives and lay midwives), the Domiciliary

Midwives Society could have little clout.[104] Their influence increased significantly when they succeeded in winning over the NZNA Midwives' and Obstetric Nurses' Section which for so long had opposed homebirth.

The second half of the 1980s, during which Guilliland and Pairman assumed senior positions within the Section, saw a sea change for the organisation. The NZNA itself was changing with the times, with its professional officer Joy Bickley publicly commenting in 1988 on the oppression of women and nurses by the medical profession; and in 1990 it sent a submission to the Select Committee on the Nurses Amendment Bill in favour of midwifery autonomy (see p. 118).[105] This must have come as a surprise to some; in 1989 Pelvin encouraged homebirth advocates to send submissions on the Bill 'to counteract all the negative stuff from the medical and nursing professions'.[106]

Homebirth midwives managed to persuade some hospital colleagues that the future of midwifery was in jeopardy, pointing to the 1985 Obstetric Regulations stipulating registered nurses without midwife training could take charge of maternity wards (a measure taken in response to staff shortages and in the knowledge that all nurses had had some experience in maternity wards included in their general training since 1957). At the Section's first national conference in 1986, Donley drew on her recently published history and traced how the homebirth midwife – 'the only relatively independent practitioner' – had been legally undermined over the years with the help of the NZNA, and 'therefore, so had all midwives'.[107] This was a rallying cry to all midwives, and it appeared to work.

The NZNA Midwives' Section held its second national conference in 1988. Following another impassioned speech by Donley, it resolved to disband the Section, leave the NZNA, and form a separate college. In her speech, Donley argued this was necessary to protect domiciliary midwives, who, she said, were a dying breed. If they failed 'to grasp the opportunity presented at this conference to determine our future, then I suggest we select several of our best specimens so that in due course they will be embalmed and placed in the museum alongside that other extinct species, the moa'.[108] Midwife Tina Gilbertson later recalled the excitement of the occasion: 'Joan stood up and asked us if we were midwives or moas. What brilliant times to be in! The College was born.'[109] The HBA had also resolved that a College of Midwives be established.[110] Donley later explained to her Australian colleague Maggie Lecky-Thompson that the New Zealand College of Midwives 'grew out of the DMs [domiciliary midwives] supported by NZHBA'.[111]

The centrality of homebirth to the founding of the new college becomes clear from the contributions of British homebirth midwife Caroline Flint, author of *Sensitive Midwifery*, who was visiting New Zealand at the time. Flint contributed an article to the first issue of the *New Zealand College of Midwives Journal* in 1989, headed 'To my dear sisters in New Zealand'. She wrote, 'Until the day I die one of the great highlights of my life will always be the wonderful week I spent with the midwives of New Zealand in August 1988 – a time when I was acutely conscious of history being made and brave decisions being taken.'[112] Reporting on Flint's speech at the 1988 conference, Pelvin quoted Flint's belief that 'the absolute baseline of normal midwifery practice <u>must</u> be the woman giving birth normally in her own home'.[113] Describing Flint as a zealous campaigner for midwifery and a hero amongst her colleagues, the *New Zealand Herald* repeated her comment that, 'New Zealand women are beautiful . . . You're tall, well nourished, get lots of lovely sunshine and you all have lovely big feet. Everything I've seen so far indicates you should be able to labour successfully and without intervention.'[114] Worthy specimens of homebirth, but a stereotype that clearly did not apply to all New Zealand women. Summing up Flint's influence, Donley claimed that: 'For many of us [Flint] was both an inspiration and a turning point.'[115]

Following the 1988 conference, a working party was created to formulate the constitution, and the New Zealand College of Midwives was officially launched on 1 April 1989, holding its inaugural AGM the next day.[116] Maggie Lecky-Thompson compared this new body favourably to the Australian College of Midwives set up in 1986. The New Zealand college's 'inaugural members and strengths' were drawn from domiciliary midwives, she said, unlike in Australia, where most college members were hospital based, and 'excluded and victimised' what she called 'traditional' midwives. As a result, she said, the Australian Society of Independent Midwives was set up in 1989.[117] A later account of the Australian College of Midwives commented that it lacked cohesion, with some midwives forming their own professional associations and others continuing to rely on the Australian Nursing Federation to represent their interests, and that, as a result, midwives in Australia lacked 'political acuity and strength'.[118] The New Zealand College of Midwives was more akin to the Australian Society of Independent Midwives than to the Australian College, just as it was arguably more akin to the Association of Radical Midwives in Britain (founded in 1976) than to its parent body, the Royal College of Midwives. Whilst resembling the break-away organisations in both countries, significantly the New Zealand College of Midwives was to become the official voice of midwifery in New Zealand.

## Conclusion

Homebirth midwives were a small group in the 1980s, whose leaders through the organisational networks of the Domiciliary Midwives Society and the Save the Midwives Association largely rejected any connection with scientific medicine, hospitals and nursing. Their views continued to be contrary to many of those of the medical and nursing professions, and some midwives, as well as to those responsible for the 1983 Nurses Amendment Act. Despite representing a minority group, homebirth midwives were on the cusp of achieving legislation that would allow them to practise alone in the community, with no required nurse training and no legislative oversight. This was an extraordinary reversal in the direction of official policy and differed in many ways from the Dutch model which was so often invoked in support of homebirth.

A major coup for homebirth activists was persuading the Midwives' Section of the NZNA to disband in favour of an independent college. Joan Donley reported that Labour MP David Caygill had suggested, '[I]f the midwives were to form their own organisation, then the government would be obliged to consult them about maternity rather than the nurses.'[119] Homebirth midwives and their supporters were well versed in this kind of political strategising, having for two decades built a campaign for midwifery autonomy, the subject of Chapter 5.

# FIVE

## 'A highly focused and effective campaign': Homebirth as a political movement in the 1980s

THE 1990 NURSES AMENDMENT ACT was the result of a carefully orchestrated campaign led by Joan Donley. She later told researcher Sally Abel that she had expected a power struggle, as she had 'a political enough background to realise that any time you start changing power relations you're in for a fight'.[1] Frequently drawing on battlefield analogies, she wrote in 1986 that she was 'marshalling information' to be used when 'planning strategies, [and to aid] recognition of the traps and ambushes'. The Home Birth Association was to carry out 'guerilla tactics against a superior and powerful force', i.e., obstetricians who were 'generals in the war against normal childbirth'.[2] In 1998 she again explained that understanding factors which had 'entrenched the medical control of childbirth' enabled 'effective tactics and strategies and wise use of electoral power'.[3]

In this chapter, I explore those strategies, and argue that the success of this determined campaign by Donley and her supporters was aided by a receptive political and social climate in the late 1980s. This included a government which itself questioned medical technology more broadly, favoured competition within health services to cut costs, and supported greater community and consumer involvement, all of which suited the homebirth lobby, as did the government's support of the new women's health movement. The social climate that caused, and was heightened by, an inquiry into medical treatment at Auckland's National Women's Hospital in 1988 (the Cartwright Inquiry) also favoured homebirth midwives. The latter insisted that, as 'midwife' meant 'with women', they were in partnership with women: their practice was woman-centred and reflected what women wanted. By 'women', however, they meant Pākehā women; the movement at this time had little buy-in from Māori or the growing Pasifika community. Nevertheless, when they formed the New Zealand College of Midwives in 1989 with great fanfare, homebirth midwives and their supporters were in a strong position to promote both independent homebirth practice and direct-entry midwifery training (no prior nurse training).

## Gaining a public profile and the role of Joan Donley

During the reading of the 1983 Nurses Amendment Bill, Labour MP Michael Bassett commented that for a very small minority group, homebirth advocates had achieved some 'very effective and voluble lobbying'.[4] Much of the credit for this can go to Joan Donley, who was tireless in leading the campaign and an inspiration to those around her.

The New Zealand Home Birth Association was founded in Auckland in 1980, at a meeting attended by 150 people, only 16 of whom came from outside Auckland.[5] Auckland's predominance continued, accounting for 64% of national membership in 1982. That Donley resided in Auckland was a significant factor in this, but membership fluctuated wildly nonetheless. In 1982, the Auckland HBA boasted 475 members; that number halved the following year. At that time there were nine branches around the country, but three of them had fewer than 10 members – Northland, Thames/Hauraki, and Manawatū. One of the more active branches was Nelson, with 19 members in 1982 and 43 in 1983.[6] Over the decade HBAs came and went, with 17 in existence in 1987.[7] Many were small and shortlived. Whilst theoretically a consumer movement, the contact people for most of its branches were homebirth midwives.[8]

The glue holding local groups together was the quarterly *HBA Newsletter* (sometimes the Auckland and the national newsletters were combined into one issue and other times appeared separately, with all including news from other branches). Homebirth advocate Lynda Williams later described the newsletter as 'an extremely effective weapon in the campaign to regain control over our bodies', whilst providing no circulation figures (the October 1980 issue reported a circulation of 450).[9] An Auckland-based collective produced the newsletter, edited by childbirth educator Brenda Hinton, and Donley largely determined the content. Donley's midwifery partner Carolyn Young counted no less than 42 articles Donley penned for these newsletters in the 1980s, along with many other notices and commentaries, and there were probably many more unsigned contributions.[10]

Young summarised Donley's input into the movement as 'immense, her research notoriously thorough – she not only pulls her own weight, she pulls most of everyone else's too'.[11] She related how Donley 'peppered the local papers with acerbic and timely "letters to the editor"'.[12] Nor was Donley averse to contacting publishers themselves; for instance, in 1986 she succeeded in getting an advertisement for ultrasound in pregnancy removed from the *New Zealand Listener* by claiming the advertisement's endorsement of ultrasound as safe was false.[13]

Donley was also a major presence at the annual HBA conferences. The 1987 conference report stated that 'once again' Donley's ideas were 'central' to the gathering; and on this occasion she led the singing of the 'Midwives United Song', which she herself had composed, as delegates stood holding hands at the end of the conference.[14] She recited part of the song to an Australian friend the previous year:

> Here we come and we're united
> New Zealand midwives on our way
> to give the mother of New Zealand
> every right to have her say.
>
> Chorus: Freedom of choice, we are one voice;
> Freedom of choice, we are one voice.[15]

Newspapers were intrigued by the new movement, often featuring it in their women's pages.[16] The weekly *New Zealand Listener* carried an article on Donley in the lead-up to the first HBA national conference in 1980.[17] The HBA courted this publicity. One initiative, copied from Australia, was an annual National Home Birth Publicity Week, starting in October 1981. Donley explained that they had chosen the last week of October because in European folklore this was the month of the witches that culminated in Hallowe'en, linking modern midwifery to medieval witch-hunts.[18] As well as media releases, these weeks included street stalls and public meetings, seminars and lectures; the 1982 event in Auckland included a march down Queen Street and an address by Labour MP Helen Clark at Aotea Square.[19] Commenting on the event, the *HBA Newsletter* lamented 'media attention lacking'.[20] One attendee questioned the suitability for children on special event balloons: 'Hospitals are awful, awful, awful'.[21] Balloons continued to feature in subsequent years: in 1987 the Auckland committee printed 1,000 balloons with the logo, 'Homebirth – the Safe Alternative'.[22]

Homebirth advocates sought to assert their presence in the new women's movement. Donley presented a paper at the 1982 Women's Health Conference and organised a stall to disseminate information. It worked; the conference adopted the right to homebirth as part of its philosophy on women's health.[23] In 1985 Donley described the HBA as 'a political force to be reckoned with – not only on its own merit, but also because of its proliferation into other feminist/political organisations' such as Save the Midwives and Maternity Action.[24]

There was considerable overlap in membership between these organisations. The Save the Midwives Association's leadership included several from the HBA, such as Judy Larkin, Brenda Hinton, Judi Strid, Lynda Williams and Micky Harrower (also a lay midwife), along with Donley and others such as Karen Guilliland and Anne Sharplin.[25] In 1985 the Auckland HBA and the Save the Midwives Association helped form Maternity Action. Barbara Macfarlane, the founding secretary of the New Zealand HBA, led Maternity Action, and consumer advocate Lynda Williams was among its 14 founding members.[26] Despite this membership overlap, having multiple organisations was useful, not least because it allowed separate submissions to Parliament when issues arose, enhancing their impact. When reviewing the activism of the homebirth movement it is important to keep in mind just how small it was. It certainly punched well above its weight.

## Political activism

The 1982 HBA conference called for political action.[27] Not everyone agreed; Christchurch midwife Ursula Helem thought that homebirth required 'peace, quiet, unaggressiveness' and not 'political battles'.[28] While these divergent views contributed to the dissolution of the national HBA in favour of a federation (see p. 73), Auckland continued to run the newsletter, the first issue of which advised: 'As consumers we should educate ourselves and then challenge the system and learn to make demands on it.'[29] The following year it issued detailed advice on how to carry this out and 'spread the home birth message'. The list was not for the faint-hearted:

> Write and distribute a pamphlet; Announce your existence to Citizen's Advice Bureau, Women's Resource Centre, Parents Centre, Plunket Society, La Leche League, hospitals; Let every GP in your area know of your existence and the presence of your domiciliary midwife, by way of a circular letter; Put advertisements in your local paper in the personal column and public notices; Offer yourselves for radio talk back, interviews; Try to get on TV interviews, news; Write newspaper articles, letters to the editor; Hold public meetings, workshops; Give talks to meetings of Plunket, drop-in centres, Parents Centre etc.; Personal contact.

It also exhorted readers to send written submissions to the Maternity Services Committee and the Committee on Women, to speak up and question candidates at election meetings, to talk to their local MP, and write to their local hospital board.[30]

The Auckland HBA prepared questions for MPs to ask in Parliament, and wrote to the Council for Civil Liberties since, it declared, homebirth was a civil liberties issue.[31] At the 1982 Home Birth Week, Donley and Mary Nacey gave a joint seminar at the University of Auckland on 'The Politics of Home Birth'.[32] The following year Nacey, a consumer activist and a lawyer who stood as a Labour candidate for the Auckland City Council in the 1970s and was for a time married to former Labour Health Minister Bob Tizard, gave an address at the HBA conference, inviting members to send her personal accounts of their homebirth experience. She also urged them to petition government to increase homebirth midwives' pay, picket National's Health Minister Aussie Malcolm, send letters to and meet with their local health officer, and write letters to the press and to other MPs. She told local HBAs to be 'bold, take the initiative and organise your own action'.[33]

Henriette Kemp, who had her third baby at home in Nelson assisted by Bronwen Pelvin, and subsequently coordinated the Wellington HBA, was appointed HBA national lobbying-resource coordinator in 1982.[34] Reporting on a *Listener* article about Michel Odent's birthing clinic in France in 1983, she enthused, 'I hope lots of homebirthers will write to the editor of the Listener explaining that that kind of natural birthing is happening all around NZ!'[35] She expressed disappointment that smaller HBAs were not lobbying MPs, and encouraged them to contribute to a 'national onslaught' on Parliament so that homebirth would become a political issue at election time.[36] Donley in a similar vein instructed her supporters to prepare submissions and lobby local MPs, adding, 'If we want to maintain the home birth option we are going to have to fight for it.'[37]

In 1983, the Wellington HBA met with the National Party politician and feminist activist Marilyn Waring, who provided them with what she described as an 'insider perspective'. She explained that she was not standing for Parliament at the next election, but advised them to write to other MPs, focusing on their own experiences rather than on complicated political arguments: 'You can't quarrel with personal experience.' She told them, 'Numbers count. M.P.s have to be able to walk out of a Select Committee hearing and say to their colleagues "We have no choice – the overwhelming number of letters/submissions from the Home Birth supporters and their Association heavily outweighs submissions from opposing organisations."' She said that in a male-dominated Parliament men could effect change by having a word in the right ear, but women 'just have to keep writing'.[38]

The homebirth leadership kept up the pressure following the election of Labour in 1984. When the Maternity Services Committee was replaced in 1985 by the Women's Health Committee, and a maternity sub-committee was formed by its obstetric and nursing members, Donley urged homebirth advocates to canvas the committee to ensure they would not be 'hoodwinked' by this sub-committee. Such action may have contributed to its rapid demise (as a 1988 Health Department report explained, this sub-committee was 'in existence for only a short time').[39] In 1987 the *HBA Auckland Newsletter* announced the theme of the annual conference would be: 'Change through Consumer Action'.[40] Donley exhorted delegates to continue lobbying decision-making bodies (including Treasury, and the Departments of Health, Education, Women's Affairs, and Consumer Affairs) and to demand the removal of medical obstruction to midwifery through legislative change.[41]

That same year, Waring offered further advice to the Save the Midwives Direct Entry Task Force, which Donley reported in full.[42] Waring suggested that, even though the task force's remit concerned midwives' education, they should frame it as a feminist issue and not an educational or health issue, as that gave it a broader political base, 'guaranteeing that feminist groups will rally to the cause'. It was, she said, essential to network with all women's organisations at the local and national level, including Māori women's groups after learning their protocols. She advised them to 'attend all women-oriented AGMs (watch supermarket notice boards, local papers), get on the committee – they're always looking for workers – put forward your remit'. Once the remit had been passed, she added, 'you don't necessarily have to attend any more meetings'. She explained that her inspiration was former GP obstetrician Doris Gordon's book *Backblocks Baby-Doctor* (1955), in which the latter outlined her strategy of 'pressure politics', representing 'petticoat government at its best and it is a system seldom known to have failed'. Gordon had worked closely with leaders of major women's organisations who would then 'indoctrinate thousands of women in hundreds of branches', leading to strong deputations to appropriate ministers at election time.[43] Waring admitted that Gordon was 'pushing for doctor oriented maternity services', whilst the modern goal was to reverse that trend, but she nevertheless considered it a model strategy.[44] Sally Pairman later acknowledged that Waring provided strategic advice for a campaign that was 'highly focused and effective'.[45]

In 2004 midwife Jacqui Anderson, who helped set up the College of Midwives in 1989 and was on its board of management, reflected on the 1980s: 'There was a real feeling that we had to get midwives in everywhere where there were women's health issues . . . There was a lot of lobbying, a lot of politicising.'[46] The minutes of a meeting of the College in April 1989 on the impending reform of the Nurses Act recorded, 'The Ministers consider 22 letters on one subject as a trend therefore all midwives need to write.'[47]

Guilliland and Pairman later reflected on that lobbying. After Guilliland took over as chair of the Midwives' Section of the New Zealand Nurses' Association in 1987, she encouraged members of the Section to lobby widely for legislative change to midwifery. Midwives spoke at meetings of the Federation of University Women, Women's Studies Associations, the Society of Research on Women, the Catholic Women's League, Business and Professional Women, and Toastmasters International. Women's branches of male service clubs like Rotary and Lions were also receptive. Some midwives joined political parties, as Waring had advised, and the Section developed a strategy for lobbying politicians to gain cross-party support. It identified every MP and his or her constituency, and delegated them to the appropriate Midwives' Section region, which then sent letters and visited MPs to inform them about the 'need for legislative change'. According to Guilliland and Pairman, most of these midwives reported that 'politicians were delighted to be involved in a positive, and from their point of view, non-controversial lobby'.[48]

In 1989 Strid claimed that politicians were 'often totally unfamiliar with the midwifery predicament and most supportive of what needs to be done once enlightened'.[49] This impression is supported by government files which show, for example, Invercargill's National MP Rob Munro writing to Katherine O'Regan as chair of the Women's Caucus: 'I gather all MPs are being lobbied at the moment concerning midwives' independence. Not unexpectedly, I know little of it! Could you fill me in on the political aspects of this matter as soon as possible?'[50] Timaru National MP Maurice McTigue likewise wrote to O'Regan for advice, explaining, 'I have been approached by the midwives in my electorate seeking our support.' O'Regan responded, 'We should support them.'[51]

## Engaging with Māori and Pasifika women

While the movement gained traction with Pākehā women's groups, it was not so successful in reaching out to Māori, despite Waring's advice.[52] Before 1990, Māori were notably absent from the movement, both as mothers choosing homebirth, and as consumer activists, as Rea Daellenbach observed in her PhD study of the movement.[53] Nor were there any Māori members of the Domiciliary Midwives Society.[54] Instead, Māori were involved in their own activism, inspired by international civil rights movements and demanding a greater level of self-determination and cultural revival, with a renewed focus on the meanings of the 1840 Treaty of Waitangi with the British Crown. The nursing profession was at the centre of a new cultural awareness, under the guidance of nurse educator Irihapeti Ramsden. She would only later become a major influence in midwifery education (see p. 196).

In 1989 the HBA held its first bicultural conference in Taranaki called 'Conceptions and Creations – Te Aitanga Me Te Putanga Aa Tangata Aa Hinengaro'. Despite this impressive title, biculturalism formed only a small part of the meeting. The conference report referred to 'the Maori session', consisting of a presentation by Parihaka kuia Marjorie Rau-Kupa on Māori healing, and another by psychiatric nurse Bob Elliott and co-workers at Tokanui Psychiatric Hospital on Māori concepts of health. The conference also included three workshops on 'the Maori perspective' at which 'Maori women shared moving and horrendous experiences of childbirth, past and present, within the callous Pakeha maternity system'. At the close of the conference, delegates were encouraged to become familiar with biculturalism before the next gathering in Whangārei where there was to be a 'session on racism'.[55] In her history of the HBA, Donley included a chapter entitled 'Biculturalism', which began by referring to this Taranaki conference; the chapter was just three pages long and most of it focused on the politics of the homebirth movement without reference to Māori or biculturalism.[56]

The next HBA conference in Whangārei in 1990 congratulated Health Minister Helen Clark for introducing the Nurses Amendment Bill to Parliament, and the conference report declared, 'We recognise autonomous midwifery as a step towards enabling Maori women their birthing options as guaranteed under the Treaty of Waitangi.'[57] However, the meeting did little to enhance relations between the homebirth movement and Māori. Indeed, the conference was almost abandoned owing to a 'misunderstanding'. While promoting a bicultural conference the HBA had overlooked an essential element of biculturalism – partnership – because the planning committee was totally Pākehā and it did not consult local Māori.[58] Newsletter editor Brenda Hinton reported that '[o]ne bright spot in the otherwise disappointing conference in Whangarei' was the keynote address by Lynda Williams, but her talk made no mention of Māori.[59]

If Māori women were absent from the homebirth movement, so too were Pasifika mothers, even in Auckland. People from Tonga, Samoa, Niue, the Cook Islands and Fiji had arrived in large numbers in the 1950s and 1960s to fill shortages in manual labour in prosperous times. By the 1970s, Auckland was said to be the largest Polynesian city in the world. Pacific peoples brought their traditional healing practices with them, but also sought access to the Western models of care available in their new home. With a great respect for authority, they valued their relationship with GPs in childbirth and chose to birth in hospital.[60] A 1999 maternity report confirmed that 'a high proportion of Pacific women wish to give birth in hospital with access to specialist care', and that Pasifika women overwhelmingly wanted their GP involved as their primary caregiver in pregnancy and birth, rather than a midwife.[61] Very few appeared to embrace the homebirth movement.

Despite largely failing to attract Māori and Pasifika mothers to the cause, the campaign for public recognition of homebirth and midwifery autonomy was waged with tremendous zeal in the 1980s. The following sections examine the outcome of their considerable efforts on the political scene, at both national and local levels.

## National politics 1980–1984

The conservative National Party governed from 1975 to 1984. Aussie Malcolm, Minister of Health from 1981 to 1984 and a father of four, was an outspoken critic of homebirth. In 1982 Lyn McLean met him on behalf of the Domiciliary Midwives Society, primarily to discuss homebirth midwives' fees. Henriette Kemp attended as note-taker, and she reported that Malcolm said he had 'no hysterical objection to home birth but wishes there weren't any'. He spoke of the letters he received from homebirth parents that, he maintained, focused on the advantages for mothers but did not consider the child.[62] The *Parents Centre Bulletin* later reported him saying that, while giving birth was a natural process, it was the most dangerous time of a child's life, and that, with advances in obstetrics, 'some mothers started saying, "it may be much safer for baby, but it's not much fun for me"'. He believed this had spurred the homebirth movement.[63]

Those opting for homebirth resented the implication that they did so lightly and selfishly, and turned to Labour Opposition MPs for support. The latter were much more receptive to their advances, particularly its female members. In 1982, under the heading 'Labour Women MP's Support Home Birth', the HBA reported the receipt of a press statement from the Labour Party Caucus Committee on Women's Issues, written by Christchurch MP Mary Batchelor. It stated that Labour's female MPs were concerned about the Minister of Health's 'opinionated and unsubstantiated' view that homebirths were trendy, and claimed that, under a qualified midwife and with a doctor's supervision, it was the preferred choice for some women. Batchelor added, 'Already two Labour women MPs, Ann Hercus and Helen Clark, have received a considerable amount of correspondence from people greatly concerned with the Minister of Health's insensitivity on this issue.'[64] Homebirth advocates had been busy.

The HBA reported positive responses from female MPs across the political spectrum. Kemp successfully lobbied two National MPs, Marilyn Waring and Ruth Richardson. The Wellington HBA established a relationship with Labour MP Fran Wilde who agreed to give the opening address for the 1982 Home Birth Week. The Christchurch HBA contacted Labour's spokesperson on health Ann Hercus, who also agreed to address the HBA on 'politics and home birth'.[65] In 1983 the Labour Party Caucus Committee on Women's Issues reaffirmed its support of homebirth in a press statement, and invited Mary Nacey to talk on homebirth at its Women's Policy Conference.[66] Labour MP Annette King opened the 1986 HBA annual conference, declaring her support for the homebirth option.[67]

Homebirth advocates sought the support of male MPs, too. Labour MP Michael Cullen was invited to address the 1982 HBA conference, and spoke of the 'powerful mystique which reinforces the high social status of doctors, and therefore their political power', and of the 'increasing incidence of iatrogenic (doctor-induced) disease'. His views were in accordance with the anti-doctor sentiment that seemed to be building within the Labour Party. Cullen complimented the homebirth movement for 'operating in a liberal/radical framework which calls for choices and community organisation', as opposed to the current childbirth practices based on 'conservative social ideologies'. Again, this reflected the Labour Party's growing commitment to community partnership and 'choice' in an open market. According to the Auckland HBA, Cullen suggested they ask Helen Clark to refer the 1982 anti-homebirth Maternity Services Committee report to a select committee for public submissions.[68]

In the meantime, the 1983 Nurses Amendment Bill was introduced into Parliament and a select committee set up. Homebirth advocates were not slow to respond. As Lynda Williams later reflected, 'In Auckland, we mothers were of course being educated and pushed and prodded into writing submissions' by Donley.[69] Labour MP Michael Bassett was, as noted earlier, impressed by the result, and pointed out that very few MPs had not received correspondence from them.[70] The *HBA National Newsletter* described the activities of the new Save the Midwives Association:

> Within a fortnight of the Bill's initial reading, press statements had been issued, pamphlets distributed and a public meeting encouraging members of the public and midwives to send in submissions against this Bill, had been organised. This public meeting was a huge success. It was well attended by midwives

and mothers. Speakers urged those present to send submissions to the Select Committee and a letter writing campaign to the local papers was instigated.[71]

The HBA congratulated itself that over 230 submissions had been received by the select committee.[72] While this figure was somewhat inflated (National MP Robin Gray counted 209 submissions in total), its members had been busy and succeeded in amending the Bill (see pp. 73–74).[73] As Kemp reported in 1983, 'Probably just about all MPs have received correspondence from people who have had home births.' However, she admitted that they had more success with Labour MPs than National, apart from Ruth Richardson and Marilyn Waring.[74]

## The Fourth Labour Government 1984–1990

The homebirth movement was afforded another lobbying opportunity in 1986 when the Labour government set up a taskforce to review the health system, with a goal of achieving 'improved efficiency and equity'; it was chaired by economics professor Claudia Scott.[75] The report, *Choices for Health Care: Report of the Health Benefits Review*, pointed to the growing influence of a small but vocal homebirth movement, noting that, while there were fewer than 40 midwives claiming the domiciliary midwifery benefit, and homebirth represented less than 1% of all New Zealand births, it featured in many submissions. It stated: 'The ability of pressure groups in this area to make some headway against the medical establishment demonstrates their growing influence.'[76] Donley congratulated the homebirth lobby: 'All the hard work and numerous submissions are finally having an effect.' She listed six HBAs (Auckland, Nelson, South Hokianga, Southland, Wellington and Whangarei) which sent submissions, along with Save the Midwives, the Domiciliary Midwives Society, and certain individuals.[77] The review's final report supported homebirth as an option, and suggested that midwives could offer competing services for 'straightforward childbirth', though this would require legislative change. However, diverging from the message of the homebirth submissions, it also suggested: 'An alternative approach – and one which we favour since it emphasises teamwork – is to encourage "firms" of midwife and doctor combinations to tender for providing a range of services.'[78]

The new Labour government offered other lobbying opportunities for the homebirth movement. In late 1984 it established the Ministry of Women's Affairs, setting its policy agendas after holding women's fora around the country. Homebirth activists were not slow to respond and succeeded in getting homebirth declared a policy priority in 1985.[79] Pairman and Guilliland later commented on the political and strategic advice midwives received from the Ministry, which saw midwifery as a women's health issue.[80] Notably, too, in an article for the UK journal *Midwifery* following a study tour of New Zealand in 1987, Canadian Professor of Nursing Peggy Anne Field wrote:

> The Honourable Ann Hercus, Minister of Women's Affairs . . . noted that at the United Nations World Conference for Women, WHO drew a clear distinction between the female scenario for the future of health and society, described as sane, humane and ecological (SHE) and the hyper-expansionist (HE) scenario, standing for unconstrained technological development. She made the point that the goal of health for all by the year 2000 belongs very firmly to the female scenario.[81]

Field's short list of references for the article included 'Donley J 1989. Current Activities and Issues in New Zealand (mimeographed paper). Auckland, New Zealand'.[82]

While the homebirth movement gained traction with the Ministry of Women's Affairs, their lobbying of the Ministry of Health initially did not go well. In 1983 the HBA reported that Labour MP Michael Bassett had 'made statements in the press in support of home birth and asked questions in the House'.[83] However, when the Wellington HBA wrote to him as Minister of Health (1984–87) about restrictions on midwives practising independently under the 1977 Nurses Act, he replied that the government envisaged no change to the legislation at that time.[84]

Following approaches from midwives' lawyers, Bassett was open to suggestions that the homebirth midwives' pay be increased.[85] As part of these negotiations, he set up a review of the services, which was conducted by Jennie Nicol, the Health Department's senior advisory officer for women, children and family, and an invited speaker at the 1987 HBA conference.[86] Nicol explained that her report was based on interviews with domiciliary midwives and other homebirth advocates.[87] From these she concluded that it was 'very clear that the current demand for homebirth far exceeds the availability of the services', and that 'caseloads would be instantly doubled if there were the professionals available'.[88] This was wishful thinking on the part of the select group she interviewed, as would become clear later, but was useful ammunition for the homebirth cause. Donley wrote to Nicol, congratulating her on her report and wondering how she got 'such a radical document past the conservative bureaucrats'.[89]

David Caygill, who followed Bassett as Minister of Health from August 1987 to January 1989, appeared more receptive to the midwives' advances. Three Christchurch midwives, including Guilliland, met with him in late 1987. Caygill apparently told them he knew little about midwifery, but Guilliland reported that he became 'excited about the prospect of reducing the doctor "gatekeeper" role in maternity services'.[90] In January 1988 Caygill informed Guilliland that he would be very interested in any research she had on midwives as the providers of cost-effective primary healthcare, as she had suggested.[91] He also asked the Health Department to evaluate the legislative restrictions on midwives practising in the community. Its report stated:

> The Department of Health does not consider the removal of the restriction . . . to be appropriate at this time. There are significant deficiencies in the continuity of safety for mother and infant in the domiciliary (home births) midwifery service. The present practice of the medical practitioner taking responsibility for the patient provides the continuity for safety in homebirth services.[92]

In light of this, when lobbied by Lynda Williams, Caygill explained that the current legislation was designed to ensure mothers received a 'safer service' as it provided for medical supervision and nursing services 'at a defined level of competency'.[93]

Caygill was open, however, to the idea of increasing the use of homebirth for low-risk pregnancies, as indicated in his reply to a question in Parliament from Labour's Birkenhead MP Jenny Kirk. When Opposition deputy leader Don McKinnon then asked him about ensuring the quality of homebirth midwives, Caygill responded: '[T]he overwhelming number of submissions I have had on the matter suggests that, in general, there are no fears about the quality of midwifery, only its scarcity'; he did not elaborate on where that overwhelming number of submissions had come from.[94]

In January 1988, Guilliland met with Labour MP and prominent lawyer Geoffrey Palmer (later prime minister 1989–90) and reported that he too appeared very receptive to changing the law relating to midwives' independence. However, he also warned the Health Department would be antagonistic. Guilliland wrote:

> We discussed O & G's and their monopoly on childbirth; the 'terrible business at National Women's' [this was six months before the Cartwright Report was published]. He and Caygill he said were very interested in any information that would change this monopoly . . . He said he'd never had a midwife in to see him before and was delighted to have talked. I assured him it would not be the last time – we are now fighting for our survival. He said yes there wasn't many of us left was there?

Guilliland ended her report with one word: 'Promising!'[95]

But the real coup for the homebirth movement came when Helen Clark took over as Minister of Health in February 1989. In her PhD thesis on the 1990 Nurses Amendment Act, former midwife Sally Abel, who interviewed Clark for her research, pointed out that the latter had been Donley's local (Mount Albert) MP for a number of years and that Donley had always kept her well informed of the issues.[96] This was not only through correspondence; Pairman later commented that Donley had met Clark 'on several occasions to discuss direct-entry midwifery and gain her support'.[97] Describing midwives' autonomy as one of her 'causes', Clark herself later reflected that Donley had been a 'tremendous support' for her over the years.[98] On the thirtieth anniversary of the 1990 Act, Clark recalled that as a young backbencher she had been approached by Donley, who explained that midwives did all the work and GPs signed off and got the credit, and that midwives were a 'sub-species' in the health profession, a situation Clark said, 'just wasn't acceptable'. She determined that if she got into a position of power, she would do something about it. Seven and a half years later she became the Minister of Health.[99]

Clark's support for Donley is evident in their correspondence. When Donley expressed concern about the composition of the new Committee on Women's Health in 1985, Clark thanked her for outlining her work with midwives and homebirth, and added, 'We will have to watch very carefully to see that that committee does not become a vehicle for anti-midwife and anti-home birth advocates.'[100] In her editorial for the April 1989 *HBA Auckland Newsletter,* Donley referred to a personal letter she had received from Clark on 13 February 1989 asking her for suggestions about 'priorities for action'. Donley ended her editorial: 'Helen Clark, we welcome you as our Minister of Health and look forward to working with you.'[101] The Domiciliary Midwives Society also congratulated Clark on her appointment, thanking her for her commitment to women's issues, 'and in particular the encouragement and support that you have expressed for home birth in New Zealand'.[102]

Two months into her term, on 30 April 1989, Clark asked her staffers to provide information about 'the midwives' campaign for autonomy', which she wanted to see progressed.[103] Sheryl Smail, a registered nurse with a Diploma in Nursing Administration, and the Health Department's Chief Nursing Officer from 1988, responded with a position paper. She pointed out that the department had always been concerned with the safety of mothers and infants which was why it recommended that legislation remain in its present form 'until other measures to guarantee the safety of mothers and babies were fully developed'.[104] Clark was not convinced. She informed her staff in June 1989 that she wanted them to speed up preparation for legislation on midwives' autonomy so that it could be introduced to Parliament before Christmas and passed before the government's term of office ended in 1990. In yet another report, Smail set out the department's support for 'a degree of interdependence between midwives and medical practitioners so that childbirth services are coordinated and cost effective'. Clark wrote in the margin, 'That is debatable.'[105]

The homebirth activists had at last found a receptive ear in Parliament. Bronwen Pelvin also reported on a 20-minute conversation with Clark when she came to Nelson to open an independent nursing practice in 1989:

> and she said how supportive she was of the option of home birth and she felt DMs [domiciliary midwives] were appallingly low paid and that she felt women had to be more assertive with their doctors about the things they wanted. We then went on to talk about how we both didn't like very premature babies and questioned the economics of very high-tech neonatal care!! It confirmed again for me that the time of the midwife is here and we have to do all we can to ensure our place in dealing with normal childbirth. We have some strong allies in high places and we must move before they disappear in the next elections.[106]

This questioning of 'high-tech neonatal care' was at odds with a 1982 Board of Health report which had devoted a section to addressing 'Some popular misconceptions about special care for the newborn'. These misconceptions included the units' costs (less than for an adult patient in an ordinary acute medical or surgical ward), and the idea that health depended on socio-economic factors and lifestyle rather than medical intervention. The report claimed that there was evidence to show that properly directed interventions in neonatal care could save lives and reduce the risk of brain damage.[107]

Clark later explained in a speech to the College of Midwives that her long-standing interest in midwifery had not arisen from personal experience, for by choice she had not become a mother. Rather, it emerged from her interest in how women's occupations were valued and given status, and from her concern that the treatment model had come to dominate health services. Both were broad principles, related to work and medicine, and not predicated on an in-depth study of maternity services. However, she also said she was 'personally strongly supportive' of the homebirth option and, taking on board Donley's counsel, she believed that a personal relationship with a midwife would mean women were likely to need fewer antenatal admissions, would feel more in control of their labour, and would need less narcotic analgesia and less medical intervention in labour and in birth. She regarded homebirth as a sensible cost-effective service, which led her to find 'some unusual allies' in Treasury, she explained. Cost-effectiveness was, however, secondary to her concerns about pay equity and the possible ill effects of high-tech medicine.[108]

Clark's views reflected a more general distrust of modern medical technology shared with many of her generation. In 1989 she told the New Zealand Nurses' Union, 'Our health services have been focused traditionally on institutions, a fascination with technology, and a treatment-oriented model of health care.'[109] Guilliland expressed this in relation to childbirth in 1990 when she referred to 'high-tech "toys-for-the-boys" obstetric care'.[110]

## Consumers and health policy

Consumer advocates in the 1980s appeared to be growing in confidence. Commenting on his attendance at the select committee on the 1983 Nurses Amendment Bill, homebirth representative Geoff Bridgman said he felt it a tremendous advantage to have representation from homebirth advocates; in comparison, he said, to the 'staid bureaucracies' of the Nursing Council, the Nurses' Association and the Public Service Association, 'the hodge-podge people who were there on the home birth side must have shown we cared about the issues: that real people having real babies wanted to have options'.[111]

The political and social climate was ripe for consumer involvement in health policy, as the Scott report recognised.[112] The Area Health Boards Act 1983 was indicative of the changing face of the health system. It facilitated the conversion of hospital boards to area health boards. The aim was to amalgamate hospital and public health services and make the boards more community focused. As Rea Daellenbach, who was involved with the Christchurch HBA, later noted, this suited the HBA.[113] In 1985 the Nelson HBA enthused that the philosophy of the area health board was 'entirely in harmony with that of the Homebirth movement' in that it envisaged healthcare being less institutionally oriented and that more responsibility and decision-making would be devolved to local communities.[114]

In 1988, the Labour government changed the enabling feature of the Area Health Board Act 1983, and Helen Clark as Minister of Health from February 1989 oversaw the replacing of hospital boards with 14 area health boards. Donley announced that these new bodies allowed more community participation in decision-making, but she added that Clark 'says these new boards will have to be encouraged to relinquish some of the power to community health committees'.[115] Labour's rhetoric of self-responsibility also suited the homebirth movement. In his 1989 policy document, *Health, A Prescription for Change*, Clark's predecessor as Health Minister David Caygill expressed his government's strategy 'to give people the knowledge and the power – to take greater responsibility for their own lives and to influence the environment around them'. The HBA pronounced that was precisely the goal of the homebirth movement. Moreover, they claimed to be in tune with this neoliberal government since 'home births and midwives are cost effective!'.[116] Homebirth midwives in Northland were delighted to note that the Northland Area Health Board Strategic Plan included women identifying and defining their own health needs and taking responsibility for their own healthcare: 'Assuming responsibility is the essence of home birth.'[117]

The HBA urged its members to become involved in local maternity services. As noted, Auckland homebirth lobbyists were the driving force behind Maternity Action, set up to prevent the closure of small maternity hospitals. Maternity Action secured a permanent position to advise the

Auckland Hospital Board on maternity services and claimed that it had managed to reverse a decision by the Obstetric Review Committee on hospital transferrals.[118] The Auckland Women's Health Council, set up in 1988 to provide a voice on health issues for women in Auckland, found itself in demand on committees such as the Auckland Hospital Research Ethical Committee and district committees of the area health board.[119] The Wellington Area Health Board invited the local HBA to comment on its policy on ultrasound in pregnancy and to help compile information for clients.[120] Health bodies were seeking consumer input in policy and practice, and homebirth advocates were more than happy to oblige.

This also applied to the Health Department itself. The Women's Health Group within the Health Planning and Research Unit set up a Working Party on Safe Options for Low Risk Pregnancy in April 1989. Among its members were representatives from the Domiciliary Midwives Society, Wellington Maternity Action, the Auckland Women's Health Council, the HBA, and of course the New Zealand College of Midwives.[121] Guilliland was the College of Midwives' representative and Pelvin represented the Domiciliary Midwives Society. Guilliland and Donley were invited to join the working party's technical group.[122] Not surprisingly, the working party, as Clark publicly declared on 8 November 1989, 'endorsed the removal of the restriction on midwifery practice'.[123] Midwives and their consumer supporters had an effective lobbying machine, but they were greatly assisted by the receptive political climate in which politicians had their own agendas for reforming the health system.

## Midwifery, feminism and the Cartwright Inquiry

In announcing the founding of the New Zealand College of Midwives in 1989, midwives claimed to be responding to consumer demand, and linked their profession to the advancement of women's rights. The GPs' magazine, *New Zealand Doctor*, declared, 'New Zealand midwives have formed a professional organisation in response to a call by women for more control over their birth experiences.'[124] Bronwen Pelvin, as editor of the *Domiciliary Midwives Society Newsletter*, also made this connection, maintaining that midwifery independence would lead to 'a strong independent voice for the mothers and their babies'.[125]

The College prided itself on including consumers within its ranks. The latter were not broadly representative, however, but closely linked to the homebirth movement. Karen Guilliland reported that the working party to establish the College had included representatives from the HBA, Maternity Action Alliance and Save the Midwives.[126] The College's national committee initially included three consumer representatives from the HBA, the Maternity Action Alliance and Parents Centre. Sharron Cole from Parents Centre was the first consumer representative. A passionate advocate of natural childbirth, she had been a childbirth educator since 1984, having attended a workshop by British homebirth activist Janet Balaskas.[127] Christchurch HBA member Rea Daellenbach, who wrote her PhD thesis on the homebirth movement, was a consumer representative on the national committee from 1992 to 1997. Both Cole and Daellenbach were later consumer members of the Midwifery Council, set up in 2004.[128]

In stressing partnership with women, the College aligned itself closely with the feminist movement, as Waring had advised, turning midwifery into an issue about women's rights. This perspective was considerably helped by the 1987–88 government-initiated inquiry into medical practice at New Zealand's major maternity hospital, National Women's Hospital, chaired by Judge Silvia Cartwright. Guilliland later said of the 1988 midwives' conference at which the decision to set up the College was made: 'Significantly, the opening of this conference fell on the day the Cartwright Report on the Cervical Cancer Enquiry was published.'[129]

Details surrounding the Cartwright Inquiry and events at National Women's, dubbed 'The Unfortunate Experiment' in *Metro* magazine, have been explored elsewhere.[130] What is significant here is how the inquiry escalated into a broader attack on the male medical profession. In Northland, for instance, the local press announced that a group of women were marshalling forces to protest the possibility of a male doctor being appointed as women's health service advisor for the Northland Area Health Board. A representative of the women claimed that, in the aftermath of Cartwright, it was 'appalling that the board could even think about appointing a man'. The Cartwright Report, she said, showed clearly that male medical professionals could not be trusted to act in a way that safeguarded women's health.[131] The Ministry of Women's Affairs joined the fray, expressing its regret that 'women's reproductive health was dependent on the attitude and skills of men who dominated medicine, in policy-making and practice'.[132]

Nurses were also given a bad press at the Cartwright Inquiry. Announcing that midwives had broken away from the Nurses' Association and set up their own organisation, the expatriate *NZ News UK* explained, 'Guilliland said the Cartwright report had made a lot of midwives accept that a separate body [from the Nurses' Association] was needed.'[133] Cartwright had castigated those nurses who did not speak up against Associate Professor Herb Green, the doctor at the centre of the inquiry, describing them as 'less than brave'. They had, she said, failed in their role as patients' advocates, and she assumed this was because they were 'sufficiently intimidated by the medical staff' not to speak up.[134] This elicited an angry response from nurses who rejected the claim.[135] Hospital nurse Barbara Smith later said that she did not believe she and her colleagues were 'less than brave', claiming that the nurses at the hospital 'would speak out all right and they would speak out loud and clear if they thought anything was going wrong'.[136] They saw the situation for what it was — a medical dispute about how interventionist to be in response to a positive cervical smear and minor cellular changes, and they described Green as a doctor who cared deeply for his patients — a description shared by many of his patients, as Cartwright found.[137] Yet the less-than-brave label persisted. A group of midwives including Guilliland wrote to the *Nursing Journal*:

> Why is it that as soon as someone makes any criticism of the medical profession, there always seems to be a nurse who jumps up to defend them? As one of New Zealand's most powerful political lobby groups, they are quite capable of defending themselves . . . We would have been more impressed to have seen letters to the editor by nurses giving support to the women involved in the unfortunate experiment at National Women's rather than to its perpetrators.[138]

While these nurses were branded as traitors, or doctors' handmaidens, publicity surrounding the Cartwright Inquiry and the wholesale condemnation of male doctors (not only those based at National Women's Hospital) also silenced many doctors nationwide. As journalist Jan Corbett later said, to speak up in this environment would have been to look 'foolish, defensive and chauvinistic'.[139]

This suited the homebirth movement very well, and both Clark and Donley saw the inquiry as an important precondition for the 1990 Nurses Amendment Act. In an interview with *Time* magazine, Clark explained that the inquiry politicised women's health issues, encouraged a questioning of the medical model, and facilitated the Act that reined in over-intervention in childbirth. Donley was even more forthright, declaring, 'the Cartwright inquiry changed the climate because it undermined the status and credibility of the obstetricians and gynaecologists and made it easier for this [legislation] to happen'.[140] Five years later, *North & South* magazine carried an article titled 'The politics of childbirth' in which journalist David McLoughlin described the Cartwright Inquiry as a defining moment for midwifery. Noting that the Cartwright Report made it politically acceptable to question the medical establishment, he maintained that: 'Among its many repercussions, it gave impetus to the home birth movement's calls to allow midwives to practise without a doctor's supervision.'[141] Similarly, historian Philippa Mein Smith argued that the natural childbirth movement in the 1980s and 'the Unfortunate Experiment' at National Women's influenced Clark's introduction of the 1990 legislation.[142] The Cartwright Report itself was a response to, and contributed to, consumer and feminist activism, and as such significantly aided homebirth advocates in their call for autonomy from the medical and nursing professions.

## On the eve of reform

The Nurses Amendment Bill was introduced to Parliament in November 1989 and was passed in August 1990. Whilst homebirth and midwifery autonomy were being debated in the House, events outside the debating chamber meant homebirth was very much in the public eye. This included Donley's being awarded an OBE in the 1990 New Year's Honours list. Carolyn Young spoke of this as a triumph for homebirth and homebirth midwives broadly, a recognition of homebirth as an accepted choice, with Donley, 'the symbolic midwife', selected as the individual recipient of this recognition.[143]

Further endorsement came with the extensive publicity surrounding the New Zealand College of Midwives' first national conference in August 1990, which coincided with Parliament's final reading of the Bill. Helen Clark opened the conference, attended by 170 delegates, and was made an honorary midwife in appreciation of her efforts in 'midwifing' the Bill through Parliament.[144] She received a standing ovation at the beginning of her speech.[145] Two days after the conference ended, the Bill passed into law.

Another speaker at the conference was Marsden Wagner who had lent his considerable weight to the cause. He railed against the high intervention rates in childbirth in New Zealand, and declared, 'The single most important thing to change all this is to put midwives in charge of all normal pregnancies and births.'[146] As Guilliland later wrote, his support of midwifery 'came at a politically expedient time. His lecture tour preceding the conference had been enthusiastically received by women and midwives and well covered by the media.'[147] National MP Katherine O'Regan referred to his conference talk when she spoke in Parliament in support of the Bill.[148]

'Women in Partnership' was the theme of the conference, a powerful motif at a time when midwives were attempting to influence political debate. Conference conveners Sally Pairman and Danielle Cameron (a consumer member of the committee, mother of two and a future direct-entry midwife) summarised the conference in the College's journal. The concept of women in partnership, they wrote, 'struck a chord, as together we reclaim midwifery for women'. They quoted Wagner's statement that in the countries where midwifery was a strong profession there were also strong women's groups. They declared that women who were protected in childbirth by midwives would in turn protect midwives, and that women and midwives were brought together by their need for self-determination. In other words, they were positioning themselves as so much more than health professionals. The 170 delegates formed a 'cohesive group of women' who at the end of the conference embraced one another and sang:

> Woman am I,
> spirit am I,
> I am the infinite within my soul,
> I have no beginning,
> And I have no end,
> All this I am.[149]

Whilst Donley and other midwives, backed by homebirth activists, had orchestrated the campaign for reform, this was now presented as midwives responding to consumer demand. Guilliland said in her speech as inaugural College president that midwives 'took up the women's call for a more women-centred service'.[150] Two Australian midwives later claimed that the 1990 legislation resulted from a 'consumer-led and midwife-supported drive for change'.[151] A 2013 research essay also asserted that 'it was a consumer-led drive for change that pressured Parliament to enact the Nurses Amendment Act . . . New Zealand women wanted what midwives had to offer – the provision of primary maternity services without medical intervention.'[152] What Clark had described as the midwives' campaign for autonomy, 'driven by the very determined midwives who worked with me out of the Mount Albert area, led by the late Joan Donnelly [sic]', had been very successful.[153]

## Conclusion

In their entry on the history of Home Birth Associations in *Women Together: A History of Women's Organisations in New Zealand/Ngā Rōpū Wāhine o te Motu*, Joan Donley and Brenda Hinton stated that the 1990 Nurses Amendment Act resulted from the combined work of the College of Midwives, a courageous Helen Clark and the homebirth associations.[154] As they pointed out, consumer support for the new midwifery system derived directly from the homebirth movement. But to what extent did this movement represent women more broadly? This chapter has charted a very determined, persistent and effective campaign by homebirth midwives and their supporters to reach this point. Just how Clark 'midwifed' the legislation through Parliament and whether it really was consumer-driven will be explored in Chapter 6.

# SIX

## *The 1990 Nurses Amendment Act and midwife autonomy*

ON 9 NOVEMBER 1989 Speaker of the House Jonathan Hunt announced to Parliament that 'Two or three minor Bills are ready. One Bill of three clauses – the Nurses Amendment Bill – will be introduced today.'[1] In fact, this Bill only had two clauses, as Minister of Health Helen Clark explained when she introduced it. She added, however, that it had 'considerable significance for the delivery of childbirth services and the practice of midwifery'. Clark explained that, under Section 54 of the current Nurses Act, it was an offence for a midwife to provide a service unless a medical practitioner had undertaken responsibility, and that the goal of the amendment was to place a registered midwife in the same position as a medical practitioner in childbirth services, or 'to allow the registered midwife to undertake sole responsibility for the care of the patient'.[2] As Labour MP Jenny Kirk told Parliament, '[T]he Bill is very simple. It merely adds three words – "or registered midwife" – after the words "medical practitioner" to section 54 of the principal Act.'[3] Clark described it in her speech to the College of Midwives as 'a simple two clause bill'.[4]

This chapter traces the passage of the Bill through Parliament. Drawing on parliamentary debates, submissions to and the report of the select committee, and other correspondence and Health Department files relating to the Bill, it interrogates the goals of the legislators, the support base for the Bill, and concerns around it. In doing so, it will be argued that the Bill was far from simple or minor, and it will address how and why it morphed into something much larger than initially suggested.

## Homebirth and the Nurses Amendment Bill

A short amendment to the 1977 Nurses Act allowing midwives to take sole responsibility for births seems straightforward. Midwives should be trusted to manage normal births without medical involvement, and to know when to call in a doctor for complications or emergencies. Opposition spokesperson for women's affairs Katherine O'Regan said during the introductory debates, 'Midwives will look after healthy mothers and babies, and any problems will be referred to a doctor. They wish to assure the nation that they are not trying to take over from doctors.' But she also looked back to a golden age of midwifery before hospitalised birth, describing midwifery as 'an ancient craft that for centuries has played a major part in assisting women in the delivery of their babies . . . technology has taken over and mothers have been left out. The Bill will turn the tide back to where it should be.'[5]

Homebirth was central to the Bill. As Manawatū homebirth midwife Ruth Martis said in her submission, 'Homebirths have to be cited to support the change of the act as it is in this area only in New Zealand where midwives are able to practise more or less as independent practitioners.'[6] Joan Donley too stated, 'The only place a midwife can work with any real independence is in the community.'[7] Just as the 1971 legislation introducing doctors' oversight of childbirth services did not affect daily practices in maternity hospitals, so this proposed legislation would have little apparent impact on hospitals, where teamwork prevailed. The current affairs magazine *North & South* reported in 1993 that: 'Clark says she changed the law to promote home births, which she viewed as more cost-effective than hospital ones.'[8]

Homebirth advocates had been very keen to draw attention to cost-saving benefits. As homebirth midwife Celeste McCoy said in her submission, 'Midwives are certainly an economic proposition. The reduction to the Health quota will be substantial – without a reduction in expertise in maternity care.'[9] The Domiciliary Midwives Society cited a British study to support this viewpoint.[10] In its submission, the National Council of Women claimed an 'uneasy feeling' that the proposed law change was simply another cost-cutting measure in the guise of acquiescence to requests by various professional and community groups. It noted 'with alarm' the reference in Clark's introductory speech to Treasury and 'to a number of other references in her speech on the money-saving benefits of the amendment'.[11]

Cost-effectiveness was not Clark's only motivation, however. As noted in Chapter 5, she was persuaded that homebirth had advantages for women, and she stressed in Parliament that this was what women wanted. Introducing the Bill, she cited the New Zealand Planning Council's 1985 report, chaired by sociologist Peggy Koopman-Boyden. This report had predicted that the number of homebirths would likely rise if mothers were given the choice.[12]

Arguments in Parliament drew on the current ideological rubric. Jenny Kirk explained how technology had 'placed doctors – mostly male – at the centre of the birth and in control', which she considered 'an uncomfortable and distressing experience for the woman involved'.[13] By contrast, 'childbirth in a home environment means a relaxed pregnant woman in labour, a relaxed baby being born, and often there is no need to carry out tests that result from a baby born under stress through the use of forceps or through Caesarean operations'.[14] The implication was that such interventions served no useful purpose and were stressful to mother and baby. Clark herself appeared dismissive of doctors' involvement, as illustrated by her correspondence at that time with Nelson GP obstetrician Bryan Hardie Boys. The latter, who had long been involved in homebirth, wrote to Clark stating his belief that the doctor's presence need not interfere with midwives' autonomy. Querying the need for a doctor's presence, Clark responded that, 'Midwifery is focussed on the woman', implying that doctors were not. She added for good measure, 'Midwifery is an ancient and honourable profession. It is unfortunate that it ever lost its autonomy.'[15]

There was little dissension during Parliament's opening discussion of the Bill, and Clark, summing up, said she welcomed the bipartisan support. The only interrogation of the Bill came from Opposition deputy leader and National Party Health spokesperson Don McKinnon who 'asked several questions relating to the scope of the work of midwives'.[16] When he posed those questions, Labour MP Anne Collins interrupted him. 'Stop waffling!' she said. 'Is the member for or against the Bill? Wiffle-waffle!' McKinnon replied, 'I said very early on that the Opposition does support the Bill.' Collins responded, 'Hooray!'[17]

The tenor of debates in Parliament was in marked contrast to those that had occurred when homebirth was discussed just six years earlier. In 1989 there were fewer qualified expressions of support than there had been in 1983 when, for example, Labour's Margaret Shields said that homebirth should be available but only for second births and 'low-risk patients'.[18] Nor did any member in 1989 raise the argument about the child's interests, as did Peter Tapsell in 1983.[19]

## Submissions

When parliamentary discussion recommenced on 29 May 1990 following the select committee process, the two-clause Bill had morphed into a 24-clause document that altered five Acts of Parliament and six sets of regulations. Don McKinnon said it should be returned to the select committee to allow proper consultation and 'to begin the entire proceedings cleanly once again'.[20] Clark disagreed and explained that the government was proposing to move a supplementary order paper to deal with the changes. She criticised McKinnon for neglecting to mention in his speeches 'the many, many people who appeared at the select committee or wrote to it expressing full support for the principles of the Bill'. She added, 'If the Deputy Leader of the Opposition wants to take on the women of New Zealand – and, indeed, many male parents in New Zealand – he will be the loser. There is much public support for the Bill.' McKinnon intercepted, 'Never would I take on the women of New Zealand.' Clark continued:

> [He] would be wise not to take them on. There were 99 submissions – I understand that they were all in support of the Bill. That shows how broad the public support for the measure was. It is broad support because most people welcome the concept of women and their partners having a choice about where the birth of their child occurs. Under the Bill more women are likely to choose to have their births at home . . .[21]

This claim of all-encompassing support can be tested by an analysis of the submissions. These fell into four broad categories: (1) Home Birth Associations (HBAs) and consumer homebirth advocates; (2) homebirth midwives and their organisations, including the Nurses' Association; (3) women's groups who were not homebirth advocates; and (4) other health and medical professionals and their organisations.

In the December 1989 *HBA Newsletter*, Donley encouraged members to send submissions, and provided an address and guidance on what to write. She told readers that it was important to support the Bill 'with a deluge of submissions. Also lobby your MP. Go for it!'[22] While they did not necessarily follow Donley's detailed instructions on what to write, their submissions flowed in. Advocacy groups who sent submissions included five HBAs (Eastern Bay, Auckland, Nelson, Tauranga and Canterbury), the Save the Midwives Association (based in Auckland), and Women's Health Collectives or Councils (two in Wellington, one each in Kāpiti, Whāingaroa/Raglan and Waikato). These were generally short submissions, reaffirming that childbirth was a natural process, that midwives were guardians of natural birth, and that women should have the option of homebirth.

Forty-nine individual 'consumers', some of whom were also members of those organisations, sent submissions in favour of the Bill. Most of these were brief. The very first submission was from a homebirth mother residing in Donley's own area, Mount Albert.[23] Three submissions were on postcards, and one of these simply read: 'dear [sic] Committee Members I support the autonomy of midwives', followed by a signature.[24] Almost all individual submissions described or referred to their own homebirth experiences, as Marilyn Waring had advised.

Nelson and the Tasman region had a particularly active lobby group for homebirth, with two-thirds of the 49 individual submissions coming from this region alone. Among these was a submission from consumer and birth-educator Heather Marr, who identified herself as a member of Nelson HBA and treasurer of the Nelson branch of the College of Midwives, both of which also put in submissions. Motueka Women's Electoral Lobby, describing itself as a feminist group, also sent a short submission in favour of the amendment.[25] Nelson's enthusiastic response could be attributed to Bronwen Pelvin's engagement in homebirth there since 1979, and/or to its significant number of alternative-lifestyle residents. While homebirth remained a minority activity, accounting for 4% of births in Nelson (49 home births in 1989), its lobbyists were particularly active.[26] Four of the 12 oral submissions also came from this region, including from Pelvin, Marr, the Nelson HBA and the Domiciliary Midwives Society led by Pelvin. With the Nelson Area Health Board presenting as well, Nelson and its surrounds made up nearly half of the oral submissions.[27] Addresses on written submissions from Nelson indicate most came from outlying districts, including from communes such as the Riverside Community in Lower Moutere, where Pelvin resided; the Graham Downs Community, Motueka; and the Tui Community in Golden Bay. Other known destinations for alternative lifestylers also featured, with one submission from Auckland's Waiheke Island and three from Coromandel. However, no other area compared with the enthusiastic response from Nelson.

The College of Midwives and eight of its branches around the country sent submissions, along with the Domiciliary Midwives Society, the Midwives of Opotiki, and at least six individual homebirth midwives including Bronwen Pelvin. The Domiciliary Midwives Society submission came from the Riverside Community, written by Pelvin with additions by Donley and Auckland midwife Mary Hammond. Donley and Hammond also sent in a submission on behalf of the Auckland Domiciliary Midwives.[28] Karen Guilliland presented the submission of the New Zealand College of Midwives as its president. Not surprisingly, all supported midwife autonomy and homebirth. The New Zealand Nurses' Association submission was penned by its professional officer Joy Bickley, under whose guidance the Association had done a complete flip-flop from its stance a decade earlier. Bickley opened her submission with the statement, 'Ripples of pleasure emanated from the membership of the New Zealand Nurses' Association when this Bill was introduced to the House on 7 November 1989.'[29] She brought a feminist perspective to bear, commenting elsewhere on midwives' powerlessness under the current system.[30]

Consumer views were also reflected in the submissions from the Women's Division Federated Farmers and the National Council of Women. Strangely, Parents Centre, traditionally the guardian of natural birth, was absent from submissions apart from the Wairarapa branch, although Sharron Cole, Parents Centre representative on the national executive of the College of Midwives, wrote directly to Clark in July 1990 supporting the Bill.[31]

The Women's Division Federated Farmers, with 8,500 members, urged caution. It believed in the right of the prospective mother to choose, but only after her medical status was assessed, emergency procedures had been discussed, and she had given informed consent. Its submission stressed the importance of midwifery training, registration and annual review so that midwives kept conversant with current practices. It 'wish[ed] to have these safeguards built into the new legislation as women may be given false assurances that the midwife is competent and that a doctor does not need to be involved in her obstetric care'.[32] In other words, the Women's Division did not support the Bill as presented.

The National Council of Women, claiming to represent a quarter of a million women through its 36 branches and 48 national affiliated societies, viewed itself as a watchdog for proposed legislation affecting women and children. In its detailed submission, the Council expressed concern that under the new arrangement women might be deprived of access to medical care, since giving midwives sole responsibility might mean removing the existing maternity benefit to doctors. It believed this could seriously disadvantage women on low incomes and/or with a high-risk factor, and their babies. This also concerned the Salvation Army Women's Organisation, while others raised concerns around midwives' training in recognising rarer pathological conditions in pregnancy. The National Council of Women favoured the Dutch system involving medical assessment of pregnant women and referral to a midwife if appropriate. Like the Women's Division Federated Farmers, the Council wanted '[c]lear guidelines, even rules and regulations . . . after consultation with representatives of midwives, obstetricians, hospital and area health board authorities, and consumers of both home birth and hospital services, before this amendment is enacted.'[33] It did not support the Bill as it stood.

Five of the 14 Area Health Boards (Canterbury, Northland, Nelson, Auckland and Wanganui) sent submissions. The strong anti-homebirth sentiment expressed in this sector in the 1980 submissions was not evident here. They were perhaps more wary of responding to what was framed as a feminist issue in the post-Cartwright environment. Nevertheless, the sector did express reservations about the proposed amendment in its current form. Wanganui Area Health Board wanted an initial medical assessment of pregnant women to assess their suitability for homebirth, referring to Clark's media release the day before the legislation was introduced to Parliament in which she affirmed doctors' skills in recognising medical problems. A submission from the Waikato Area Health Board came from its nurses and midwives, drafted by the board's Director of Nursing Practice Maureen Lawton. The submission cautioned that 'without any controls, inexperienced midwives could set up in domiciliary practice or could practice in small maternity hospitals where there is minimal supervision'. They expressed concern about oversight and auditing of standards, and did not believe the consumer-driven domiciliary midwives standards review committees were enough of a safeguard; rather, they believed a senior midwife should oversee services.[34]

As in their 1980 submissions, the major medical organisations were not averse to the development of homebirth services but wished to see safeguards in place (see p. 52). In its 1990 submission, the Royal New Zealand College of Obstetricians and Gynaecologists stressed the need for an improved team concept in homebirth, and urged that midwives be subject to systems of quality assurance, continuing medical education, and time-limited contracts, as medical practitioners were.[35] The New Zealand Medical Women's Association's submission was presented by Dr Diana Edwards, president of the Canterbury branch.[36] It expressed concern about allowing midwives to practise alone in the community, and referred to Britain where all births had two attendees and a flying squad available, and where a professional team assessed every case before a homebirth was attempted.[37] Standards of training and back-up support were also a focus of the New Zealand Medical Association's submission. It wanted midwives to meet the same conditions as GPs practising obstetrics set out by the obstetrics standards review committees. It urged caution:

> Maybe, prior to making any amendment to the Nurses Act to increase the independence of midwives in New Zealand, it is more important to look at the support systems that do exist, the current levels of training, the need for peer review and quality assurance. Once assurances can be given that these factors have been addressed, then it may be more appropriate for the midwives to be given greater autonomy.[38]

In short, the submissions did not support Clark's claim of 'many, many women' writing to support the amendment. Of the 49 individual consumers who wrote to the committee, at least 33 came from the Nelson-Tasman region and could not be regarded as representative. Nor did all 99 submissions support the amendment, as Clark suggested, although it is true that they supported it 'in principle', but only after their concerns had been met. Professional groups and prominent lay organisations issued stern warnings that safeguards needed to be in place before the legislation was passed, and they stressed the importance of ongoing education of midwives, team efforts, and prior medical checks on women before homebirth was considered. Their submissions did not support midwife autonomy without additional safeguards. Clark acknowledged the overriding concern about safety, declaring without addressing the individual points:

> The 96 [sic] submissions received by the select committee were, I understand, supportive of the principle of the autonomy for midwives. The major concern identified in the submissions was whether the safety of the mother and child could be ensured. In removing the restrictions on the practice of midwifery it is essential that the safety of women and babies remain paramount. I am satisfied that the Bill, when enacted, will bring about improvements in birthing services for women and babies.[39]

In her talk to the College of Midwives the previous day, Clark had spoken of reservations about the adequacy of midwifery training and accountability, and said, 'While these concerns would merit serious attention if they were well based, it is my judgement that they are not.'[40] She did not elaborate on how she had reached that judgement.

## Social Services Committee and Supplementary Order Paper 66

Labour MP Judy Keall chaired the Social Services Select Committee and reported to Parliament on 29 May 1990. She explained:

> During the hearings of evidence on the Bill it became clear to the committee that, for registered midwives to provide comprehensive services and to ensure the safety of mother and child, it would be necessary to permit midwives to perform the range of related services referred to in submissions. They would include the administering of medicines commonly used in low-risk pregnancies and childbirth, the ability of midwives to call for routine diagnostic laboratory tests and to claim associated social security benefits, and the ability to transfer patients to an obstetrician or to a hospital, if necessary.[41]

Safety was therefore to be ensured by giving midwives a greater range of powers, not through training, regulations, accountability or even back-up services. Strangely, the need for these 'related services' listed by Keall had not been a primary focus for many of the submissions either in support or critical of the amendment. Rather, homebirth advocates tended to stress their right to natural childbirth, and professional organisations and other consumer groups emphasised the need for a team approach, midwifery training, and medical assessment and flying squads for homebirths. Above all else, the submissions focused on homebirth. As Rea Daellenbach explained, homebirth advocates and medical professionals alike considered the Bill to be about homebirths, and this accounted for the latter's relative lack of opposition provided that safeguards were put in place; major women's organisations took a similar view.[42] Daellenbach concluded, 'Neither the leaders of the medical profession nor home birth activists anticipated the profound consequences that the 1990 Nurses Amendment Act would have for the arrangements of maternity services.'[43]

As noted, Don McKinnon was critical of the initial two clauses morphing into a 24-clause Bill following the select committee process, with no public consultation about the proposed changes. Others shared that concern. Katherine O'Regan, herself a member of the select committee, thought it 'an abuse of the House and its procedures'. She quoted Prime Minister Geoffrey Palmer's words in his book *Unbridled Power*: 'Law-making should be a solemn and deliberate business.'[44] Opposition MP Murray McCully also quoted Palmer's assertion that law-making should allow people to 'have a chance of knowing what is happening and making representations about it if they wish'.[45] Their concern was the lack of due process. Jenny Kirk responded that they were 'quibbling over a minor technicality'.[46]

Throughout the process, the Opposition insisted it supported the Bill.[47] Even McKinnon assured Parliament in August 1990 that he had supported the Bill since its introduction.[48] The 'quibbling' over procedure had given the Opposition an opportunity to attack the government without risking the loss of women's votes. After all, they had been told that 'the women of New Zealand' supported the measure. Murray McCully claimed to be 'disappointed' when he received a letter from a midwife who told him that 'Opposition members had not been supportive of her profession and of the measure promoting the advancement of her profession'. He was puzzled as to how she had gained that impression, and reassured Parliament that the Opposition supported the Bill; it was just the process they did not support.[49]

To appease concerns about process, a special two-hour sitting of the select committee was agreed for 18 July 1990.[50] The prescribing of drugs was a major focus of this meeting. This had apparently elicited little discussion during the original select committee process, because Clark had responded in the negative when McKinnon asked during the first reading whether midwives would be able to prescribe drugs for mothers and mothers-to-be.

She stated unequivocally, '[M]idwives will not prescribe drugs, because that point is reached after complications have appeared, and such complications are more properly handled by medical practitioners.'[51] Press coverage of the debates repeated Clark's response; journalist Simon Collins reported on 10 November 1989 that: 'Helen Clark replied [to a question by McKinnon about prescribing drugs] that the bill would not change the normal work of midwives, which included . . . not prescribing drugs. That would remain the work of a doctor.'[52] The select committee explained that while it proposed that midwives should be able to prescribe certain specified drugs, it found, on the advice of the Health Department, it was not possible to define appropriate drugs, and so midwives were to be given equal prescribing rights to medical practitioners. The two-hour special session in July, at which this was discussed, was well attended by both medical and midwifery organisations. The College of Midwives later reported that Donley, Pairman and Guilliland addressed the meeting and that 'once again the Select Committee was impressed with the soundness of our arguments'.[53]

Major medical groups continued to have misgivings and expressed these in writing following the special session. The New Zealand General Practitioners' Association, a branch of the New Zealand Medical Association, wrote to the select committee chair. It pointed out that, as had been made clear at the hearing, the major medical organisations – the New Zealand Medical Association and Medical Women's Association, and the Colleges of Obstetricians and Gynaecologists and of General Practitioners – were now 'more resolutely opposed to the amendments than was the case in their original submissions'. They explained that these organisations had not opposed 'greater autonomy' for midwives but were now concerned that with the introduction of the supplementary order paper, midwives were being given even greater autonomy than was originally envisaged. They believed that introducing these changes 'in haste and without proper discussion with consideration to the safety and quality assurance aspects, can only be detrimental'. In particular, they expressed amazement that it was not possible to restrict prescribing lists for midwives under the legislation. They noted that midwives were seeking greater autonomy for dealing with low-risk obstetrics, which should not necessitate extensive use of drugs.[54]

The select committee had sent a list of potential prescription drugs to the New Zealand Medical Association, which reported back after reviewing this document: 'It is apparent from the comments on many of the drugs in the attached list that medical practitioners do not work in isolation, and often require the input and support of hospital staff, and specialists, and that this should also apply to midwives.' They added that, to ensure the welfare of mother and baby, the approach to obstetrics should be 'of the highest standard, and conducted in a supportive, team environment – not in isolation'.[55]

The College of Obstetricians and Gynaecologists explained that the education of medical practitioners in pharmaceuticals was extensive, far exceeding the training that midwives received. They wrote: 'If Parliament decides to extend prescribing rights to midwives, the women of New Zealand are entitled to clear assurances that the midwives are fully registered, are under contract to the Area Health Boards and are competent to deal with adverse effects.' Their letter concluded with a statement that many issues in the supplementary order paper required further study by health professionals, and that there needed to be clear guidelines to area health boards and practitioners involved in maternity services. Their College would welcome the opportunity to be involved in further discussion.[56]

Director of Nursing Practice at the Waikato Area Health Board Maureen Lawton, who had fronted a submission on the Bill, sent a letter to Clark in July on behalf of her nurses and midwives. She acknowledged support for independent midwifery on the grounds that childbirth was a normal process and was being unnecessarily medicalised. But she was also concerned about the risk of complacency developing, drawing attention to the potential dangers of homebirth in the absence of adequate emergency services, such as a flying squad.[57] Clark invited Karen Guilliland, another recipient of the letter, to respond. Guilliland told Lawton, 'The resistance to this change from Medical and Nursing Managers is not unexpected as it threatens traditional hierarchys [sic].' She maintained that Lawton's statement about the dangers of homebirth could be challenged by evidence 'easily found in any medical or nursing library'. She responded to the flying-squad concept by claiming that in Britain, where it was practised, homes were without telephone and transport, and midwives did not carry emergency equipment as they did in New Zealand.[58] In fact, 87% of UK households had landline telephones in 1990 and 85% of passenger kilometres were by private vehicle in the late 1980s. Nor did emergency equipment carried by midwives in the New Zealand and the UK significantly differ.

The National Council of Women also protested the lack of discussion and consultation on the supplementary order paper. Council secretary Lois Robertson later wrote to Labour MP and Speaker of the House Jonathan

Hunt, pointing to her organisation's substantial written and oral submissions, and advising him of the Council's considerable dismay that it had not been given an opportunity to express an opinion via the select committee process. The Council appreciated that a situation could arise where a select committee process might reveal the need for ancillary legislation but believed 'this should have been foreseen in the preparation of the legislation'.[59]

Judy Keall continued to insist that all of the provisions in the supplementary order paper were in response to submissions.[60] Clark responded to Lois Robertson that it became clear to the committee during the hearing of evidence that these additions were necessary.[61] She repeated this in a press release, and told the College of Midwives in her speech just before the Bill's passage that it had become evident to her 'earlier in 1990' that the simple two-clause Bill could bring about autonomy in principle, but that additional Acts and regulations were needed to create real autonomy.[62]

## Unforeseen amendments?

The National Council of Women objected to the late addition of changes not subjected to public scrutiny, and thought they should have been anticipated in the Bill's preparation. In fact, evidence suggests the changes had been foreseen. Nine days before the Bill was introduced to Parliament, the College of Midwives had sent the Health Department a long list of changes to enable midwifery autonomy, including access to drugs, laboratory services, hospitals and maternity benefits.[63] The department had been aware of these requirements for some time. In her report to Clark on 20 June 1989, more than four months before the Bill was introduced to Parliament, the department's chief nursing officer, Sheryl Smail, had identified six 'consequential amendments' to Acts of Parliament to give effect to the Nurses Amendment Act.[64] Another memorandum written in September 1989 on the necessity of amending further legislation stated: 'Minister was advised of this in May 1989 and reference to it has been made since in subsequent paper. She has noted these accordingly.'[65]

Not only had Clark's advisors identified the need to amend other legislation and regulations to effect the change but they had also expressed some disquiet about the Bill in the planning stage. In advocating for midwife autonomy, Clark was at odds with her department. In a report on 22 June 1989, Smail wrote: 'Cost effective childbirth services require a co-ordinated approach. Medical practitioners and midwives must work together so that the service provided meets the needs of the clients, is of high quality, and promotes a healthy outcome for mother and child.' Clark underlined 'Medical practitioners and midwives must work together', appending a question mark in the margin.[66]

Dr Bob Boyd from the Health Department's Primary Health Care Unit wrote a memorandum on the 'Autonomy of Midwives' in early October 1989, a month before the Bill was introduced to Parliament. In this he wrote: 'I have yet to learn where in the world this autonomy exists to the degree that appears to be proposed.' He noted that the department's Working Group on Safe Options for Low-risk Pregnancy and Childbirth supported the amendment, but said that the group's major reference point was a system in Britain called 'Know your midwife'.[67] He rightly pointed out that this scheme was 'far from being a story of midwife autonomy'; it was run out of a hospital with the backing of hospital obstetricians, who provided initial assessments and two routine consultations, along with others if required. He also noted that the 'Dutch home-confinement system' was a midwife–doctor team approach.[68]

Chris Harrington, assistant manager in the Health Department's Medicines and Benefits Unit, had previously compiled research for the 1986 Health Benefits Review. Three weeks before the 1989 Nurses Amendment Bill was introduced to Parliament, Harrington presented a report headed: 'Further changes required to give effect to autonomy for domiciliary midwives'. He claimed that prescribing drugs represented a 'major policy change', and not the minor one as it was later introduced to Parliament. His report also shows that there had been discussion about prescribing rights even at this early stage.[69] Harrington expressed concern as to whether domiciliary midwives currently had sufficient knowledge about medicines in pregnancy, and if they would be aware of contra-indications and possible adverse reactions. He was uneasy not only about their training in pharmacology but also their ability to interpret laboratory tests. He wondered about their aptitude to make paediatric assessments at birth and at six weeks and asked, 'Is the midwife to take full responsibility for form H661 which details foetal abnormalities. If so, what is their training to carry out this?' He queried the criteria to be used for deciding which problems were to be considered pregnancy-related and which should be referred, giving the examples of back pain, haemorrhoids, varicose veins, deep vein thrombosis, hypertension and diabetes. He raised concerns about making 'controlled drugs' (such as narcotics for pain relief) accessible to midwives, adding, 'It is not sufficient to say that the current domiciliary midwives rarely if ever administer narcotic pain relief.' He also raised 'policy issues'. Given that it had 'always been stated' that domiciliary midwives' practices would be restricted to low-risk pregnancies, then the definition of low-risk pregnancy must be clear, just as it must also be clear how that assessment would be made and whether it would involve a medical assessment. He noted that nothing in the proposed legislation referred to low-risk pregnancy. In addition, he identified issues for area health boards. If domiciliary midwives were to be given hospital-admitting rights, the relationships between midwives and medical and specialist practitioners in hospital must be clarified.

'The change to autonomous maternity practice by domiciliary midwives is a major one with far-reaching implications for benefits administration. It is vital that important issues are resolved before implementation occurs in order to avoid significant administrative problems at a later stage,' Harrington warned.[70] Teenah Handiside, the Health Department's acting chief nursing officer and a former nursing lecturer at Nelson Polytechnic, expressed a similar view in a memorandum to Clark on 19 December 1989:

> The change to autonomous maternity practice by domiciliary midwives is a major one with far-reaching implications. The department believes that it is vital that the policy issues are resolved before the Bill comes into force, and that there must be adequate opportunity for consultation and discussions with consumers, midwives, nursing and medical groups and area health boards.

Handiside suggested that, because the Bill was 'controversial', any further drafting should be halted until the end of submissions to the select committee the following March. Delaying until the end of July would, she said, allow for, amongst other things, 'the implementation of safety measures'. Clark responded with margin notes: 'No, please proceed – I want the Bill passed by 1 April so all relevant issues must be addressed a.s.a.p. – or at least by Easter if at all possible. See comment at end. 31 July seems too far off.'[71] It appears she had made her mind up before receiving submissions.

Those supporting the Bill had expected medical opposition, as Guilliland told *Listener* journalist Pamela Stirling.[72] Clark had informed the Cabinet Social

Equity Committee (one of the two Cabinet committees involved in major administrative and legislative changes) back in mid-1989 that the medical profession was likely to oppose the relaxation of restrictions on midwifery practice.[73] Around the same time, she told fellow MPs that she had consulted widely about the proposal: 'Comments have been sought from a wide range of interested groups and organisations including the Nursing Council of New Zealand, Nurses Union, Nurses Association and College of Midwives.'[74] Notably absent were any medical groups. When, in the opening parliamentary debate, McKinnon asked Clark if she had consulted the New Zealand Medical Association, she replied, 'Such consultation was not specifically sought on the Bill.'[75] According to Pairman and Guilliland, Clark was dismissive of the concerns expressed by the medical profession in any case. She had told the College of Midwives that 'she believed the lobbying by doctors stemmed from their opposition to sharing the gate-keeping role to maternity services with midwives'.[76]

Whether medical practitioners were consulted or not, their views did not seem to carry any weight in this debate. Doctors expressed reservations in their submissions to the select committee and in correspondence following the introduction of the supplementary order paper, but these were ignored. On prescribing rights, Katherine O'Regan explained that as a member of the select committee she was

> convinced at the end that midwives will know when and when not to prescribe. Midwives do not usually prescribe much, anyway. They believe in assisting women in a natural fashion . . . The midwives told us that they rarely used or needed to use any major drugs. That information led us to believe that midwives should have the power to sign prescriptions.[77]

Select committee member Jenny Kirk stated during the Bill's first reading that the midwife was skilled in establishing whether the woman in labour needed pain-killing drugs, or whether such drugs were 'unnecessary if other more natural means of relaxation' could be used.[78] Putting aside the fact that her comment throws into question the concept of women's 'choice' of childbirth practices if midwives were to decide, the argument that midwives would not prescribe much was an odd justification for allowing them access to prescription medicines. This had been Harrington's point, too.

## The 1990 Nurses Amendment Act and midwife autonomy

Katherine O'Regan told the House on 24 August 1990, 'The committee was convinced, after considering submissions from midwives, that the standards of practice will be enhanced with the passing of the Bill.'[79] She announced during the final debates, 'I congratulate the New Zealand College of Midwives and the Domiciliary Midwives Society of New Zealand on the manner in which they brought their submissions to the committee. They were good-humoured at all times, they were patient, and they were certainly very civil. I congratulate them on that.'[80]

The last word in Parliament before the Bill passed into law went to Jeff Grant, National MP for the Southland electorate of Awarua, who had joined the Social Services Committee after it delivered its report in May. He told the House that his interest stemmed not only from his own child's recent birth and also because 'of all of the Bills that have been introduced in recent times I do not think that there has been one on which I have been lobbied so much by the parties involved'.[81] He said, 'If there is one message that Parliament wants to give to the public and to those who are involved in providing the professional service to mothers it is that the House regards childbirth as natural, and, therefore, women should have a choice.'[82] The Bill passed into law on 28 August 1990, one month before Labour lost the general election to the National Party. The reason for Labour's demise lay elsewhere, but Clark had succeeded in her goal of passing this legislation before that demise.

### Direct-entry midwifery training and Supplementary Order Paper 67

There was one more late addition to the legislation, introduced within 24 hours of Parliament's final debates (the second and third readings) on 21 August 1990. Introducing the second reading, Helen Clark outlined details in Supplementary Order Paper 66, and then referred to a further paper, number 67, which, she said, related to the approval of experimental training programmes by the Nursing Council following the recent transfer of nursing education to tertiary institutions. In her introductory overview she did not mention direct-entry midwifery training, which was the subject of clause two of Supplementary Order Paper 67.[83] This clause proposed an experimental programme of midwifery training which did not require prior nurse training, unlike existing midwifery courses. As they had for Supplementary Order Paper 66, Opposition members such as Don McKinnon and Murray McCully focused primarily on process and not substance when addressing the new addition. The latter argued that Clark should have been more 'up-front' about the proposal and allowed proper consultation to take place. He asked:

> When we are considering making important changes to the powers of midwives, which the Opposition supports, why was a supplementary order paper sneaked in – an important measure . . . which relates to the training of midwives and their professional qualifications? Why did that happen one day before the debate on the second reading but after the introduction and the select committee process?[84]

In its submission to the select committee, the National Council of Women had declared its support for nursing education as a prior requirement for midwifery training.[85] The Council later criticised the lack of public consultation about the proposal relating to midwifery training, pointing out that midwifery education was on the agenda for discussion at a meeting they were planning for October 1990. They claimed to be deeply concerned about this curtailment of public comment through the supplementary order paper process on issues of major importance to consumers.[86] Whilst direct-entry midwifery training was something for which homebirth midwives and their supporters had long lobbied, its inclusion at the eleventh hour, Pairman and Guilliland later noted, took all parties by surprise.[87]

Nurse training had frequently been invoked in debates in the House about the safety of autonomous midwifery practice. Introducing the report of the select committee on 29 May, Judy Keall had pointed out that the New Zealand Medical Association, the Royal New Zealand College of Obstetricians and Gynaecologists, some area health boards, and the National Council of Women had not opposed the principle of autonomy for midwives but expressed concern about the need for sufficient training to ensure safety. She continued:

> By comparison, midwives maintained that they had sufficient training. Strong submissions received from the New Zealand College of Midwives, the domiciliary midwives, and the Nurses Association stated that midwives were trained appropriately, receiving midwifery training after spending 4 years training as nurses. Therefore, they felt that they were competent to do the job.[88]

The submission of the New Zealand College of Midwives, which Guilliland presented, began by addressing 'Knowledge and Safety to Practice'. She affirmed that New Zealand midwives had considerable education behind them, having undertaken a three-year course as a registered general and obstetric nurse or registered comprehensive nurse, and then undergone midwifery training.[89] Midwife Ruth Martis also made the point in her submission that medical practitioners had just upgraded their obstetric diploma time from six to nine months, whilst midwives trained for 'one year postgrad', in recognition of midwifery as a postgraduate nursing course.[90]

Throughout the parliamentary debates, supporters of the Bill constantly invoked nursing training when addressing issues relating to the safety of independent midwifery practice. During the opening debate on 9 November 1989, McKinnon raised the issue of patient safety, and Katherine O'Regan replied, 'Personally, I trust midwives to know when things are going wrong. They have 4 years' experience as general nurses, and then a time specialising in midwifery. They are trained.'[91] This refrain continued during the Bill's second hearing. Addressing safety issues on 29 May, Jenny Kirk claimed that training for midwives consisted of '2 years of further training after the 3 years of general nursing training; a total of at least 5 years'.[92] She repeated this on 21 August 1990, presenting this nurse training as an endorsement of safe practice after Clark had introduced (unopposed) the proposal for direct-entry training. Kirk was seemingly unaware of the contradiction.[93] Moreover, after direct-entry training had been introduced and the amendment agreed to, Judy Keall reassured Parliament of the safety of midwives administering drugs, pointing out that midwives took a basic nurse course first and then a postgraduate midwifery diploma, and that they had pharmacological training in both courses.[94]

The supplementary order paper was incorporated into the Bill after minimal discussion in Parliament. Section 39 of the Nurses Act 1977 was amended to allow the Nursing Council to establish direct-entry midwifery pilot courses with the approval of the Minister of Health. But was this simply an afterthought? Save the Midwives had been advocating for direct-entry midwifery training since the mid-1980s. In 1987, its taskforce chair Judi Strid sent a letter on the subject to Minister of Women's Affairs Ann Hercus, who raised it with Sally Shaw, the Department of Health's chief nursing officer. Shaw replied that the department did not support direct-entry midwifery training, explaining that childbirth is an episode in a woman's life and that a 'broadly based nursing education provides the knowledge and skills to practise a holistic approach to health'.[95] Around the same time David Caygill, then Minister of Health, replied to a query about midwifery training by stating that 'midwifery will continue to be an advanced <u>nursing</u> preparation. Direct entry courses are not seen as being appropriate.'[96] In his meeting with Guilliland in December 1987, Caygill had told her that the Department of Health was strongly opposed to direct-entry midwifery training.[97]

The Health Department made its position on direct-entry midwifery training clear to Helen Clark early in her tenure as Minister of Health. Chief nursing officer from 1988, Sheryl Smail told Clark in May 1989 that some midwives saw direct-entry midwifery training as an 'integral part in their campaign for autonomy', but that the department did not support it.[98] At the same time Gayle O'Brien, from the department's Advisory Committee on Women's Health, told Chief Health Officer Karen Poutasi that the department did not support the College of Midwives' request for direct-entry training for midwives. She added, 'A paper had gone to the Minister on this issue and there has been no indication that she has different views from the department.' Two days earlier, Clark had written 'Noted' in the margin following the comment, 'Note that the department does not support direct entry midwifery'.[99]

Sheryl Smail reiterated to Clark the department's 'policy for all nursing preparation to be broadly based at a basic level, and for specialisation to occur after registration as a nurse'. Clark underlined this and wrote in the margin: 'we'd need to see pros and cons of that', and 'not everyone accepts that view'.[100] The real disagreement between Smail and Clark occurred in February 1990, in relation to a draft policy paper for the 'Review of the Nurses Act'. At this time, direct-entry midwifery training was not being considered by Parliament as part of the Nurses Amendment Bill. Smail noted in her paper that Clark had asked her to redraft her policy paper 'in a more balanced way inviting discussion', which she claimed to have done. Clark responded that the new draft was 'more unbalanced and biased than the first', and proceeded to rewrite it, deleting whole sections. One of those deletions was the recommendation that midwives who were not trained nurses should be on a separate register, with restrictions placed on their practice.[101]

Smail was not the only one to have concerns about direct-entry training. In her July 1990 letter to Clark, Maureen Lawton affirmed that the nurses and midwives she represented in Waikato believed midwives used their general nursing knowledge 'a great deal in assessment of the pregnant women' to detect underlying conditions which required medical referral.[102] This view was not shared by the College of Midwives, but Lawton maintained that the College did 'not necessarily reflect the opinion of the majority of midwives in New Zealand'.[103]

Reflecting on Clark's role as a minister in the 1980s, biographer Brian Edwards cited Geoffrey Palmer's view that Clark 'would make officials do what she wanted. She was pretty hard on them even then.'[104] Elsewhere Palmer described Clark as a 'micro' minister.[105] She certainly disregarded Smail's advice in 1990, and later joked about 'some divine intervention' when her staffer (Smail) went on maternity leave; by the time she returned, the Act had passed.[106] A press release reporting Clark's speech on the occasion of the Bill's passage through Parliament stated, 'The Minister said she had not seen any evidence to persuade her that direct entry training was neither feasible nor desirable, and objections to it appeared to be based on belief rather than reality.'[107] In her speech to the College of Midwives she also expressed her view that objections were 'doctrinally and not empirically based'.[108] Many hospital midwives and others would disagree.

## The 1990 Act and the meaning of autonomy

The 1990 Nurses Amendment Act significantly changed the legislation relating to maternity services. The sum effect was to reverse the direction of legislation and regulations over the previous 20 years, and to allow homebirth midwives to practise alone in the community with no oversight from, or accountability to, public health, hospital, nursing or medical professionals. Introducing direct-entry midwifery education in the tertiary sector with no prior nurse training also aimed to limit nursing or medical influences on midwifery practice. This was no minor legislation, as had been recognised by Helen Clark's Health Department advisors before the amendment was introduced to Parliament.

The assertion that midwives would be involved only in low-risk pregnancies was often made in support of the Bill. Clark did so when introducing the Bill, saying that it was 'appropriate that midwives are able to provide a low-technology childbirth service to meet the needs of low-risk women'.[109] She also spoke of the skill of midwives in recognising the limits of their professionalism, and in accepting that their role was with low-risk births and healthy mothers likely to experience normal births.[110] Summing up at the end of the parliamentary debates Judy Keall too declared, '[T]he midwife can be autonomous at a low-risk birth.'[111]

This became a common perception of the 1990 Act. As Rea Daellenbach later wrote, the Act enabled midwives to attend "normal" births without medical supervision'.[112] In her 1997 analysis of the Act, Sally Abel claimed, 'The intent of the Bill was to enable midwives to provide total maternity care to low-risk women experiencing normal childbirth.'[113] Similarly, the Department of Health prefaced its 1990 *Information for Health Providers* pamphlet with the explanation that the Act enabled midwives 'to provide all maternity services including delivery, for normal pregnancies, without the supervision of medical practitioners'.[114]

Yet one commentator reflected in 1991 that, while she had always understood that the 1990 Nurses Amendment Act enabled midwives 'to provide all maternity services including delivery, for normal pregnancies without the supervision of a medical practitioner' (her underlining), the word 'normal' appeared nowhere in the Act.[115] In fact, nothing in the legislation specified that midwives would be restricted to caring for low-risk pregnancies; nor were they directed to provide low-technology childbirth. On the contrary, they were given the same access to technology and specialist services as medical practitioners. It was a leap of faith that midwives would engage only with 'normal' births, and that they would be able to define or predict a normal birth. As Guilliland and Pairman later pointed out, 'It is often assumed that midwifery practice is restricted to normal childbirth, but there is no legislative requirement for this.'[116]

Another argument for pivoting childbirth services away from hospital birth to midwifery care in the community had been the benefit for women of getting to know their midwife before the birth, establishing a relationship that would continue in the immediate postnatal period. Yet, as Sally Abel noted, there was nothing in the 1990 Act that ensured continuity of midwifery care; it merely took away obstacles to it.[117] With no regulations built into the legislation, the functioning of the new service was based on trust.

The words 'midwife autonomy' were frequently used to describe the outcome of the 1990 reform. Autonomy, as it applied to midwifery, was later defined in the preface to a 2006 midwifery textbook, edited by Sally Pairman among others, and described as the Australasian equivalent of the leading international Myles textbook (then in its fourteenth edition):[118]

> [Autonomy occurs] when a midwife provides care to a woman and her baby on her own responsibility. As autonomous practitioners, midwives have the knowledge and skills to provide care independently without a requirement to refer to another health professional. This does not mean that midwives practise alone; rather, midwives work in partnership with midwifery colleague(s). Nor are midwives independent of women, because all midwifery professional judgements emerge from midwife/women relationships.[119]

In other words, autonomous practice did not mean working alone, but the only admissible partners were to be other midwives and mothers. Pelvin also explained in this book that the concept of autonomy meant midwifery had its own distinct body of knowledge, its own worldview, and was self-determining in its educational pathways, philosophy, ethics and standards. Sally Pairman and her colleague Judith McAra-Couper further explained that autonomy involved 'a specific philosophy and body of knowledge, together with the ability to practise without reference to another discipline'.[120] What that philosophy meant in practice as the new system was rolled out after 1990 will be explored in the following chapters.

## Conclusion

During the final reading of the 1990 Nurses Amendment Bill, Katherine O'Regan said, 'Perhaps there could be a birth notice that would read thus: "Delivered legislation heavier than was thought and slightly delayed, but now doing well. Thanks to midwives, officials, and members of Parliament."'[121]

Health Minister Helen Clark had indeed very successfully 'midwifed' the Bill through Parliament. The Opposition expressed some misgivings about the late inclusion of wider powers for homebirth midwives through the supplementary order paper process than had been anticipated, including direct-entry midwifery training, but it seems they were more concerned with process than with the substance of the reforms. Perhaps they were persuaded that to resist the Bill would be to lose the women's vote; after all, a general election was looming. Whether women were as united in favour of the change as parliamentarians assumed will be addressed in the following chapters. Moreover, as Chris Harrington had forewarned, many unresolved issues were left to subsequent administrations to grapple with, even following the supplementary order paper process. This lack of detail suited homebirth lobbyists in their goal for autonomy. Those who had long campaigned for midwife autonomy were delighted by the Bill's passage. As Lynda Williams later said, their sense of elation was 'mixed with a sense of surprise and disbelief at such an overwhelming victory on all fronts'.[122]

# SEVEN

## *Midwifery autonomy and partnership in the 1990s*

THE 1990 NURSES AMENDMENT ACT gave homebirth midwives and the newly formed New Zealand College of Midwives much cause for celebration with their new-found independence. Yet, independent practice in the community – or 'autonomy' – did not equate to a rise in homebirths. The College of Midwives sought to rectify this, upholding the ethos of the homebirth movement, and defining the New Zealand midwifery profession as rooted in feminism and partnership with women. However, as this chapter will explore, not all mothers felt like equal partners in their relationship with midwives, particularly when things went wrong. Rumblings of discontent led to the formation in 1995 of a new small consumer group, Parents for Safe Birth, and from 1996 consumers started to make use of a new complaints mechanism through the Health and Disability Commissioner. Nor did all midwives accept the partnership model; hospital midwives in particular felt alienated from, and unrepresented by, the College and its definition of midwifery. Māori midwives chose a separate path and did not work in partnership with the College, despite the latter claiming that the Treaty of Waitangi informed the midwifery partnership. The 1990 Act was celebrated as a great achievement for women, but it appears that women were not as united as had been assumed by MPs and others during the Act's passage through Parliament.

## Celebration of autonomy and of Joan Donley

Speaking at the College of Midwives' 1996 annual conference, Helen Clark reflected on the midwives' 'remarkable achievement' in 1990: 'Had the dominant forces in the medical profession had their way in this country, midwives would have been permanently subjugated.' Instead, 'Joan Donley and her sisters dared to think the unthinkable . . . It was a change whose time had come.' She remarked that what had happened to midwifery in New Zealand was attracting worldwide admiration, and that College representatives were sought after at international meetings.[1]

Others shared that elation. At the 1997 International Midwives Day, Sandy Grey, an Auckland midwifery coordinator and future College president (1997– 2002), declared that New Zealand midwives were 'further down the track than any other women' in the world and a 'shining example' internationally.[2] This had been a common theme from visiting speakers throughout the decade – and would continue into the next. At the College's 1992 annual conference, London midwife Alice Coyle said she felt honoured to speak in New Zealand with its system of domiciliary midwifery; Britain, she said, was 'way behind'.[3] In 1995 Lesley Page, the first midwife to be appointed to a chair of midwifery in Britain (in 1992), described the New Zealand College as a world leader.[4] Expatriate New Zealander Diony Young of the International Childbirth Education Association (see p. 42) wrote an editorial for the Association's journal *Birth* on New Zealand midwives' great achievements and lessons for other countries; her first reference was Donley's *Save the Midwife*.[5] Beverley Beech, childbirth activist and chair of the UK Association for Improvements in the Maternity Services, stated in a 1998 address to the New Zealand College that its midwives were the envy of the world, and that the ground-breaking 1990 legislation gave 'enormous hope and encouragement' to those campaigning elsewhere to move away from medical-centred childbirth services.[6] In 2001 a recently arrived midwife from the UK, Sarah Stewart, published an article in a UK midwifery journal entitled 'Midwifery in New Zealand: A Cause for Celebration'. She believed that New Zealand's pioneering model of maternity care challenged midwives worldwide to reflect on their own practices.[7]

As Clark intimated, College representatives were in demand at international meetings. Donley was an invited plenary speaker at the 1990 International Confederation of Midwives conference in Kobe, Japan, which hosted 6,000 registrants from 43 nations. One of the 12 New Zealand delegates spoke of their pride at hearing Donley present her paper, 'The Midwives' Dilemma'. She said that many midwives from other countries envied the New Zealanders' new-found autonomy.[8] A publication from this conference featured articles from three New Zealand midwives including Donley.[9] Karen Guilliland and Sally Pairman reported on the next International Confederation of Midwives conference in Vancouver in 1993, claiming that New Zealand's story was met with great excitement and that they received 'much congratulation' on their achievements. Joan Donley was already in Canada at the time of the conference, having been invited to advise its Health Ministry on the establishment of a College of Midwives, help define midwives' standards of practice, and set up a direct-entry midwifery training course.[10] She gave a press interview at the conference, and, along with Guilliland, was part of a television documentary.[11] Donley remained a revered figure in the homebirth movement at home and abroad. The front cover of a *Home Birth Association Newsletter* in 1993 depicted her as Mother Mary holding baby Jesus.[12]

The College of Midwives made Donley its first honorary member in 1990, 'in recognition of her political acumen and midwifery vision'.[13] Seventy-four years of age in 1990, Donley had no intention of resting on her laurels, and she continued to play a role in College affairs. In October 1989 the College had agreed to invite her to attend all future national committee meetings 'as a resource person with full speaking and voting rights'; in later years this position evolved to 'Elder and Mentor'.[14] Her 'untiring energy and clear vision' was, Sally Pairman said in 1996, an inspiration to them all.[15] In 1997 Donley was awarded an honorary Master's degree in midwifery from the Auckland Institute of Technology, one of the first two tertiary institutes to introduce a direct-entry midwifery training programme.[16]

From 1990 to 1999, Donley produced 12 political commentaries for the College's journal, as well as another 13 papers on various other topics, averaging two or three articles per year.[17] The College republished *Save the Midwife* in 1998 under a new title: *Birthrites: Natural vs Unnatural Childbirth in New Zealand.*[18] The College also set up the Joan Donley Midwifery Research Collaboration in 2001 as 'the evidence or research arm of the College', holding biennial fora from 2003.[19] By then Donley's influence over College affairs was waning owing to ill health, and she died in 2005, aged 89. Her enduring presence in College affairs in the 1990s, her extensive writings and the College leaders' high esteem for her 'midwifery vision' meant that her views continued to matter, not least because they aligned with the views of those leaders.

## Homebirth and Donley's vision in the 1990s

Donley predicted after the 1990 Act that midwifery independence would lead to a witch hunt against homebirth midwives.[20] Her forecast seemed to be borne out by a 1992 *Frontline* TV programme covering bad outcomes in two homebirths. Donley had just attended the second International Homebirth Conference in Sydney, which Marsden Wagner had addressed. She reported his description of 'the battle raging throughout the western world between the medical and midwifery model of childbirth . . . [which was about] freedom of choice versus totalitarian repression'. Wagner argued that, to maintain their power, doctors used the issue of 'safety' to generate fear and uncertainty, and Donley claimed this was happening in New Zealand, as evidenced by the cases featured on *Frontline*.[21]

The first case was the death of a baby four hours after being delivered at home in Wangapeka, about an hour's drive from Motueka (in the Tasman region), by midwife Maggie Matthews on 2 March 1991.[22] Matthews, who had practised homebirth since 1985, was the sole practitioner at the birth. This case was brought to public attention not by doctors but by Nelson coroner Dale Hunter, who called for a review into homebirth.[23] In his inquest report, Hunter drew attention to the 1988 Coroners Act, which stated that one purpose of an inquest was to allow the coroner to make recommendations to avoid a repetition of circumstances like those in which the death occurred. With that in mind, he outlined the circumstances. He began with the home environment. He did not believe that, despite strong representations to the contrary, a house-truck that lacked running water and electric power was a suitable place to deliver a child. He considered it fundamental that a midwife check the location in advance for its suitability, particularly in respect of hygiene and convenience for homebirth, and this midwife had not done so. Secondly, he referred to the mother's drug habit, pointing out that, while there was no firm evidence that this contributed to the child's death, the fact that the mother admitted intravenous use of heroin, most recently less than two months before the birth, should have alerted the midwife to the need for a hospital birth. Thirdly, he was concerned by the considerable distance from medical support services. Finally, and above all, Hunter thought there should have been more than one practitioner present, providing two pairs of skilled hands in case of an emergency. Hunter commented that while a homebirth might be the mother's wish and be acceptable to the midwife, 'the unborn babe is the one at greatest risk'. In his view, 'If home births should result in only one avoidable death throughout the whole of the country then in my belief that is one death too many.' As a result, he thought the greatest fault uncovered by the inquest was that the law permitted homebirths to take place in the presence of a sole practitioner, and he intended to recommend to the Minister of Health that the law relating to homebirths be reviewed.[24] This was just one year after the 1990 Act. Commenting on the case, Donley wrote that the midwife had since challenged the coroner in the High Court with the support of the College of Midwives. But, as she later admitted, the judge found in the coroner's favour.[25] Nonetheless, she continued to dismiss criticism of homebirth practices as a witch hunt.

Hunter was not the only one concerned about midwives practising alone after 1990. In June 1991 Dr Diana Edwards, president of the Canterbury Branch of the Medical Women's Association, forwarded the Association's 1990 submission to Katherine O'Regan, now Associate Minister of Women's Affairs. Edwards claimed the Wangapeka case reinforced their concern about the safety of sole practitioners.[26] Donley rebuffed such concerns as a medical ploy to maintain control.[27] Elsewhere, she also rejected using perinatal mortality rates as 'the yardstick used to assess "safety"', claiming it was based on 'the fetus [being] seen to take precedence over the "selfish" mothers'.[28]

Despite the deep concerns of the Nelson coroner and others, the Nursing Council's disciplinary process exonerated Matthews. She continued to attend homebirths until 2007 when, following the death of another homebirth baby under her sole care in Motueka, she was suspended from practice, following claims by other professionals that she presented a risk of 'serious harm to the public'.[29]

The second homebirth midwife featured in the 1992 *Frontline* programme was Sian Burgess. On 1 August 1990, before the Nurses Amendment Act was passed, Michelle Witten's son Llewellyn was transferred from home to hospital with fetal distress, and was born asphyxiated and severely brain-damaged with cerebral palsy. The parents laid a complaint against Burgess, alleging she had ignored signs of distress such as meconium in Witten's ruptured waters following artificial rupture of the membranes, and failed to get Witten into hospital in good time. Unlike the Matthews case, the issue here was not sole practice, as GP Leone Dillon was also present. Rather, it involved interpretation of warning signs. According to the Medical Disciplinary Committee which investigated Dillon, the latter had suggested transfer once meconium was present but there had been a 'divergence of views' between doctor and midwife.[30]

The case was discussed in the College of Midwives' journal by Bronwen Pelvin. A central figure in the College, she helped to draft its first *Handbook for Practice* (1992), ran workshops on the code of ethics and for the midwifery standards review committees, was later appointed midwifery advisor to College members in 1997, and in 2002 was granted life membership of the College for her work with the midwifery standards review process and the Domiciliary Midwives Society, including its integration into the College.[31] In her review of the case, Pelvin stated that the significance of meconium-stained liquor was 'extremely contentious', and 'each midwife will make a decision and give information based on her own experience and her assessment of what is safe practice'.[32]

Others regarded the presence of meconium in the amniotic fluid as a significant warning sign. Interviewed for a 1993 article, GP obstetrician Allan Sutherland called certain non-interventionist practices promoted by natural childbirth adherents 'dangerous'. These included 'not regarding a leak of meconium . . . during labour as a sign of distress'.[33] Much later, Sutherland's views were endorsed by an Australian study which recommended transfer to hospital 'when a planned home birth is complicated by the presence of meconium stained liquor'.[34] Meanwhile the respective disciplinary bodies exonerated both practitioners.[35] Burgess was subsequently invited to give a keynote address to the College of Midwives' 1992 national conference.[36]

In the event, it was not a witch hunt against homebirth midwives that exercised Donley after the 1990 Act; rather it was the behaviour of some new so-called independent midwives and their failure to embrace homebirth. 'Independent midwives' were those who set up practice in the community as general practitioners did, and who, following the 1990 Act, could claim from the government the same rate of pay as GPs (see p. 158). Just after the Act was passed, there were about 40 independent midwives, mostly homebirth midwives. This number increased to 64 by the end of 1990 (compared to 1,448 hospital-employed midwives); 150 a year later; 350 by 1994; and 500 by 1995.[37] Most of the new independent midwives ended up accompanying their clients into hospital, which the new system allowed. Reviewing the statistics for 1994–95, journalist Cate Brett found that of the 58,000 babies born in New Zealand that year, independent midwives were involved in delivering about 21,000 of them; they worked in a sole capacity for about 9,000 births and with GPs for 12,000. Almost all the babies were born in hospital, including those in the sole charge of independent midwives. In 1989, before the law change, there had been around 900 homebirths; in 1991 there were 1,148 planned homebirths (of which 947 were born at home); in 1992 there were just over 1,000 (2% of all births). In 1995 planned homebirths dropped to 937, of which 845 occurred at home.[38] Brett concluded, 'So much for the government's hopes that liberating midwives from the shackles of the hospitals and doctors would mean an upsurge in budget (cheap) home births.'[39] In his 1993 *North & South* article on the politics of childbirth, David McLoughlin also pointed out that, despite the intentions of the Act, the great majority of babies delivered by independent midwives were born in hospital, a development which irked the HBA.[40] He remarked that Helen Clark admitted surprise at the outcome.[41]

Even Donley's homebirth partner, Carolyn Young, moved into hospital practice in the mid-1990s. She later explained that the demand for homebirths had started to decline once women could receive one-on-one care from their midwife at home and in hospital, and that many women preferred the latter. She also thought that the birth experience in hospital had 'improved out of sight'.[42] In 1995 the HBA advertised in its newsletter that midwives were taking bookings for planned hospital births. The same newsletter reported from Auckland, 'We have stopped running Home Birth Preparation classes anywhere in Auckland because of the lack of demand.' Only six people attended the Auckland HBA AGM, two of whom gave their valedictory speeches. Editor Brenda Hinton despaired: 'Too few families are experiencing the benefits of home birth – we have an advertisement which travels around Auckland on the back of a bus – has anybody seen it?'[43]

Donley was not impressed by the trend, claiming that, after 50 years of medical dominance, it would take time for women to overcome their fear-based medical dependence and regain control; but she primarily blamed midwives. She explained that women who had been conditioned to be 'under the doctor' would be 'easy prey' for the 'nice' midwife who offered them options 'as defined by her'. She advised women to join an HBA to learn about their real options, and about the difference between the medical and midwifery models of childbirth.[44] In 1994 she commented on the 'surprising' number of women under midwifery care who had routine ultrasound scans, polycose tests (for diabetes in pregnancy), epidurals and oxytocins. She described these midwives as 'paralysed agents for the medical model' and asked whether they feared birth or obstetrical criticism, or 'is it in their economic interests to gather the crumbs from the obstetric table?'. It is unclear what she meant by this latter statement, since going into hospital did not increase the midwives' funding.[45]

Others too expressed concern. Midwife Valerie Fleming explained that she had undertaken her PhD thesis in 1991 on a feminist perception of midwifery practice because: 'I felt that some midwives were turning out like doctors, that some were abusing what the fight was all about when we gained the right to practise independently.'[46] Maggie Banks, another highly respected homebirth midwife within the College of Midwives and a contributor to its journal's 'Practice Wisdom' column, concurred. In her PhD thesis, she explained that her study was motivated by the fact that many midwives who left the 'obstetrically-dominated hospitals' for the community took hospital practices with them. She found mounting anecdotal evidence from 1992 onwards that increasing numbers of midwives, 'bereft of the understanding and experience of natural and healthy (physiological) childbirth', were providing homebirth services within a medicalised framework.[47]

Some consumer advocates also complained that many independent midwives were taking the medical model into the community. One of them was Judi Strid, who believed that some midwives were too interventionist and were not offering continuity of care. In an interview with researcher Sally Abel, she lamented, 'Midwives, having finally gained the status, autonomy and pay fought for by a few for so many years, had forgotten their history and the original intent of the Act.'[48] She relayed this message forcefully in a talk to a College of Midwives' national conference in 1994 and again in 2000, arguing that midwives had benefited more than women from the 1990 legislation and subsequent changes. These changes, she said, had provided opportunities for midwives to position themselves well in the maternity marketplace, whilst ignoring the former partnership with homebirth advocates that had 'helped to make them strong'.[49] Her scathing attack in 2000 was not mentioned in the College's journal but was reported in *New Zealand Doctor*.[50] At the same conference, in her presentation on homebirth, Donley argued that midwives were being 'colonised'.[51]

Denise Black, a homebirth midwife since 1982, also criticised independent midwives in a letter to the College's journal in 2001. She wondered why, with 70% of women having a midwife as their primary caregiver, intervention rates were going up. The answer was, she said, that 'more and more midwives are aligning with the medical pathway'. She declared, 'We can quote/theorise all we like about the midwife/woman partnership, but this is just not the reality which is happening. Compliant medically motivated midwives have failed to see the bigger picture.'[52]

If choice of birthplace had community support, as Clark had suggested in 1990, this did not translate into more homebirths after 1990.[53] There were only 1,013 recorded home births in 1992 (1.7% of the births that year), rising to 1,620 recorded births in 1997 (2.8% of all births).[54] Homebirth midwives complained that many of the new independent midwives did not live up to the so-called midwifery model and were becoming over-medicalised, and they wondered whether the 1990 Act had been so liberating after all. Meanwhile, the College of Midwives was doing its best to reverse this trend, emphasising natural birth and honouring the promised partnership with women.

## The College of Midwives, feminism and partnership

In a 1995 international publication on midwifery, two New Zealand midwives declared, 'The New Zealand College of Midwives has stated categorically that midwifery is a feminist profession.'[55] Karen Guilliland, its first president and later coordinator, was 'not bashful' about describing midwifery as a feminist profession. There was, she said in 1996, 'no escaping the fact that the battle for control of birth is a battle of the sexes'. She claimed that when she '[had] this argument with establishment people . . . they just snort and accuse me of reducing everything to gender. But that's precisely what this is all about.'[56]

Karen Guilliland and Sally Pairman said in a 1994 College presentation that, through its political and personal involvement with women, midwifery accepted its responsibility as an 'emancipatory change agent'. As a feminist profession, they argued, midwifery was a force for social change.[57] In other words, midwives were not just health professionals; their involvement with women was both personal and political, as was the feminist movement itself. Guilliland expanded on this in 1999, asserting that the 1990 Act had given midwives, GPs and obstetricians 'equal status in the provision of services around childbirth'. This equality was a triumph for women in general and provided a role model for other countries in their fight against gender inequities. By contrast, she saw institutionalised childbirth as a tool for the suppression of women.[58] Others within the College agreed. Maggie Banks saw midwifery as so much more than a form of healthcare. She explained that midwifery's philosophy shared the three basic principles of feminism: the valuing of women, recognition of their oppression, and a desire to bring about social change.[59]

In their 1994 College presentation Guilliland and Pairman affirmed that midwives were to partner their clients.[60] As president in 1997, Pairman repeated this call when discussing the College's strategic plan.[61] She explored the concept of midwifery partnership as part of her Master's degree, and would do so again in her Doctorate of Midwifery at the University of Technology Sydney (2005). In the introduction to this thesis she stated unequivocally: 'Midwifery partnership with women is the philosophical foundation to midwifery in New Zealand.'[62] But not all midwives agreed. One was Joan Skinner, a midwifery lecturer at Victoria University of Wellington, who had experience in homebirth.[63] In 1999 she reflected on whether 'partnership' was the right word. She supported partnership with consumers in midwifery's professional organisation, but struggled to see herself as partnering her clients who were 'predominantly poor, dispossessed and non-Pakeha'. She argued that attempting to be partners at a practical level could be 'dangerous for the practitioner and misleading for the mother', as it did not recognise inequalities in power and in access to resources, and was culturally elitist.[64]

In response to criticism of their partnership model, Pairman and Guilliland claimed their detractors misunderstood the concept of partnership, and added somewhat patronisingly, 'Midwifery has undergone a transformation of a magnitude seldom achieved by a profession. Such changes will always be accompanied by uncertainty and very often "hurt" as people slowly accept and redefine the old and the new.'[65]

A careful reading of the partnership model shows that it was not new, however, but rather a repackaging of the homebirth ethos. Pairman later explained that partnership involved midwives encouraging women to make decisions and to take responsibility for them, with the goal of building confidence as mothers.[66] The goal of the partnership model, like homebirth, was women's empowerment.[67] Pairman and co-author Nicky Leap stated in 2006, 'Confidence in her body and in herself [in childbirth] will stand a woman in good stead as she takes on the complex role of mother that is central to the healthy functioning of a family.'[68] They even saw the uncertainty surrounding natural birth as important for a woman's future development, explaining that: 'Grappling with uncertainty is an ongoing process in life that is central to the challenges of becoming and being a mother.'[69]

In 1996, Barbara Katz Rothman, a visiting American sociology professor with an academic interest in childbirth, gave a presentation to the College and was praised by Pairman for her 'very clear understanding'.[70] Rothman referred to the midwifery philosophy which saw birth as not just about making babies but about creating strong, confident mothers. She contrasted midwifery's aim of nurturing the mother's strength with the medical model which was about the efficient removal of a fetus, and which stripped a woman's sense of herself and undermined her knowledge of her own body.[71]

Partnership meant encouraging women to make decisions. In 1989 Donley had explained that midwifery care was 'advice-oriented', allowing women themselves to be the decision-makers. But she also questioned women's capacity as decision-makers when she lamented that 'under the present medical controlled system there was too much conflicting advice'.[72] Similarly, Pairman and Leap saw huge advantages for women in taking responsibility for decisions, but also told midwives to be wary of women's conditioning: 'This might mean persuading the woman of the safety of home birth, for example.'[73] Such sentiments throw into doubt the very concept of partnership.

But perhaps most significantly, partnership involved sharing responsibility for any adverse outcome. Referring to the Witten case, Bronwen Pelvin said it must be assumed that the midwife had explained the way she practised, and that the woman 'made a clear decision to opt for midwifery care rather than the medicalised care she would have received in hospital'. In her words, 'One of the basic issues about choosing home birth is the woman and her family accept responsibility for the choice that they make.'[74] Michelle Witten did not see it that way, and in 1995 she along with four other families with children who had suffered preventable brain injury at birth formed a lobby group called Parents for Safe Births.[75] There was nothing straightforward about making decisions on birth choices when professionals themselves disagreed about issues of safety, as was evident in the different interpretations of the presence of meconium in the Witten case. Pelvin's final comment on this case was: 'Tragedies *do* occur at birth and less than perfect babies *are* born. The complaints procedure should be one that increases our understanding of these events and not one which seeks to apportion blame'.[76] This would have been little consolation to Michelle Witten.

Another member of Parents for Safe Births was Lisa Mannion, whose baby had died following a brain injury at birth.[77] She was critical of those who perpetuated what she described as the dangerous notion that all women should strive for a natural birth at the expense of more commonsense concerns for the baby's safety. Mannion said that her midwife shared that 'natural' birth bias, and had admitted at a disciplinary tribunal that she 'was aware of warning signs but did not disclose them to me'.[78]

When things went wrong, mothers were more likely to see themselves as unequal in their relationship with the midwife. During an inquiry after a baby died during a homebirth in Christchurch in 1996, the mother claimed that the midwife had informed her only about 'the good side' of homebirth. Coroner Richard McElrea found that the parents had assumed back-up would be available, but it took 20 minutes for an intensive-care team to arrive. The parents were unaware that their midwife did not have access to Christchurch Women's Hospital and that her access to St George's Hospital had been suspended following an incident which resulted in her being charged by the Nursing Council for professional misconduct.[79] They did not feel like partners in this experience. Nor did the woman whose story was featured in an article in *Next* magazine in 2000. Her first child had died during a homebirth. She urged parents to be wary of any midwife who had an 'I know best' attitude and would not consult a doctor. In her case, she said, the midwife dismissed her requests for a transfer to hospital as unnecessary, and did not seek a second opinion despite signs of fetal distress.[80]

When homebirth midwives were asked about indemnity insurance in the lead-up to the 1990 Act, they had argued that in a partnership model this was not an issue (see p. 83). It is true that it was not an issue, but not because of the partnership model. Rather, under legislation passed in 1974, the Accident Compensation Corporation (ACC) provided for government compensation for accidents, including those within medical practice, regardless of the cause of the accident. Under this scheme, claimants were effectively barred from suing a registered health professional, and so midwives were largely protected from civil action or lawsuits.[81] A study of midwifery in Britain in the 1990s noted that the Royal College of Midwives provided indemnity insurance for the 100 or so private practising midwives (that is, working outside the National Health Service), but, following two claims brought against these midwives, the insurance company serving the College increased their premium significantly. The implication for independent practice was 'immense', the study noted, since most independent midwives did not earn enough to pay an individual indemnity premium, and it was unknown whether the College would continue to support them.[82] In Australia, a later article discussing why independent midwifery had not taken off in that country noted that 'the prohibitive costs of personal indemnity insurance for midwives working outside the public hospital system' was one of the disincentives.[83] From 2002, Australian midwives were not required by law to take out indemnity insurance as other health professionals were, but they still had to disclose to their clients that they were not indemnified.[84] ACC in New Zealand made independent practice an altogether more viable option.

From 1996 there was another complaints procedure in place in New Zealand. The 1993 Health and Disability Services Act was followed by the 1994 Health and Disability Commissioner Act, and by 1996 the Commissioner had set up a Code of Health and Disability Services Consumers' Rights. These included the right to services of an appropriate standard, the right to effective communication, and the right to be fully informed and to give consent. If these were breached, the Commissioner could require the caregiver to apologise to the consumer and could pass the case to the appropriate disciplinary body, at no cost to the complainant. The Commissioner also had discretion to make recommendations about healthcare. Unlike the Patient's Charter in Britain, the New Zealand system was enshrined in law and, according to a review of the system, the Commissioner's opinion was 'not taken lightly by the providers of health care services'.[85]

Donley complained that the Health and Disability Commissioner used a punitive rather than a mediation process. She argued that in maternity a significant number of interventions were opinion based rather than research based, and that the Code did not support the client/patient-centred or partnership model of care. The Code had been used very effectively against midwives, she claimed, aided by obstetricians and other doctors who encouraged parents to bring complaints. She added that the media did its part, featuring sensational stories to question the 'safety' of midwifery care.[86] Lynda Williams, a homebirth advocate and coordinator of the Auckland Maternity Services Consumer Council set up in 1990, was similarly concerned about the Commissioner's influence. She told Ron Paterson, who was appointed Commissioner in 2000, 'Whether you like it or not you do seem to have become an invisible presence in the birthing room. And it does not seem to be a presence that is supportive of women being able to decide for themselves how and where they choose to give birth.' In his response, Paterson reminded her there was no need for concern if midwives complied with the Code.[87]

While Parents for Safe Births accused midwives of sometimes holding doctrinaire views, mothers too could be insistent in their expectations. In 1996 Pelvin described a 'woman who went four weeks past her due date but still wanted to stick to her homebirth in the water pool – nothing to give me, as a midwife, any inkling that I would have to deal with this'.[88] She did not say what happened. Another homebirth mother related experiences that, whilst not resulting in a bad outcome, had forced her to reconsider her views. Lucinda was a self-professed natural birth advocate who ran antenatal yoga classes. When she became pregnant in 1992 she planned a homebirth, but ended up in hospital after 12 hours of labour and with the baby in posterior presentation. In hospital she had an epidural and 'all sorts of other things' before a healthy baby was born. She commented, 'The pressures on women to Do It Right – meaning drug, forceps and episiotomy free – are enormous.' She thought women needed to be more flexible in their expectations. Yet she also admitted to later wondering whether she had somehow failed. 'I have always taught women to trust their instincts, to use their breath for pain control,' she said, but 'I am a lot more humble now.'[89]

The partnership concept appeared very woman-centred and a continuation of the empowerment argument long used to advocate for homebirth. But the concept was fraught with inconsistencies. Those espousing it also insisted that women had been conditioned to believe homebirth was unsafe and needed to be persuaded otherwise. Others claimed that women needed to take responsibility for deciding to birth at home, even when it went wrong. But, as the Women's Division Federated Farmers had wondered in 1990, did all women have the knowledge base and objectivity to make those decisions? As midwife Joan Skinner suggested, the concept did not recognise power inequalities.

## Hospital midwives and partnership

Sally Pairman claimed that partnership was the philosophical basis of midwifery in New Zealand, but, as a rebranding of the ethos surrounding homebirth, what did this mean for hospital midwives? In 1995, Auckland midwife Barbara Clotworthy responded to Guilliland and Pairman's concept of partnership. Pointing out that she dealt with women in the high-risk category who required medical and midwifery help, she said she was disappointed to read that she was not practising midwifery. Midwifery was 'dependent neither upon where I work, nor upon whether I fit into someone else's theory'.[90] Palmerston North midwife Edna Rose categorised Guilliland and Pairman's description of midwifery practice as narrow and restrictive. She argued that the partnership model took no account of the large number of women who chose hospital care, that it denigrated the midwife employed in a hospital setting, and was elitist and politically motivated. In her view, 'For the College of Midwives to support a paper that suggests that midwives practising in hospital settings are not practising midwifery, is at best irresponsible and at worst downright dangerous.' She felt their paper confirmed that the College was focused on the independent practitioner, and that there was 'no recognition or acknowledgement of the work and commitment of the many midwives who work in hospitals'.[91]

Kim Wheeler from Wellington also insisted that as a hospital-based midwife she did practise midwifery. She asked why an effective partnership could not be formed between a midwife and a woman transferred to emergency care or a woman who found herself in the care of a hospital-based midwife. She believed the term partnership was a superficial construct in any case, 'coined to justify the lack of substance engendered by the dogma of a small group that signify what midwifery has become in New Zealand'. She entered a plea that midwives be called midwives wherever they worked.[92] Dunedin midwife Barbara Churcher argued that a long-term acquaintance with the mother was not a prerequisite for partnership, pointing to the need to form a relationship very quickly in hospital: 'To form such a relationship quickly and under conditions of stress is to be celebrated, not denied.'[93]

Hospital provision was categorised as primary, secondary or tertiary, depending on the level of available facilities. Primary care was provided in birthing units with very limited facilities for dealing with emergencies; secondary care was provided in general hospitals; and tertiary institutions were those hospitals with specialist facilities. A group of midwives from the Delivery Unit at Auckland's Middlemore Hospital, a tertiary hospital, complained in 2002 that the College of Midwifery's philosophy placed them automatically in the medical model, with only those working in the community or in birthing units viewed as practising the midwifery model. Pointing out that most hospital births occurred in a secondary/tertiary hospital (less than 12% of hospital births in 2001 were in primary midwifery-led units and 3% at home), they asked, 'Who said the big institutions belonged to the medical profession?' Addressing the higher rate of caesarean sections in secondary and tertiary care, they reminded readers that they cared for many high-risk women with diabetes, other medical problems, premature labour, cardiac complications and other high-risk indicators. They explained that 1.5% of women who arrived at Middlemore Hospital in labour had not booked and had a very chequered obstetric history, and that many who had booked experienced little or no real antenatal care. Reminiscent of the hospital midwives pre-1990, they stressed teamwork. At their hospital, they declared, 'out of necessity and aligned with a group of fairly hard-nosed midwives, a unique relationship has evolved between the midwifery and medical teams which has proved to have advantages for both'. They believed in both a sound medical/midwifery teamwork environment in which each respected the skills and values of the other, and the importance of good working relationships between registrars and charge midwives. Such a relationship was required for the safe and effective functioning of the unit. They were, they insisted, still midwives.[94]

Donley herself persisted in categorising hospital midwives as second-rate, telling her Australian colleague Maggie Lecky-Thompson in 1996 that there were still 'quite a number' of midwives with the 'obs [obstetric] nurse mentality who are prepared to work on slave labour contracts under their masters'.[95] The same year, Guilliland wrote an article for *Kai Tiaki: Nursing New Zealand* titled 'Viewpoint: Learning from Midwives', in which she demanded support and 'allegiance' from the nursing profession for midwifery autonomy. She complained that some midwives and nurses had 'opted out of their obligations in favour of a dependent, and in their view, less threatening role' – that is, they had chosen to work in a hospital. She found it disheartening in their women-intensive profession that some midwives and nurses 'accept the doctors' position and then use it against their own profession/s. Some have joined doctor groups and publicly disassociated themselves from their colleagues and the college's stance.'[96] She informed dissident midwives and nurses that, if they believed that the medical profession was more concerned about their interests than were the nursing and midwifery professional bodies, then they were 'astonishingly naïve and display[ed] oppressed group behaviour'. Their failure to stand up to the medical profession was a denial of women's struggle for autonomy.[97] Pairman referred in similar vein to the media backlash against the 'unsafe' practice of some midwives, and wrote of her dismay that '[t]he backlash also comes from our own colleagues, often midwives now in managerial positions'.[98]

There were ongoing tensions between hospital midwives and those practising in the community, as Sarah Stewart noted in her 2001 article celebrating New Zealand's independent midwifery system. She explained that hospital midwives often felt devalued and regarded as second-class citizens, and that the midwifery professional body did not support them. However, Stewart herself fuelled these tensions when she wrote that hospital midwives were 'losing their fundamental midwifery skills in the normal'.[99]

## The College of Midwives and partnership with Māori

In their 1994 address to the College of Midwives, Karen Guilliland and Sally Pairman claimed: 'The bicultural nature of New Zealand has evolved a practice and profession of midwifery in a way which is unique in the world . . . Women's understanding of partnership under the Treaty [of Waitangi] has facilitated their understanding of, and their demand for, midwifery as a partnership.'[100] Not everyone was convinced by this interpretation. In Joan Skinner's view, the premise that the Treaty of Waitangi taught midwives about partnership was incorrect. She explained, 'I certainly do not mean to denigrate the vital importance of the Treaty for New Zealanders, both Maori and Pakeha, but to see it as one of the origins of midwifery partnership is, I think, mistaken.'[101]

Skinner was right. The concept of midwifery partnership originated within the predominantly Pākehā homebirth movement. There is no evidence that tikanga Māori (Māori custom) or the 1840 Treaty of Waitangi played a part in that movement, despite the growing recognition of the Treaty's significance to politics and society from the 1970s (as discussed in Chapter 5). The homebirth movement had its roots in Western notions of feminism and counterculture, and there was no significant involvement in it from Māori women as activists or as clients. When Māori women did become involved in advocacy for maternity services in the 1990s, it was through their own networks and in response to a Māori cultural revival which had gained strength since the 1970s. Nor is there evidence that Māori played a part in the passing of the legislation in 1990. Significantly, the word 'Maori' did not appear once in the parliamentary debates leading up to its passage. The reforms appeared to do little to address health discrepancies between Māori and non-Māori, as will be discussed later.

In her speech at the first conference of the College of Midwives in 1990, Karen Guilliland addressed consumer partnership, which she said was unique to New Zealand; she did not mention Māori or the Treaty in relation to that concept.[102] Her only mention of Māori and Pacific women was the suggestion that the new programme of direct-entry midwifery training should attract them to the profession; she rightly noted that they were 'poorly represented in the nursing and midwifery fields yet their health statistics are the poorest'.[103] As discussed in Chapter 4, the Save the Midwives Direct Entry Task Force had suggested that a bonus of direct entry would be the recruitment of Māori and Pacific women to the profession. In 1991, Guilliland and Pairman drew attention to the 'desperate shortage' of Māori and Pacific midwives, stating that the direct-entry training programmes gave them the opportunity to introduce a bicultural model for childbirth, and explaining, 'The philosophical base of Direct Entry more easily allows for different cultural definitions of childbirth.'[104] That philosophical base will be further discussed in Chapter 9. Significantly, the courses still struggled to attract Māori and Pasifika applicants.

The College's national committee initially included three consumer representatives elected from the HBA, the Maternity Action Alliance and Parents Centre; all were Pākehā.[105] In 1991, the College sought advice from Māori nursing educator Irihapeti Ramsden on establishing consultation with Māori. Ramsden's advice was to contact the National Council of Maori Nurses (established in 1983) and the Ministry of Maori Affairs (Manatū Māori). In 1992, Mina Timutimu from the Council of Maori Nurses joined the College's national committee as its first Māori representative (and later, in 2004, she was appointed to the Midwifery Council).[106] Timutimu, of Te Ātiawa and Ngāti Mutunga, had graduated as a nurse in 1951, worked for the Plunket Society, and trained in midwifery at Wellington's St Helen's Hospital in 1961. She also had a long association with the Maori Women's Welfare League, which had not sent in a submission on the 1990 Nurses Amendment Bill. In 1995 Timutimu set up Taranaki's first Māori community maternity service, Nga Puna Ora Te Atiawa, and other support networks including a kaumātua group in Waitara. In 2016, shortly before her death, she became a Member of the New Zealand Order of Merit in recognition of her efforts.[107] The obituary Guilliland wrote for *New Zealand Doctor* called Timutimu a 'wise woman' who 'graciously bridged worlds of Maori and midwifery profession'.[108]

*Midwifery autonomy and partnership in the 1990s*

Developments in Māori midwifery came not through College activities but rather from Māori themselves. Apart from Timutimu's service in Taranaki, other initiatives for Māori women included a marae-based maternity service, Te Hiiri Hauora, at Papakura in South Auckland in 1992, which initially employed a Pākehā midwife owing to the shortage of Māori midwives.[109] Another was a Māori midwives' collective (Puea O Pua) in Auckland, which offered an independent Māori midwifery service primarily to Māori women. In 1996 this group received funding from the Maori Development Division of North Health to establish a comprehensive service for Māori and Pacific women in South Auckland, an area with a high Māori population.[110]

In 1994 the first Māori midwives' hui was held at Waikato Polytechnic to formalise a national group of midwives formed the previous year and known as Nga Maia, or Nga Maia o Aotearoa me te Waipounamu (later known as Ngā Maia Māori Midwives Aotearoa).[111] According to Māori midwife Hope Tupara, this was a representative body for some but not all Māori women. Other partners, she said, included the Maori Women's Welfare League, urban Māori health authorities, and government agencies for Māori development such as Te Puni Kōkiri (Ministry of Māori Development) and Te Taura Whiri i te Reo Māori (Māori Language Commission).[112] She did not mention the College of Midwives as a partner.

Nga Maia remained separate from the College of Midwives, although in 1996, at a meeting of the College's national committee, the first to be held on a marae and attended by four Nga Maia midwives, the College provided the latter with some funding. At that meeting Timutimu and Donley were appointed College kuia (elders). Nga Maia set up its own midwifery standards review process, to be held on a marae, with a stronger focus on cultural aspects than the College provided.[113] From 2004 Nga Maia had representation on the new Midwives' Council.

The College of Midwives facilitated Nga Maia's presence at the Asia-Pacific Region of the International Confederation of Midwives Conference in 1998 in India, funding two of the four Māori midwives (including Timutimu) who attended.[114] Guilliland claimed that Nga Maia was the first professional midwifery organisation of Indigenous midwives in the world.[115] One of the Māori attendees who addressed the conference was Joanne Rama (Ramamanga) of Ngāti Apakura. She was a homebirth midwife in Auckland and had been mentored by Donley. She worked with Māori mothers across three health boards, as far as Te Awamutu (some 150 kilometres south of Auckland),

and developed the first marae-based pregnancy and childbirth and parenting programme in 1993, running this for the next 22 years and working closely with teenage mothers in particular. She was later described as 'passionate about empowering Whanau through wananga and sharing traditional birth knowledge and wisdom'.[116] Māori were dealing with childbirth in their own way, but the number of Māori midwives did not significantly expand in the 1990s, despite the existence of Nga Maia.[117]

## Conclusion

The College of Midwives' leaders, including Donley, had a clear vision of what the 1990 Nurses Amendment Act meant to them and what was expected of the new independent midwives. The College wanted its members, in contrast to the medical profession, to be woman-centred and to work in partnership with women. They were concerned that some of the new midwives were too immersed in the medical model, and expressed disappointment at the failure of homebirth to take off as expected.

The College of Midwives' understanding of partnership involved much more than a contractual arrangement in healthcare. It was a political statement and a continuation of the ideologies of the feminist and homebirth movements. As the homebirth movement had before it, College leaders continued to frame arguments about safety as simply a ruse for medical control by doctors in particular. The partnership model was best suited to low-risk and white middle-class women who had in the past been aligned to homebirth, and not everyone bought into the reframed concept. Some mothers, particularly those who experienced a bad birth outcome, did not feel like partners in the relationship. Hospital midwives resented the implication that they were not real midwives. Māori set up their own initiatives and networks, and in the mainstream services it remained to be seen whether the legislative changes and the partnership model would meet the needs of Māori mothers.

Despite dissension from within the midwifery profession itself, the College remained the official voice of midwives, and its views enjoyed considerable support from the government and its health agencies. A major outcome of this was the exodus of GP obstetricians from maternity care. This process and its consequences form the subject of Chapter 8, which addresses the politics of maternity care after 1990.

# EIGHT

## *The politics of maternity services and 'shared care' after 1990*

IN A 1995 INVITED editorial in the *New Zealand College of Midwives Journal*, UK-based midwifery professor Lesley Page complimented the 'fierce pride in the unique nature of midwifery in New Zealand' but posed the question: '[W]ill you be able to achieve a mutually beneficial collaboration with the medical profession?'[1] She received no answer, for a good reason. This was not on the College's agenda, at least not as far as collaboration with GP obstetricians was concerned.[2] Rather, College president Karen Guilliland told *North & South* journalist David McLoughlin in 1993 that she looked forward to the time when 'almost all babies are delivered by midwives. "We'd be like GPs are today," she enthuses.' She proceeded to explain that in childbirth a woman needed a midwife but not a doctor – 'We are just waiting for society to catch up with that.'[3]

The 1990 legislation introduced a competitive environment by giving midwives equal status with GPs as primary caregivers in childbirth. Following the National government's reforms in the mid-1990s, midwives increasingly replaced the latter as providers, just as Guilliland had hoped. This chapter seeks to explain how and why this happened. It will also show that not all midwives and consumers favoured sole-midwifery care; many preferred a system of shared care and sought ways to continue this model. It was the next Labour government, elected in 1999, that put an end to these shared-care initiatives, and ensured a mass medical exodus from primary maternity services. This chapter explores the politics of primary maternity care after 1990.

## 1990–1996: Teamwork between midwives and doctors in maternity care

Liz Carlaw, a homebirth midwife since 1988, described the early 1990s as a golden age of choice for childbearing women, because they were able to access both GPs and midwives. She herself worked with GPs at the St Andrews Medical Centre in Hamilton.[4] Such collaboration was to prove expensive for the government, however, as the funding system had not been designed to accommodate the 1990 changes. Challenged in 1991 for introducing a system that was not cost-effective, Helen Clark responded that it was up to the Health Department to 'tidy up all the complexities [which had resulted from] a very simple law change'.[5] Yet, the situation was far from simple.

Following the introduction of free maternity care in 1939, GPs had been paid under the Maternity Services Benefit schedule, while domiciliary midwives were contracted to the Health Department. The first goal of the Domiciliary Midwives Society set up in 1981 had been to lobby the Health Department to increase homebirth midwives' rates of pay.[6] At that time they earned a maximum of $141.75 per birth (including antenatal and postnatal care). They also suggested a $75 donation from homebirth parents to supplement the fee.[7] Under the Labour government from 1984 they received pay increases, employing an industrial lawyer in 1986 to argue their case with the help of the Home Birth Association which raised $3,000 for that purpose.[8] From 1985 to 1988 their fee for attendance at the birth (for six hours) rose from $54 to $225, a 400% increase; over the same period doctors' fees (for one and a half hours) rose from $185 to $285, a 40% increase.[9] While the gap was reducing, this pay disparity nevertheless persisted until the 1990 Nurses Amendment Act, after which both could claim the same amount.

Before the law change, the doctor's fee was intended to cover the time he or she normally spent at the birth, with a half-hourly rate thereafter intended to cover complicated births. Homebirth midwives spent much longer with the mother even for normal births, so paying them at the same hourly rate as doctors would considerably boost their incomes. In 1993, journalist David

## The politics of maternity services and 'shared care' after 1990

McLoughlin used Health Department records to show that the average payment to doctors per birth was $1,198 and for midwives $2,023. He found that the five top-earning midwives earned an average of $203,862 each during a 10-month period, 'considerably more than the prime minister', he added for good measure. The new funding system allowed women to choose both midwifery and medical care, which he said was a popular choice; both midwife and doctor could claim the maternity benefit, significantly increasing the cost to the taxpayer.[10]

In 1992, the New Zealand Medical Association suggested a tribunal to review payments to maternity-care providers, a procedure required under the 1964 Social Security Act if the negotiating parties (now the Medical Association, the College of Midwives and the Department of Health) could not agree to a schedule. Joan Donley claimed that the Medical Association aimed 'to put [midwives] back where they are seen to belong . . . as soyabeans are used to extend hamburger meat', a metaphor she had borrowed from American sociologist Barbara Katz Rothman.[11] The tribunal's terms of reference specified that payments should be fair, equitable and economical. The Medical Association argued that midwives should be paid under a separate schedule. The College of Midwives argued that doctors and midwives provided the same care (albeit in a different manner) and, having equal value, deserved equal payment. The tribunal agreed and, in its 1993 recommendations, suggested a reduced hourly rate of $52 per hour and a $338 birth fee. Following a submission from panel member Sally Pairman, Minister of Health Bill Birch raised the hourly rate to $90.80 and reduced the birth fee to $313.50.[12] Midwives celebrated both the increased hourly rate and the tribunal's acceptance of their work as equivalent to that of a GP.

Shared care, in which all parties – midwives and doctors – could claim the benefit, added to the cost of maternity care. The government's maternity bill soared from $47 million in 1989–90 to almost $90 million by 1993–94.[13] This growing expenditure on primary maternity care was, as journalist Bruce Ansley later wrote, 'a red rag to the new order' of neoliberalism under the National government that had come to office in 1990.[14] *Consumer* magazine found in 1994 that most of the estimated 11,000 women contracting an independent midwife continued to use their doctor as well, and most gave birth in hospital. The desire to involve doctors, it explained, was because women had an established relationship with them, and saw pregnancy as part of their normal family healthcare.[15] GPs continued to be involved in homebirths as well. Commenting on a 2004 newspaper article, Auckland GP obstetrician William Ferguson wrote: 'What was not mentioned in the article on home birth is that in the 1980s and early 1990s, when home birth was in its ascendancy, this often involved an excellent working partnership between GPs and midwives.'[16]

It is evident from the pages of the *HBA Auckland Newsletter* that GPs continued to be involved in homebirths after 1990. These newsletters contained birth notices, providing details of deliveries by midwives, and included a column for any other attendant. While the law no longer required midwives to involve a doctor, they often chose to do so, or their clients requested it. Homebirth midwife Carolyn Young's high regard for GPs she had worked with since 1974 was noted in Chapter 3. The birth notices show that in the early 1990s she continued to work with doctors.[17] After homebirth doctor John Hilton died in 1994, Young described him as 'an inspiration and a father figure and mentor' to many doctors who practised homebirths.[18] Hilton's name often appeared alongside midwives' in the Auckland HBA birth notices.[19]

Increasingly, however, midwives worked alone. Liz Carlaw said in 1993 that a GP was present at about half of her homebirths; for the rest she was the sole practitioner, or was accompanied by another midwife.[20] The HBA birth notices reveal that in Auckland in early 1993 midwife Sian Burgess attended five homebirths alone, but for three of these she listed a doctor as 'backup'. In the same issue, midwife Veronica Muller, who had often worked with Hilton, recorded a homebirth with no other professional present.[21] The practice of midwives working as sole practitioner or with other midwives appeared to be more common amongst newer recruits. The first six midwives listed in Auckland's autumn 1993 newsletter worked with another midwife or alone, but never with a doctor.[22] Similarly, in 1995 the first 13 midwives listed worked solo or with another midwife.[23] In fact there appeared to be peer pressure on midwives not to work with doctors; Sally Abel noted in 1997 that 'those midwives who did only or largely shared care felt judged by those who did mainly midwifery-only care'.[24]

This attitude may have been encouraged by the College of Midwives itself, which did little to foster good relations between the two sectors. In 1993 Jo Coco, coordinator for the Auckland region, dismissed GPs' pleas to be involved as gatekeepers in maternity care as demeaning to women and upholding the old stereotype of 'doctor knows best'.[25] She was responding to a 1993 article by West Auckland GP obstetrician Philip Rushmer, assisted by Drs William Ferguson, John Hilton, Alison Denyer and Lannes Johnson. Rushmer argued that GPs' gatekeeper role meant they made a unique contribution, being able to evaluate the pregnancy in the context of the patient's general health, family dynamics or other ongoing issues. By contrast, the midwife's care of the woman started and stopped with the pregnancy.[26]

Teamwork had been a catch cry amongst doctors during discussions around the 1990 legislation, and was still invoked, for instance at a 1995 meeting of interested parties on the proposed new funding system. At the meeting, GPs argued that neither they nor midwives should attend childbirth alone, as both skillsets were important. They explained that they were trained to deal with emergencies, which could happen even for low-risk pregnancies. Paediatricians at the meeting expressed concern about midwives' training in postnatal conditions.[27] Sandy Grey, the spokesperson for the College of Midwives at the meeting and later College president, dismissed these concerns as an over-reaction and a failure to recognise midwives as competent, autonomous practitioners.[28] Her view aligned with that of the Auckland HBA which insisted that the midwives on its list were 'competent to provide full care for women and their babies during the entire childbearing cycle from early pregnancy to six weeks after birth'.[29]

## Setting up the new Lead Maternity Carer scheme 1996

These debates occurred at a time when a new funding model was under discussion following the 1993 Health and Disability Act. This Act aimed to make New Zealand's health services more efficient and accountable through a purchaser/provider split. Four regional health authorities (RHAs) were created as purchasers of healthcare throughout the country. The current 14 area health boards were replaced by 23 Crown health enterprises, which operated as hospitals or community trusts, competing with private providers to run health services. Payment systems for primary-care services, such as the General Medical Benefit, Maternity Benefits, and pharmaceutical and laboratory services, were to be changed from fee-for-service to budget-holding by individual or group practitioners. Maternity services were caught up in a broader restructure of the delivery of healthcare.

In 1993, the RHAs set up a joint Maternity Services Project, which commissioned consulting firm Coopers & Lybrand to provide a framework for the restructuring. The firm summarised the problems in maternity services as 'fragmentation of funding, fragmentation of care, differing philosophies, inequality of access, lack of balanced information; and lack of statistical data'.[30] In response, it suggested dividing maternity care into four modules, which RHAs would purchase from contracted providers. Under this system, a woman would choose a lead carer, who could be a midwife, GP, private obstetrician, or a hospital (Crown health enterprise). The lead carer would hold the budget and coordinate the maternity care but would not necessarily provide it all themselves, subcontracting parts to others.

Cabinet approved these proposals in April 1994. However, fraught consultation between the various parties (particularly the College of Midwives and the Medical Association) meant that it took another two years to come into effect. Eventually the Lead Maternity Carer (LMC) scheme began in July 1996 with the publication of the Section 51 Maternity Notice, setting out the new system. While doctors initially boycotted the scheme, it went ahead with the approval of the College of Midwives. As Abel explained, '[T]he new arrangements worked in favour of midwifery autonomy and recognised the equivalency of midwifery and GP skills for normal childbirth.'[31] Journalist Bruce Ansley explained that, while GPs objected on the grounds that it inhibited teamwork and offered a financial incentive to midwives to hold on to patients longer than they should, 'in an odd alliance, regional health authorities, crown health enterprises and midwives by and large supported it'.[32] GP obstetrician Helen Rodenburg, a member of the Medical Association's negotiating committee for the reform, later reflected that, 'from a doctor's point of view it was a no-win situation'; she believed the changes were 'politically driven'.[33]

This viewpoint seemed to be borne out by the College of Midwives' conference in August 1996, just a month into the new scheme. Two senior women politicians attended that conference: Jenny Shipley, the National government's Minister of Health 1993–96, who oversaw the new arrangements; and Labour's Helen Clark. Senior health reporter Kathryn McNeil wrote in *New Zealand Doctor* that these two 'political rivals' were united in their praise for the determination of midwives to improve maternity services and choices for New Zealand women, and that '[b]oth also took the opportunity to knock doctors for their stance in the maternity benefits debate'. Shipley, who also held the portfolio of Minister of Women's Affairs 1990–96, reassured her audience that no Parliament would change the 1990 maternity legislation and that the government supported midwives as 'equal maternity caregivers'. She claimed that doctors had advanced 'many myths' during the recent negotiations, and she believed that their argument for patient safety was a code for: 'I don't like these changes, I am not recognised to the extent I would like to be, or I am not being paid sufficiently.' Midwives, she said, never used such tactics. She boasted that, for the first time, those negotiating the legislation were dealing with a Minister of Health who had had babies herself.[34]

In her conference opening address, president Sally Pairman complained how the media continued to 'buy into the doctors' unsubstantiated and misleading claims that their concerns over the new LMC scheme are to do with safety', whereas the underlying issues were in fact power, control and gender. She described the doctors' worldview as 'patriarchal and positivist' whilst the midwives' philosophy 'sees multiple realities and takes a feminist perspective'. She complained that even when midwives provided scientific evidence to support the safety of their practices, doctors disregarded this. She added, 'Interestingly for a "scientific profession" they were never able to provide evidence for their claims. But with the arrogance born of years of unchallenged control over maternity services, this did not seem to worry them. Instead anecdotal and unsubstantiated stories were given great weight.' She also alleged that many midwives were subjected to personal abuse by their medical colleagues.[35] She presented midwives as eminently reasonable and their views as scientific, and GPs as self-interested, irrational and even abusive.

Karen Guilliland, now College of Midwives national director, wrote an in-depth article for the College's journal on the LMC scheme the following year. She argued once again that, regardless of doctors' expressed concern about safety, their real concern was about control. In her words, 'Fighting Section 51 [the LMC scheme] buys doctors time to claim back the total maternity budget, thus disenfranchising midwifery.' There was no suggestion in the negotiations that doctors were attempting to 'claim back the total budget'. Guilliland's use of the word 'disenfranchising' depicts midwives as a disadvantaged minority group fighting for civil rights. Indeed, she ended her article with a citation from civil rights champion Nelson Mandela's 1994 inaugural speech as President of South Africa: 'As we are liberated from our own fear, our presence automatically liberates others.' This, she declared without explanation, 'says it all'.[36] For as long as midwives saw themselves as an oppressed minority in a civil rights battle, there was little prospect of collaboration.

## The LMC scheme in practice

Under the new system, if the LMC was a midwife or GP, they were required to provide services free of charge to the woman, whilst an obstetrician as LMC could charge an additional fee ranging from $300 to $2,000. The LMC held the budget and received a total sum (then $1,300) per birth to cover prenatal, birth and postnatal services to six weeks. It was theoretically possible to have shared care, or more than one provider, but the capped budget inhibited this.[37] The system favoured midwives who could technically provide all the services themselves; it did not favour GPs for whom childbirth was just part of their medical practice and who therefore had to contract some services to midwives. Indeed, the new system 'required doctor LMCs to have midwifery support services during labour and birth and for the required five to ten postnatal home visits', significantly reducing their fee.[38] One Kaipara GP noted in 2000 that the LMC scheme 'cover[ed] costs but that is all'.[39] Nor did it encourage midwives to work with GPs, as this would mean forgoing some of their payment. Dunedin GP obstetrician Tony Fitchett later said of the LMC system, 'A system which financially disadvantages primary carers who seek consultation or help is a bad system, however ethical that carer tries to be.'[40]

While the new scheme favoured midwives whose sole job was providing maternity care, many GPs continued to be involved. The Auckland HBA birth notices indicate that homebirth GPs still practised alongside midwives after 1996, suggesting that some midwives valued collaboration or that women continued to request it. Of 97 homebirths attended by Auckland midwives in 1997, 37 also listed a doctor and 52 another midwife. In a further eight cases the midwife was the sole practitioner, as the law permitted. Carolyn Young continued to work collaboratively, with just over half her 1997 listed births shared with a doctor and the rest with another midwife. Of her 20 homebirths over seven months that same year, Sian Burgess carried out 17 with an accompanying midwife, one with a doctor, one as sole practitioner, and one with the assistance of the woman's partner.[41] While some midwives continued to involve doctors, many did not, and the system did not encourage it.

Many of the homebirth doctors were women; Auckland had at least 10 in the 1990s.[42] However, even the College of Midwives' strong gender rhetoric did not lead it to embrace these women doctors. One of them was

Diana (Di) Nash, who had graduated in medicine in 1969. She explained in 1999 why she was leaving obstetrics. In an article headed 'Dejected GP quits babies', she mentioned the lack of funding but said it was not just about the money; it was also about the fact that GPs' contribution to obstetrics was no longer valued. Health authorities and midwives misrepresented GPs, she said, as the ones who 'run in and catch the baby'. She found the stance of the midwifery profession 'exceptionally galling', as she had strongly supported its development, and had indeed written the preface to Joan Donley's book, *Save the Midwife*.[43] Involved in homebirths since 1977, Nash had pleaded with the audience at the 1987 HBA conference to 'Please treat Drs as people not as Adversaries'.[44] But she also insisted that 'the idea that midwives and doctors are interchangeable is absurd'; what was important was teamwork.[45]

In 2003, Dr Margaret Shanks wrote an article for the *New Zealand Herald* explaining that she was a mother of six and the only remaining female GP obstetrician in central Auckland. She lamented the pending closure of National Women's Hospital, 'a positive, woman and baby-friendly place' for her and her clients.[46] But she also commented on the 'erosion of funding for GP obstetricians without acknowledgement of the role of the family GP in the continuity of care of the whole family'. She insisted:

> The essence of a good birth experience for the mother, and a good outcome for the baby, is a welcoming, safe environment and the knowledge that the person qualified to care for her is able to handle any emergency that may arise. Without this, more postpartum depression and complications will ensue.

She continued to practise obstetrics despite the disincentives, she explained, because she was passionate about caring for families.[47]

Helen Holden was said to be the last GP in Dunedin still practising in childbirth services when she opted out in 2004. She had initially quit in 2003 but was persuaded back by a client to deliver her fourth baby. This mother spoke of her attachment to Holden during her pregnancies, and of how much she valued the 'cradle to the grave tradition'. It was a relationship of trust, she said, with Holden as emotionally involved in the birth as she was. Holden found giving up obstetrics hard; it had been part of her practice for 13 years. She had delivered about 1,000 babies and considered it an honour to be involved in families' lives in this way. She said in 2004 that it had taken her the previous five years to accept that GPs no longer had a place in obstetrics. She hung in purely for the love of it and the misguided hope that things might change.[48] Another female GP, Jackie Mills, who provided maternity services until 2003, reminisced in 2005 about a midwifery conference she attended in the late 1990s at which Helen Clark in a speech 'deeply celebrated the fact that GPs were back in primary care and out of obstetrics. She got a standing ovation.' Mills was devastated, adding, '[T]he working relationship [between GPs and midwives] had been so good and offered astounding care for women. We sure didn't want to give up.'[49]

Nor did it appear that consumers were entirely happy. A *New Zealand Listener* article lamented in 1999 that the so-called choice of providers offered to women by the 1996 changes had been illusory, as having a doctor as lead carer was no longer an option for most women.[50] Labour's Health spokeswoman Annette King was also reported as saying that choice was disappearing for pregnant women.[51] Discontent among women had been mounting since 1997, just a year into the new system. Karen Guilliland expressed concern in mid-1997 at midwives' flagging consumer support. Referring to a recent article by health columnist Sandra Coney, she lamented, 'If feminists like Sandra Coney cannot see our issues then what hope has the average person when regaled by biased and inaccurate reporting.'[52] *New Zealand Doctor* reported a survey by Parents Centre representing 11,000 women, which found that women were unhappy and wanted the option of shared care.[53] Guilliland complained that the low returns in the survey invalidated its findings, adding condescendingly, 'Parents Centre has been a naïve partner in the political campaign to undermine women's trust in the normal process of birth, and the midwifery services that attend them.'[54]

Another consumer organisation called AIMS (Action to Improve Maternity Services), set up by Janne Witt in 1996, expressed its concerns about the GP exodus. Witt spoke of the many complaints she received, including one from a woman who had contacted 73 GPs in a 'fruitless search for someone to deliver her baby'.[55] GP obstetrician Lynda Exton, writing about the changes from 1990, cited a 1999 National Council of Women survey with 1,245 respondents which found that many women wanted shared care between GP and midwife, and were unhappy this option was not available.[56] Others too reported consumer dissatisfaction with the loss of GPs and shared care as options.[57] Consumer activist Lynda Williams was secretary to the Auckland Maternity Services Consumer Council set up in 1990 to 'enhance the consumer lobby' in maternity services.⁵⁸ She told *New Zealand Doctor* in 1999 that since the introduction of the new scheme in 1996 the Council had fielded hundreds of calls from women or their family members. Issues included the inability to access the LMC of their choice – or any LMC for that matter. Another concern was inadequate postnatal care and support.⁵⁹ The Plunket Society, which was then contracted by the government to oversee babies from six weeks of age, had been picking up the pieces, attending to babies less than two weeks old.⁶⁰ Williams supported an AIMS petition to increase postnatal care.⁶¹

Postnatal care was at the heart of Whakatāne GP obstetrician Tim Insull's decision to quit maternity services in 1998. When his clients approached him for postnatal care, he discovered that, as he was not their LMC, claiming payment from the LMC system was a bureaucratic nightmare.⁶² Insull was the last GP practising obstetrics in Whakatāne; there had been 11 when the LMC scheme was introduced. In 1998, Taumarunui doctor Upali Manu explained that he had been a GP obstetrician since 1973, but had quit the system prior to the 1996 reform, owing to an environment of hostility and competition. But he added, 'I continue to give some services, sometimes unpaid, because I have known the patients.'⁶³ Auckland's Dr Lynn Coleman told a reporter in 1997 that she had provided unpaid maternity care for three women during the past week: 'I will service these women because they are my patients but I can't do it forever for all my patients. I can't afford to lose my practice.'⁶⁴

By May 1999, *New Zealand Doctor* reported that the number of GPs registering as LMCs had 'crashed dramatically' from almost 3,000 in 1996 to just 325 nationwide.⁶⁵ Dr William Ferguson said GPs' morale was 'at rock bottom', especially in rural areas. In response to the National Maternity Services Coordinator's claim in 1997 that the drop was because maternity no longer suited the GPs' lifestyle, the New Zealand General Practitioners' Association (a branch of the Medical Association) conducted a survey to which 360 GPs responded. Fully 94% of those believed maternity care was an important part of general practice.⁶⁶ Lynda Williams urged GPs to take the issue up with the government rather than 'punishing women' with co-charges, as a group had attempted to do on Auckland's North Shore.⁶⁷ The Medical Association agreed, and reported in 1999 that after trying for a few years they had finally managed to achieve a review of maternity services.⁶⁸

## 1999 National Health Committee Review

In 1998 National's Health Minister Bill English ordered the National Health Committee to carry out an inquiry after what he described as an increasing number of reports about problems with maternity services, including the GP exodus. Television garden-show host and future MP Maggie Barry, who was a lay member of the committee and a new mother, chaired the review, and in 1999 the new Minister of Health Wyatt Creech confirmed its terms of reference, including that its recommendations were to be within current funding levels.[69] *New Zealand Doctor* declared that consumers and GPs 'hoped for confirmation GPs were needed and desired in obstetric care', explaining that they wanted the government to recognise their skillset as different from and complementary to that of midwives, and to make provision for more shared care.[70]

In its final report, the committee pointed to 'poor and insufficient data to assess quality of outcomes' owing to a lack of a coordinated perinatal database and 'a lack of comprehensive assessment of provider performance' which, it said, impeded the ability of the government to identify quality and safety problems. It also noted that there was no consistent mechanism requiring providers to review and monitor outcomes.[71] The committee's own findings were based on a consumer survey, with a questionnaire published in the magazines *Little Treasures*, which targeted new parents, and the *New Zealand Woman's Weekly*, and given out at meetings and hui around the country. It generated about 11,000 (anonymous) postal responses. This was accompanied by a telephone survey, targeting women who gave birth in selected weeks in March and April 1999, with about 1,000 women interviewed.

From its surveys, the committee reported a high level of satisfaction with services among women. It did note, however, that its survey methods offered the potential for providers to selectively supply the questionnaire to women who were likely to have been satisfied with their services, though this was impossible to assess.[72] *New Zealand Doctor* noted: 'From the start, people questioned the reliability of the proposed method for gauging public satisfaction with safety and quality of services – a women's magazine questionnaire.'[73] This format drew criticism from Sandra Coney who pointed out that respondents were 'older, whiter and better off' than many women giving birth; Barry replied that the report acknowledged selection bias and included quotas for Māori and Pacific women in its telephone survey.[74]

The Māori and Pacific quota – 15% Māori, 6% Pacific – had not been reached, however, and the committee admitted that: 'Women of European ethnicity and aged 30 to 39 years were over-represented in the respondent group, while women aged under 24 years and of Māori, Pacific Islands and Asian ethnicity were under-represented.' Those who had homebirths were also marginally over-represented (7.7% of all respondents and 3–4% of births). The report also noted that respondents were more likely to come from higher-income households and that those with tertiary education were over-represented.[75]

Despite reporting overall satisfaction amongst women, the committee did also point to some significant issues. These related to access to services by those living in rural areas, and by Māori and Pasifika women. It found that women with the highest need for antenatal care were more likely to receive a lower number of antenatal visits, and that the same applied to postnatal care.[76] It criticised the system for failing to adequately respond to Māori cultural needs.[77] This was despite the attention to cultural safety in midwifery education (explored in Chapter 9). Their review also reported concerns that safe outcomes were being 'compromised by inter-professional tensions, poor communication between providers, and inappropriate and late referrals of women in labour to specialist care'. It speculated that possible explanations were financial disincentives to refer to a specialist and a 'reluctance of community providers to admit that they are unable to cope with medical complications of pregnancy'.[78] Thus it evaluated the current system as far from optimal despite reporting consumer satisfaction.

In his foreword to the review, chair of the National Health Committee Mason Durie noted that 'many women' wanted a 'return to willing co-operation between medical care and midwifery', a call which he said the committee supported.[79] Commenting on the 166 submissions it received, the committee declared, 'Most submissions from medical practitioners, consumers and advocacy groups favoured increasing women's access to "shared care" arrangements.'[80] The review concluded that it was important to 'foster an environment where midwives and doctors are able to join forces to provide maternity services'.[81] It referred to some successful shared schemes outside the LMC system (which will be discussed in the next section) and recommended that the LMC system itself should allow an entity rather than just an individual to hold financial accountability in order to encourage professionals to work in teams.[82]

The committee appeared to favour shared care but did not make concrete suggestions on how to achieve this. New Zealand Medical Association chair and Christchurch GP obstetrician Pippa MacKay declared that the review was the death knell for family doctors delivering babies. She despaired that obstetrics was hard, unprofitable work for GPs, and that the review, coming on top of the 'politics, competition and nastiness' that had entered the maternity system since government funding changes, would be the last straw for many who had been hanging on, hoping the review would improve matters. Improvement was not reliant on more money, she said, but on funding a system that got doctors and midwives to work together.[83]

Amidst this gloom from GPs about their future in maternity services, Anton Wiles, a GP obstetrician and chair of the Royal New Zealand College of General Practitioners, claimed in 1999 to see signs of growing cooperation between midwives and GPs. This was occurring, he said, despite the 'uncooperative and belligerent stance' towards GP involvement in maternity by Guilliland and others 'who hold the reins of power in the College of Midwives'.[84] The vehicle for this cooperation was schemes which did not operate through the funding mechanism for the LMCs (often referred to as non-Section 51 schemes), which emerged after 1996.

## Last-ditch attempts at shared care

In 2001, tireless GP obstetrician Margaret Shanks told a reporter that while midwives said they could manage all cases, everyone knew there was now a very high rate of referral to specialists. She believed that under the LMC scheme, GPs practising obstetrics had been worn down by paperwork and lack of pay and feelings of being undervalued but had also forgotten that maternity was a positive part of their practice. To relieve her own administrative burdens, Shanks had recently joined a collective maternity scheme in Auckland called SAMCL which employed 145 midwives, 12 GPs and 21 obstetricians.[85]

In 2000 *New Zealand Doctor* editor Barbara Fountain expressed surprise at an announcement by Barbara Browne, maternity manager to the Health Funding Authority (HFA) which had replaced the regional health authorities (RHAs) in 1998, that schemes like SAMCL were to be closed down. These schemes, Fountain wrote, had been successful in getting doctors and midwives to work together, offering women shared-care options. They involved collective rather than individual practitioner contracts with funding authorities. There were 20 around the country by 2000, providing 30% of all maternity care and accounting for 29% of the primary maternity budget. Some, such as those run by Hokianga Health and the Ngati Porou Hauora Board, operated in rural areas with access problems, and like others such as the Porirua, Hutt and Newtown Union Health Centres, combined maternity with other services such as social work. Despite the schemes being relatively cost-effective, a 2000 HFA report recommended their abolition in the interests of 'cost, equity, administration and data on maternity care'.[86]

In 2001, Labour's Health Minister Annette King pointed to a Wellington organisation called Matpro (Maternity Project) as an example of how GPs and midwives could work together.[87] Matpro had been set up in 1996, not by doctors but by a group of midwives who had formed the Association of Wellington Midwives. They joined forces with GPs and obstetricians, and contracted directly with the Ministry of Health to serve Wellington city, Porirua and Kāpiti. The company director and midwife representative on the board was Kerry Prendergast, then deputy and later mayor of Wellington. A self-employed midwife, Prendergast provided care to about 50 Wellington women per year, 70% as shared care and 30% as midwife LMC. When Matpro was first established, it included over 40 GPs, 50 midwives and two obstetricians, with 85% of its clients choosing shared care.[88] Helen Rodenburg, president of the Royal New Zealand College of General Practitioners (2001–03), described Matpro as having 'the best clinical governance framework' in the country, with a 'real commitment of providing quality care'. This service, she explained, included peer-review groups of GPs, midwives and specialists, and a system for monitoring problems.[89] But just months after King had applauded Matpro she withdrew its public funding. By 2004, with its contract withdrawn, the company considered winding up, and by 2008, its sole function was to provide a list of LMCs.[90] To Rodenburg, the decision simply confirmed her 'ongoing impression' that the Ministry made some 'very bad policy decisions with regard to maternity care', and she questioned the value it attached to mothers and babies. She reflected that while 'superficially the statistics look all right', the fact that between 9% and 12.5% of women needed to be re-admitted to hospital after they had their baby 'surely means something is amiss'.[91]

Two contracts bypassing the LMC system had also been established in Dunedin. In 1997 obstetrician Glen Blanchette set up a cooperative involving three midwives and two obstetricians called Albany Maternity and

Gynaecology, which negotiated directly with the health authorities at LMC prices. The cooperative managed over half of the obstetric care in Dunedin by 2000, and reported that many women liked the shared care offered.[92] The other scheme in Dunedin was an independent practitioner association called South Link Health (SLH), which in 1996 contracted with Healthcare Otago (Dunedin Hospital) and the RHA to provide maternity services.[93] According to the SLH director Professor of General Practice Murray Tilyard, its maternity services operated successfully with high consumer satisfaction. It expanded to other areas covering most of the South Island, and by 2000 had 284 GPs working for it, whilst staying within budget.[94]

One of those who joined SLH after the organisation extended its programme to the lower Northland region in 2000 was William Ferguson. Ferguson was excited by a development that, he said, had 'reignited the subspecialty of general practice at the eleventh hour', offering women shared care, just as the 1999 National Health Committee review had advocated.[95] He wanted to see it implemented nationally, believing it would change overnight the morale of the maternity workforce.[96] But that was not to be. Barbara Fountain believed that the success of the schemes embarrassed the government and the College of Midwives because it contradicted 'the popular myth that GPs and midwives could not work together'.[97] The government was in 'full steam ahead to dismantle these primary care success stories', ostensibly in the interests of standardising payment structures for maternity services.[98] Karen Guilliland was certainly in favour of dismantling the schemes, arguing that standardising would mean equity for women and providers. Fountain countered that several midwives spoken to by *New Zealand Doctor* felt these were the services they most benefited from and that enabled them to spend more time with women, and they were 'alarmed' at the prospect of losing them. *New Zealand Doctor* declared that maternity providers working outside the LMC framework, including GPs, specialists and midwives, were disappointed and angry about the Ministry of Health's proposal to shut these schemes down by the end of 2001.[99]

Karine Baker, an obstetrician in a group scheme in Dunedin from 1996, was one of these dismayed providers. Pointing out how she and the midwives she worked with valued shared care, she argued that the quality of their outcomes challenged the 'currently held government philosophy' that solo care was 'at all beneficial to women'.[100] The chair of Auckland's SAMCL Muriel Wormald also chided the Ministry of Health for throwing away both real choice for women and a good working relationship between GPs and midwives.[101] Other commentators queried the government's claim that the schemes were too costly.[102] Ferguson cited an accountancy firm which calculated a $37.19 additional cost for SLH, and he fumed that the Ministry of Health was 'prepared to bulldoze New Zealand's few remaining GPs out of the maternity service for a mere $37.19 per pregnancy'. GP obstetrician Tony Fitchett pointed out that the SLH operated 12 different models of care to suit different needs, and that its services and reporting exceeded that required under the LMC contracts but cost only 1.9% more. Cancelling the scheme, he added, would mean less choice for women.[103]

Despite these protests, the government cancelled contracts outside the standard LMC scheme in 2002. This affected a third of the maternity cases around the country, including the Albany practice, which caused its director Glen Blanchette to lament that its 'very old-fashioned' philosophy of shared care was clearly no longer politically acceptable.[104] Why were these supposedly successful shared-care schemes not embraced? Pippa MacKay thought it was about 'ideology and money'.[105] Others pointed to the strong influence of the HFA maternity manager Barbara Browne and Karen Guilliland.[106] Lynda Exton noted that Browne, a former midwife, did not see the GP exodus as a problem, because she believed that maternity care could be provided 'equally competently' by obstetricians, midwives or GPs.[107] Glen Blanchette commented on how effectively the College of Midwives continued to lobby the Minister of Health.[108]

William Ferguson himself had lobbied the new Minister of Health Annette King in 2000 about the value of the GP in obstetrics. He told her that normal delivery and labour should never be the primary focus of a maternity service, but rather prevention and management of complications, morbidity and mortality.[109] He also raised the issue of postnatal depression, pointing out that GPs recognised the signs and knew their patients well enough to detect changes, but women were not seeing their GPs and were presenting later with more severe cases. 'What more profoundly important thing can you do to support motherhood than provide early diagnosis and treatment?' he asked. Failure to do so, he said, destroyed marriages and relationships.[110]

King was not convinced. She explained her decision to move all LMC contracts to a standard national contract in a 2001 guest editorial in the *New Zealand College of Midwives Journal*. She saw women as partners in the management of their care, and said the change would give women certainty.

While the future of primary healthcare was to involve 'greater coordination, continuity and teamwork', she also believed it important that 'the gains that women have experienced in maternity care over the last decade must not be lost and a strong, independent midwifery profession is a key part of this'.[111] Referring to these so-called gains for women, Exton argued that King disregarded the fact that the shared schemes offered women choice of caregivers, were popular with women, and were models of inter-professional cooperation.[112] Was King keen to court favour with the College of Midwives? She certainly described Helen Clark as an 'absolute hero' to some health professionals and as 'the patron of midwives', and added, 'I haven't reached that lofty status', suggesting this might have been an aspiration.[113]

The Hokianga Health Trust had long stood out as a success story in the delivery of health services to a poor, largely rural area with a predominance of Māori. It was one of the few organisations allowed to hold a contract collectively rather than through individual doctors and midwives after these group schemes were dismantled, continuing to provide shared care.[114] The government had listened to the 1999 National Health Committee review to this extent at least. The review had advised that Māori service providers should be free to develop contracting arrangements outside the LMC system, and that 'Maori midwives, medical staff and community workers should be able to work in multi-disciplinary teams, to serve needs in areas with a high Maori population'.[115] The government clearly saw this as a special case.

Another special case was the College of Midwives' Midwifery and Maternity Providers Organisation (MMPO). This was the College's response to the group schemes. In 2003 midwife lecturer Chris Hendry explained that, in 1997, 'Concerned by the fact that midwives had no option but to join medically-run organisations to gain the commercial advantages', the College formed MMPO exclusively for its midwife members. According to Hendry, because the College was a non-commercial not-for-profit incorporated society, it 'found it necessary' to establish MMPO as 'an alternative structure to take on the contracting and budget-holding role as a commercial venture'.[116] MMPO supported the 'business side of midwifery', according to the 2006 midwifery textbook, with about 550 mostly self-employed midwives using the service by 2005, making it the 'largest non-government maternity provider in the country'.[117] What distinguished it from the other schemes that were culled was that it did not involve cross-disciplinary collaborations.

## The medical exodus after 2000 and consumer responses

In 2001 Queenstown mayor and former National Party MP Warren Cooper claimed to be 'horrified' that maternity work was no longer a viable option for GPs and that women were left with no choice of maternity providers. He demanded answers from Health Minister Annette King, and his wife Lorraine launched a petition asking the government to put incentives in place to encourage doctors and midwives to work together.[118] The same year, *New Zealand Doctor* reported that 'a large number of patients' were saddened by the lack of GP obstetricians in the town of Ōamaru, suggesting this would mean more referrals to Dunedin and Timaru hospitals.[119]

One consumer group in East Auckland, calling themselves Let Mothers Choose, asked the government in 2002 to consider allowing them to pay GPs a surcharge for maternity services to keep them in the system. 'This demonstrates the value we as consumers place on the role of GPs in obstetrics,' spokesperson Rachel Crombie explained. She added that it was their right to choose, and that paying a surcharge was more affordable than going to a specialist.[120] Referring to this failed petition, Helen Rodenburg declared that choice 'for and by women' had gone. 'Disturbingly it seems that only one perspective from "women's groups" is allowed and that perspective is anti-doctor – not so good for New Zealand's feminist traditions.'[121]

When another lay person, comedian, actor and writer Jon Gadsby, 'lambasted' the 1996 changes to maternity care, largely because they destroyed shared care in New Zealand, he found himself in deep trouble with some midwives. Gadsby had commissioned a student journalist to write an article called 'Broken Dolls' in *Avenues*, a Christchurch magazine he had founded in 2004.[122] He explained this followed another published article by the student in the *Press* on Karen Guilliland's views on maternity, which, he said, included 'outrageous claims' such as that midwives could do anything doctors could do. 'Broken Dolls' consisted of three case studies highlighting problems with midwives working in isolation and not recognising, or refusing to recognise, any need for medical involvement. Gadsby told *New Zealand Doctor* that the article was met with 'howls of outrage' from a handful of midwives who had responded with abusive phone calls and letters. He claimed they accused him of gutter journalism, bias and telling lies. One accused him, he said, of using the grief of parents who lost a baby to make his point. He retorted that as a parent he was as entitled to his views as anyone else.[123]

Protest also erupted in the Wairarapa in 2005 after a maternity services manager from Canterbury DHB was brought in to conduct a review. At the time there were only three GPs providing maternity care in the Wairarapa. The reviewer advised that paying GPs as LMCs was 'inappropriate and a financial risk' to the local board. The local mayor joined Parents Centre in protest. The latter claimed that it was vital for women to have a choice of LMC, and that the community was 'privileged to have three GPs [doing obstetrics] and their role should be valued and nurtured'. *New Zealand Doctor* did not report on the outcome of these protests.[124]

Rodenburg claimed in 2004 that the loss of maternity care from general practice continued to be a source of bitterness amongst GPs.[125] William Ferguson certainly felt bitter, resigning as maternity spokesperson for the College of General Practitioners and opting out of providing maternity care in 2005 'in despair'.[126] He took exception to Annette King's suggestion that GPs left obstetrics because they no longer wanted to work after hours, considering this an insult to a generation of dedicated GPs who had been 'cut from their subspecialty by a discriminatory and dysfunctional funding mechanism' introduced in 1996.[127] When the College of General Practitioners had examined reasons for the GP exodus in 2002, it found 'a lack of professional recognition; limited financial viability; and a stressful working environment caused by the politics of maternity care and deteriorating relationships with midwives'.[128]

In 2009, University of Otago researchers interviewed 23 GP obstetricians, past and present (they calculated there were 38 GPs practising obstetrics throughout the country, compared to 3,000 in 1990). In their report, they maintained that the dominance achieved by midwives in New Zealand was unmatched elsewhere in the Western world. They commented that, despite their interviewees' critique of the LMC system, they did not 'appear to be grieving the loss of their dominant position in the maternity market'. Rather, they mourned the loss of the social and clinical value of obstetrics to their practices, and the loss of the 'cradle' from 'cradle to grave' care which was integral to the philosophy of general practice. It was also 'one of the greatest rewards of general practice', and central to their identity in smaller communities in particular. The interviewees were adamant they had a role to play in maternity care, and that the changes had compromised maternal and neonatal safety.[129]

A few years later, in 2012, a Ministry of Health-commissioned comparison of New Zealand's maternity system with those in other developed countries put a different spin on it. Malatest International, the New Zealand company that conducted the study, pointed out that the role of the GP in primary maternity care had since 1990 decreased markedly in New Zealand, as it had in Australia, Canada and the UK, and cited reasons for the decrease: 'the funding arrangements, difficult working hours, disruption of office hours, interference with lifestyle, fear of litigation, costs of insurance and fewer opportunities to maintain competency'. Yet, as we have seen, New Zealand GPs committed to maternity care considered the advantages outweighed disruption to lifestyle and difficult hours. Additionally, while in America malpractice premiums appeared to play a significant role in family physicians' withdrawal from attending births, fear of litigation and the cost of insurance were not relevant to New Zealand because of ACC.[130] There was little sense in the Malatest International report of the context in which New Zealand GPs had left maternity services, and the attempt to draw parallels with other countries deflected attention away from New Zealand's unique reforms.[131] As midwife Chris Hendry had pointed out, GPs 'did not seem to be leaving this area of practice quietly'.[132] Pippa MacKay had explained in 1999 that maternity care was 'the cornerstone of good family practice. It's the most enjoyable and satisfying part of being a doctor.'[133] GPs' withdrawal from maternity care was not a positive decision based on lifestyle choices; rather, as Ferguson said, they left 'in despair'.

The Malatest Report told its international audience that women and their families in New Zealand could choose their LMC, that most chose a midwife, and that the number 'choosing' a GP was 'small and is decreasing'. It cited Ministry of Health figures for 2010 showing that 78% chose a midwife, 1.6% a GP and 5.8% an obstetrician.[134] The implication was that women had choice and that most rejected GPs. Yet there was plenty of evidence to suggest women were not happy with their lack of choice after the shared-care schemes ended.

Specialist obstetricians also felt disheartened by the current maternity landscape. One was Dr Vicki Robertson who attributed the decision to move her practice overseas in 2002 to the current environment. She reflected that if doctors had 'hung together more and refused to go along with the changes' they could have achieved something, but that the system had gone too far to be retrievable.[135] It is questionable whether they could have changed anything. Blanchette referred in 2003 to an obstetrician in his Albany practice who had recently left for Australia, adding there was 'little hope of attracting another obstetrician in New Zealand's current anti-medical climate', and that: 'Morale within the senior levels of the specialty is virtually non-existent.'[136]

Blanchette thought the system introduced in 1996 undervalued secondary care. Under this system, funding for secondary care was to apply only to hospital emergency services.[137] Many of the shortlived group schemes had involved obstetricians working in the community and not just providing emergency services in hospital. Researchers in a 2007 study on how to expand the role of midwives within Australian maternity services would have agreed with him. They argued that the way to expand midwifery-led care outside hospital was to involve obstetricians in birth centres. They pointed to successful local programmes, based on collaboration between midwives and obstetricians, that were reminiscent of New Zealand's group schemes in the late 1990s. The authors of the study concluded, 'It is from this basis of collaboration and cooperation that alternative models of care that are safe and effective are most likely to emerge.'[138]

## Rural women feel the pinch

Whatever the reasons for the medical exodus, women in rural areas were particularly hard hit by the trend. In December 2000, a group of women called a 'crisis meeting' to consider the rights of rural women regarding maternity care. Delegates came from 'Women's Health Action, Federation of Women's Health Councils, Rural Women of New Zealand, Maori Consumer Advocates, Parents Centre and Rural Community Health Trust'. One attendee told *New Zealand Doctor* that the gist of what women really wanted was the re-establishment of a working relationship between doctors and midwives to ensure a safe system.[139]

Don Simmers, a former Queenstown GP obstetrician and a member of the Ministry of Health's Maternity Advisory Group, was concerned that women in the small town of Wānaka would be forced into specialist care, at a cost of up to $2,000, owing to the lack of GPs practising obstetrics. He believed the Wānaka situation was typical of most rural areas. He pointed out that Pat Farry, Director of Rural Health for the South Island from 1999 to 2003, had advocated for midwife/GP teams in rural areas because of their special needs, but had been thwarted by the Ministry of Health and the College of Midwives.[140] Simmers said in 2006, 'It's high time New Zealand corrected this nonsense of having midwifery only obstetrics', particularly in rural areas. He insisted, 'There has to be a willingness from politicians to CEOs of DHBs to stop beating about the bush and admit it was wrong to get rid of doctors from providing maternity services and move quickly to reinstate the role of the GPO [General Practitioner Obstetrician].'[141] Two years later Simmers was pleased and surprised to discover that there were still 52 GPs practising obstetrics around the country. They had 'battled for a decade against bureaucratic indifference and the anti-doctor mindset of our health system', and should be congratulated and encouraged.[142]

One of the problems Simmers identified for midwife LMCs was that, while GPs could combine maternity care with their general practice in small communities, there was generally not enough work to attract LMC midwives.[143] A 2008 MMPO study into rural midwifery also raised the issue of attracting and keeping LMC midwives in rural areas.[144] This study found that most travelled out from urban centres to work. This meant that postnatal care was almost non-existent; one visit could mean a three-hour round trip. At this time birthing mothers were entitled to a minimum of seven sessions with their LMC in the first six weeks after giving birth, five of them home visits. The report noted: 'Anecdotally women claimed to miss out on postnatal care if there are no local midwives.'[145] Of 52 rural primary-care facilities surveyed in the study, two had GPs working as LMCs, and 15 had medical back-up available; the rest were reliant on midwives. The report noted that recruiting midwifery staff for these rural maternity facilities was becoming problematic.[146]

Another 2008 study of maternity care in rural areas considered the consequences of direct-entry midwifery training introduced in 1992 and the separation of nursing and midwifery. Direct-entry midwifery training was still being debated in Australia where in 2009 a Royal College of Nursing Australia submission to a maternity services review advocated nurse training as part of midwifery education 'to ensure that the midwifery workforce is not just flexible but well equipped to provide holistic family-centred services'.[147] The 2008 New Zealand study was conducted by Adele Robertson, an experienced rural nurse and midwife, and co-founder of Great Barrier Island's primary healthcare service where she had worked since 1985.[148] Robertson believed combining nursing and midwifery was particularly important for areas where a small population was spread over a wide geographical area, and health professionals needed to be multi-skilled. The midwife with nurse training, as an 'expert generalist' or 'multi-specialist', would be more cost-effective and efficient than personnel from a single profession. Yet, she lamented, the professional midwifery climate in New Zealand did not value nurses who were midwives. Referring to the College of Midwives' concept of partnership, she said that rural nurses met this prerequisite in their work with communities and provided a partnership that continued over a family's lifespan. She concluded that the introduction of direct-entry midwifery training and professional competency requirements, alongside an ageing rural workforce for both nursing and midwifery, was likely to adversely affect maternity services in rural areas. Nurses and midwives, who were able to operate across both scopes of practice, would no longer be available.[149]

Others also predicted a midwifery crisis in rural areas. In 2004, Rural General Practice Network chair Tim Malloy said his network had anticipated five years earlier that there would be a shortage of midwives in rural areas following the demise of GPs in maternity care, not least because of burnout among midwives having to take total responsibility.[150] The 2012 Malatest Report too noted that by the mid-2000s there was a chronic shortage of midwives, particularly in rural areas.[151] The disbanding of the shared schemes hit rural areas hard.

## Conclusion

By the turn of the century there appeared to be two opposing views on the state of New Zealand's maternity services. In her comments on a stillbirth at Hutt Hospital in 1999, Pippa MacKay described the system as 'dangerous, blinkered and ideological', whereas Karen Guilliland called it 'one of the best and safest in the world'.[152] In 2000 William Ferguson claimed the service was creating serious risks, pointing to the rise in obstetric intervention rates, a fall in breastfeeding rates, high antenatal and postnatal hospital admission rates, rising infection rates related to childbirth, and reports of an increase in babies transferred to a tertiary hospital with brain damage linked to delivery.[153] By contrast, a 2000 Health Funding Authority reference document on maternity services concluded, 'New Zealand is acknowledged internationally as a leader in its model of maternity services.'[154]

It was easy to make such pronouncements in the absence of hard data; as noted by the 1993 RHA Maternity Services Project and the 1999 National

Health Committee review, there had been no audit of services since the system changed. One thing was clear, however: it was not a model that everyone liked. Many parents, doctors and midwives spoke in favour of shared care between midwives and doctors during this period. Whilst expensive to the government, the shared care allowed in the period 1990–96 was a 'golden age' for maternity care. After 1996, and despite the individual contracts set up under the LMC system, group schemes flourished for a time, not just because doctors liked shared care but because many consumers and midwives did too. One of them was Joan Skinner, who in 2004 explained that she had worked in a primary healthcare team for seven years and it was one of the most satisfying times of her practising career.[155] And yet, unless there was a 'sea change', Christchurch GP obstetrician Colin Chin (who described obstetrics as 'general practice in its truest sense') told *New Zealand Doctor* in 2013, GP obstetricians 'will meet the same fate as the gold guineas those gypsies paid my grandfather long ago – becoming rare, but valuable treasures, likely never to be seen again'.[156]

# NINE

## *The practice of midwifery and the 'midwifery model' in the 1990s*

FROM 1990, AND PARTICULARLY from 1996 when the Lead Maternity Carer scheme was introduced, independent midwives became the primary carers for many women from early pregnancy to six weeks postnatally. The philosophical oversight of these carers came from the New Zealand College of Midwives, which launched its own journal in 1989, held national conferences, and provided leadership for the new midwifery training programmes from 1992. The College's discourse of the 1990s emphasised what it called the 'midwifery model' as opposed to the 'medical model', with the former defined by a midwife as a 'natural and holistic/social model' and the latter a 'technical and mechanistic model'.[1] How this discourse played out in practice under the new maternity framework (including protocols for midwives' access to hospitals, referrals and LMC responsibilities), in the new midwifery training programmes, and in the College's approaches to medical technology more broadly including immunisation, forms the subject of this chapter.

### Protocols on transfer to hospitals or specialist care

The 1990 Nurses Amendment Act, allowing midwives the right to practise on their own in the community – whether at home or in the new midwifery-run maternity units – did not set guidelines for when, or whether, they should transfer clients to hospitals or to medical specialists. Nor was a medical assessment of a woman's suitability for homebirth required, as it was in other comparable countries, and the law did not restrict midwives to conducting 'normal' births.

In her 1992 commentary entitled 'Protocols?', Joan Donley cited the Medical Practitioners Disciplinary Committee which was, she wrote, '"dismayed" at the lack of national protocols which define the respective responsibilities of medical practitioners and midwives'. The Committee's comment followed two disastrous homebirths (see pp. 140–42). One of the cases involved disagreements between the midwife and the GP attending the birth about when to go to hospital, and further conflict and delays once the patient was in hospital (it had taken three hours before the caesarean section was performed). Donley maintained that, 'rigid, medically oriented "protocols"' are a convenient way to place independent midwives under "control"'. This was, she said, an old tactic that went back to the Middle Ages. She asked facetiously if such 'protocols' would protect the public from the obstetrician whose glasses fell off into the woman's abdomen during a caesarean section. She noted that the Department of Health was considering a policy that a medical registrar should assess all transfers within 15 minutes of arrival in hospital to determine who should continue care, and she saw it as a breach of the woman's right to be cared for by her own midwife and/or GP.[2] Whilst Donley viewed this as a way for the medical establishment to take control, others saw it as a team approach working in the best interests of the mother and baby. A later account by journalist Cate Brett claimed that the case Donley was discussing provided 'a clear example of the sort of confusion and danger which can and does result when midwives, doctors and hospital teams failed to work as one'.[3]

Karen Guilliland, who held an ongoing leadership role within the College of Midwives, was also outspoken about protocols or guidelines for transfer from home to hospital. She argued in 1993 that they were based on an 'infuriating' paternalistic attitude that doctors knew best. She believed a 'risk list' simply meant a guaranteed income for obstetricians, and insisted that it was a bigger issue than doctors versus midwives; it was about the containment of women's rights and doctors controlling women's bodies.[4] She expanded on this in 1999, maintaining that protocols and rules were 'designed to reinforce women's dependence' and were based on the medical view that midwives could not make safe judgements.[5]

Guilliland explained that judgements around childbirth were not evidence-based in any case, but rather were 'best guesses'.⁶ Cardiotocography (CTG) monitoring of the baby's heart rate in relation to the mother's contractions to detect fetal distress was, she said, an example of this. Echoing the College of Midwives' rejection of the routine use of CTG in a 1991 position paper, Guilliland argued that CTG had 'a number of disadvantages and few advantages'. Disadvantages, she explained, included a greater likelihood of caesarean section or forceps delivery and the associated ill effects of these interventions, including an increased risk of infection and death.⁷ However, in the absence of other ways to assess fetal hypoxia during labour (where the fetus is deprived of an adequate supply of oxygen), this form of monitoring continued to be popular into the new century.⁸

The Royal New Zealand College of Obstetricians and Gynaecologists (RNZCOG) favoured establishing guidelines for transfers, for both midwives and GPs, and invited obstetrician Tony Baird to do so in the early 1990s. 'It's been done from the specialist viewpoint, so it will be shot down,' Baird told journalist David McLoughlin 'with a nervous laugh'.⁹ He was right. As Sally Abel noted in 1997, the RNZCOG recommendations for consultation with or referral to an obstetric specialist, including criteria for identification of at-risk patients, did not sit well with the College of Midwives.¹⁰

Abel described the interface of primary and secondary care as an 'ill-defined grey area' and highly contentious. GPs, as well as midwives, had to deal with transfers to hospital or to a specialist, and one GP told her that the relationship worked only after they had demonstrated a level of skill and developed working relations and mutual respect with those at the secondary or hospital level.¹¹ Midwives' ideological position on what constituted normal pregnancy and labour did little to engender trust, as Dean of the University of Otago Law School Mark Henaghan noted in his study of health professions and trust.¹² Nor did it help that midwives were vocal in claiming that guidelines were simply a ruse to control midwives and women, and an attack on midwives' competence.¹³

Particularly outspoken about referral criteria in the 1990s was GP obstetrician Allan Sutherland who had attended about 3,000 births since he graduated in 1966 and was a member of the Medical Practitioners Disciplinary Committee. Sutherland claimed to be aware of both doctors and midwives who did not know when to call for help, pointing out that it was more serious than the equivalent scenario for dietitians or physiotherapists, for example, as childbirth could be a life-or-death matter. He also believed that a non-interventionist philosophy clouded the judgement of those practising it.[14] Guilliland retorted that midwifery was safer than medical practice, and invoked the Cartwright Report in support, adding, 'Judge Cartwright underestimated the bravery it takes to speak out in the face of such organised opposition. Midwives are, however, unable to watch silently any more when they know there are alternatives which are safer.'[15]

Risk factors for the transfer of homebirths to hospital continued to be hotly debated. In 1998, three Australian researchers – Hilda Bastian, Marc Keirse and Paul Lancaster – investigated homebirths there, and concluded that the largest contributors to the excess mortality in homebirths were underestimating the risks associated with post-term birth, twin pregnancy and breech presentation, and a lack of response to fetal distress.[16] In New Zealand, the Christchurch Medical School carried out an audit of planned homebirths that ended up in hospital in 1997, and concluded that five of the seven women had risk factors that should have ruled out a homebirth. Guilliland described the audit as 'unadulterated rubbish'.[17]

Two contentious determinants for transfer to hospital were having a prior caesarean section and presentation with a breech birth. When guidelines for the new LMC system were under discussion in the mid-1990s, obstetricians worried that there would be no requirement for pregnant women who had previously undergone a caesarean section to birth in hospital. They considered this potentially dangerous. Women having a vaginal birth following a previous caesarean risk uterine rupture, a serious condition that can lead to neonatal death. Tony Baird explained that, while a woman who had already had a caesarean would not routinely be given another for her next birth, it was 'known that up to half of women who had caesareans would require another'.[18] In stark contrast, Brenda Hinton, editor of the *HBA Newsletter*, attributed any suggestion that a previous caesarean should be grounds for hospital birth to the 'anachronistic demands of medical specialists who want to regain control of childbirth'.[19] Baird responded that he was highly offended by the implication that obstetricians walked around labour wards 'just itching to perform a caesarean section'. Given the increased risks to the mother, he fumed, 'Who would want to do that to a woman unnecessarily?'[20] However, the 2006 midwifery textbook *Midwifery: Preparation for Practice* attributed the rising caesarean section rate to non-clinical factors, suggesting that the stressful hospital environment influenced decision-making and clinical judgement, 'so it is not surprising that all practitioners resorted to the use of technology'.[21]

Guidelines in 1998 specified that mothers who had had two or more caesareans should not have a vaginal birth because of the risk of uterine rupture. A later study advised that, if a woman planned a vaginal birth after having a caesarean, those responsible for her care must have confidence that resources necessary for management of a catastrophic complication were readily available.[22] Ultimately, the choice remained with the woman, as Commissioner for Health and Disability Robyn Stent explained in 1998. Choice, however, remained contingent on information given and, as the 2006 midwifery textbook explained, choice could be based on multiple considerations; for instance, it could be 'more about safeguarding and promoting emotional wellbeing and personal integrity [of the mother] than about avoiding physical damage to their bodies and babies'.[23]

Breech birth, where the baby is lying bottom first or feet first in the uterus rather than in the usual head-first position, was another situation that gave rise to conflicting views about management and consequent place of birth. Medical advice was generally elective caesarean section or induction of labour at 38 weeks' gestation. In 1996, midwife Maggie Banks wrote an article for the *College of Midwives Journal* advocating planned homebirths for breeches.[24] A domiciliary midwife since 1989, Banks explained in 1996 that for the past two and a half years she had supported women in home breech births. However, she complained, midwives who did so were 'very open to hostility and Nursing Council action from those operating in the medical model'. She protested that referral criteria 'covered a woman's physical experience without acknowledging her baby's birth as also being a social, emotional, spiritual and sensual experience'. In her view, 'To deny these aspects is to reduce a woman to pregnant uterus and her baby to a foetus needing to negotiate a hazardous route to the outside world.' In opposing hospital breech deliveries, she maintained that it was difficult, if not impossible, to ensure a calm and loving environment for a woman when she did not want to be in hospital. Her description of her local Waikato Women's Hospital would have deterred any woman from going there. She described it as:

> like a dungeon with neither windows in the rooms nor locks on the doors. There are doors on either side with utilitarian furniture and apparatus abounding. The dank atmosphere of calamity

and fear is often palpable. Midwives, nurses and doctors dress in camouflage and abattoir clothing. A paediatrician and anaesthetist are in the room for breech birth. This is not the environment that sets the scene for a gentle birth.

She cited American midwife Ina May Gaskin, who reported assisting 55 breech births, 37 at home. Gaskin's childbirth manual in fact listed pre-existing conditions that indicated when the woman should birth in hospital, and made it clear that a doctor should always attend home breech births.[25] By contrast, Banks advised that if a woman with a breech birth had all the information and decided she wanted to birth at home, or in hospital without being subjected to the medical model, she should be supported to do so. She believed this support was unlikely to come from anyone except midwives, who needed to 're-educate themselves, reclaim midwifery knowledge, have the courage to practise what they know and walk in an equal partnership with women'.[26] However, while she presented the relationship as one of partnership, she explained elsewhere that midwives were not simply to undertake any task which the woman requested, but rather to honour their 'innate promise' as midwives not to perform 'unnecessary interventions'.[27]

In 1997 a baby in Hamilton died following a home breech birth. The mother had opted for a homebirth despite knowing the baby was in a breech position, against obstetrical advice. Three midwives tried unsuccessfully to resuscitate the baby, as did the hospital specialist when summoned. The specialist subsequently complained to the Nursing Council that the interests of the baby should override the interests of the mother, including her desired place of delivery, but he was overruled. The coroner too was satisfied that the mother had made an informed choice to have a homebirth, while noting that the midwives had done nothing to dissuade her, and commenting that the immediate availability of emergency care in hospital would have greatly reduced the possibility of death.[28] Not to be deterred, the following year Banks published her book, *Breech Birth Woman-Wise*, in which she again complained that guidelines focused on the clinical situation and ignored birth as a 'social, emotional, spiritual and sensual experience'.[29] Midwife Sian Burgess, after attending the first of Banks's 'midwifery intensives', described her as 'charismatic and a real inspiration to midwifery knowledge'.[30]

## LMCs in charge

In 2001 Karen Guilliland enthused that the LMC scheme introduced in 1996 had further encouraged midwives' independence by permitting them to 'consult' obstetricians and other specialists rather than simply transferring their clients to secondary services.[31] Even if they did transfer, the 2006 textbook *Midwifery: Preparation for Practice* explained, the midwife as LMC could still 'provide primary, secondary and tertiary midwifery services . . . if she feels she has the capability'.[32] A later study on transfer from primary maternity units to secondary or tertiary hospitals stated: 'The New Zealand context, where physical transfer occurs but there is no change of primary caregiver, is unique'; legally the LMC remained in charge.[33]

Some specialists continued to question whether midwives had the knowledge and training to undertake this responsibility. Peter Jennings, a senior obstetrician and gynaecologist appointed to advise the coroner on a death in childbirth at Auckland's North Shore Hospital in 1996, believed that midwives often lacked the experience or expertise to do so. Amale Moore had died from a haemorrhage triggered by a ruptured uterus during an induced labour after her baby died inside her. Along with the midwife's 'other failures of judgement', Jennings referred to the failure to recognise Moore as a high-risk patient, and said that the midwife's method of induction was against specialist advice.[34] Professor Peter Stone, then head of obstetrics and gynaecology at the Wellington School of Medicine, also commented on this case, arguing that an LMC had to be experienced enough to know when to consult and, if they did, whether to accept the advice they received.[35]

Some midwives chose to exercise their legal rights to remain in charge of their clients in hospital. For instance, at Hutt Hospital in 1996, independent midwife Jean O'Neil did not alert the on-call obstetrician that an unborn baby was having problems for four hours; nor, according to the mother, did she inform her of the risk to the fetus. The baby, eventually delivered by caesarean section, was brain-damaged, and died five weeks later. Hutt specialist obstetrician Howard Clentworth, who delivered the baby, said the case was 'an example of a lack of consultation which was typical of some midwives'.[36] The Health and Disability Commissioner investigated the case in 1997 and found professional misconduct; it passed the case to the Nursing Council which still oversaw disciplinary procedures for midwives. The press reported that, following its inquiry in 1998, the Council cancelled O'Neil's midwifery registration, allowing her to continue practising as a nurse under supervision for a year before reapplying as a midwife. According to the press, Guilliland called the outcome 'exceptionally harsh' and 'punitive'.[37] Commenting on the case in the College's national newsletter, Guilliland stated that the most distressing aspect was that Clentworth had needlessly terrified many women and made them mistakenly believe the alternative to this 'unsafe' midwifery care was medicine and technology. 'This faith is categorically misplaced and is likely to have serious consequences for women's health and status in society,' she wrote.[38]

Leaving decision-making to the LMC, in consultation with the mother, could create a dilemma for obstetricians. In 2000 the *New Zealand Doctor* reported specialists' concerns about LMCs not following their advice. Dr Anne Sissons of Christchurch noted that the Royal Australian and New Zealand College of Obstetricians and Gynaecologists (founded in 1998, combining the Australian and New Zealand colleges) had recently sought a legal opinion following complaints that midwives were ignoring advice. The opinion stressed the importance of thorough documentation by specialists, and advised the latter to leave the labour ward so they could not be seen as complicit in the management of the labour.[39] This situation was obviously not ideal for the mother and baby.

Hospital midwives also questioned the capabilities of some independent midwives who accompanied their clients into hospital. Addressing this in 2002, a group of midwives from Auckland's Middlemore Hospital delivery unit, asked, 'What is our role when we find ourselves in the delivery room as support person [to an independent midwife] seeing practice that we consider less than safe?'[40] Deborah Earl and her colleagues cited the specific example of an emergency transfer. The midwife accompanying the woman consulted the hospital obstetrician, who asked her to 'put in an IV line, send off bloods, start antibiotics, provide adequate pain relief, start syntocinon and follow the primigravida guidelines in the running of the syntocinon'. Earl said the midwife 'comes to me, as charge nurse, very anxious about [those instructions]', and needing 'a little refreshing' on how to use this medical equipment. Earl said this was not uncommon in the delivery unit. She also related a story of being asked by an LMC to review a CTG trace that the latter was concerned about. Earl advised calling a consultant, but the midwife declined. Complaining about the lack of clear guidelines, Earl and her colleagues wrote:

> It is said to us that professionally and ethically we are responsible for any situation at which we are present because there is a 'duty of care' and yet how does that 'pan out' in practice? If we, as charge midwives, were so concerned about the CTG that we called the consultant to come in and review it – where would we stand? We do this on occasions but it is a horrible position in which to be put.[41]

The 1990 Act had given midwives the authority to prescribe medicines. This had been subject to much debate in Parliament when it was included in a supplementary order paper (see pp. 122–24), but MPs were persuaded that midwives received enough training in pharmacology in their combined nursing and midwifery training (even though nurses at that time did not have prescribing rights) and that midwives did not believe in prescribing much anyway. Allowing midwives to prescribe drugs continued to cause consternation among some health professionals. In November 1990, Evan Begg, a senior lecturer in clinical pharmacology at Christchurch School of Medicine, referred to the extensive training doctors underwent before being allowed to prescribe, including a six-year undergraduate course followed by postgraduate training and supervision. He explained that the pharmacology of pregnancy and lactation was extremely complex, and doctors were generally advised to get specialist help when prescribing in these areas. He did not believe that midwives currently received sufficient training to enable 'rational, safe and effective prescribing'. Among other things, he was concerned about their ability to assess the safety to the fetus of medicines that might be prescribed to pregnant women even for minor complaints.[42]

Responding to what she described as an 'orchestrated effort to challenge and discredit the prescribing ability of midwives' in late 1990, Judi Strid on behalf of the Federation of Women's Health Councils reiterated to Minister of Health Simon Upton that the College of Midwives promoted drug-free childbirth anyway, focusing on normal pregnancy and birth, and prescribing only when 'absolutely necessary and as little as possible'. She asked him to 'endorse the ability and expertise of midwives to those who have difficulty with what midwifery practice actually involves'.[43] This was not going to be relitigated. The Health Department information pamphlet made it clear that, though there was no defined list of drugs, prescribing (including of the controlled drug pethidine) was to be confined to antenatal, intrapartum and postnatal care.[44] It stated that midwives were not to prescribe for underlying medical conditions such as asthma or hypertension, and nor were they to prescribe medicines such as antibiotics. However, in 1995 the College of Midwives challenged this restriction, and the Ministry acknowledged that there was no legal basis for restricting the prescription of antibiotics.[45]

In a 2002 consensus statement, the College of Midwives agreed that midwives would prescribe only for conditions commonly associated with uncomplicated pregnancy, labour and the postnatal period up to six weeks after the birth of the baby.[46] However, this remained a grey area, as is clear from the 2006 textbook for midwives. In a chapter on pharmacology and prescribing, the head of midwifery and a senior lecturer in midwifery at the Auckland University of Technology (AUT) advised caution. For instance, they admonished that if narcotics were used in labour, 'the midwife must have the equipment and skills necessary to cope with the effects of this medication'. They advised that not all pregnancy-related conditions were suitable for treatment by midwives, and stressed the importance of midwives not prescribing 'outside their scope of practice'. Midwives should not prescribe antibiotics for neonates, for example, and prescribing paracetamol should be left to medical practitioners because of the immaturity of the neonate liver. In a section on adverse reactions, they cautioned that midwives needed to be aware of the local policy for reporting adverse reactions of medicines and 'to promptly refer women experiencing any adverse effects to a medical practitioner'. Midwives, they stressed, needed to have a 'low threshold for referral'.[47] The fact these authors felt the need to issue such cautions indicates it was an ongoing concern, but it was not subject to regulation. A legal guide to nurses and midwives explained that there was 'no specific list of medicines which a midwife may or may not prescribe, nor is there any legal definition provided of the terms "antenatal", "intrapartum" or "postnatal" care. Therefore, it is left to midwives to use their professional judgement as to what is best for their clients.'[48]

Under the new LMC system, midwives carried a heavy responsibility for their clients, yet there was also mounting concern about their ability to assume that responsibility and the effects of their ongoing disdain for the so-called medical model. What was being taught in the new midwifery schools was therefore key to the future of midwifery in New Zealand and to public confidence in the system.

## Direct-entry midwifery training

Direct-entry midwifery training, legislated for in 1990, was firmly rooted in the midwifery model of childbirth, or what midwives also described as 'midwifery knowledge'. While postgraduate midwifery diploma programmes for nurses were still available in the early 1990s, in 1991 Karen Guilliland and Sally Pairman urged their immediate abolition in favour of the new courses.[49] As the Save the Midwives Direct Entry Midwifery Task Force had done, they argued that, to be effective midwives, students needed to be socialised into their profession, and this was more difficult if they had prior nurse training.[50] Pairman explained in 1994 that, with direct-entry, students did not have to 'unlearn nursing philosophies and behaviour but are instead grounded in the New Zealand model of midwifery'.[51]

Three-year direct-entry courses started at the Auckland Institute of Technology (called AUT from 2000) and in Dunedin (Otago Polytechnic) in 1992, each with about 20 students.[52] With favourable assessments of these 'experimental' courses in 1993 and 1995, other institutions followed. Programmes at Waikato and Wellington polytechnics began in 1996, and Christchurch Polytechnic in 1997. The one-year diploma courses following nurse training were discontinued in Otago (1992), Christchurch (1996), Waikato and Wellington (both 1998), and Auckland (1999).[53] The Auckland direct-entry course, which started as a diploma, was converted into a Bachelor of Midwifery in 1995.

AIT programme leader Jackie Gunn reported on the first intake of 20 students in 1992. When Joan Donley was invited to meet them, she noted that a number of the students had had homebirths and that some had been members of the Save the Midwives Direct Entry Midwifery Task Force.[54] As programme leader at Otago Polytechnic, Sally Pairman reported on the 20 student entrants there. She commented that they had been waiting to do midwifery for a long time and were therefore very enthusiastic. About half already had children, whom they sometimes brought to class.[55] Like the Direct Entry Midwifery Task Force before them, the programme leaders valued life experience, as evidenced by the students' age distribution. Of the 180 direct-entry midwives in practice in 2000 (all of whom had been qualified for less than five years), 66.7% were between the ages of 30 and 50, and 33% were over the age of 40.[56] When Pairman reflected on the first intake as they were about to graduate in 1994, she commended the students on their 'maturity, wisdom and life experience'.[57]

## The practice of midwifery and the 'midwifery model' in the 1990s

In her report on these first graduates, Pairman deferred to Otago student Annabel Farry:

> In learning about midwifery we have all learned a great deal about ourselves . . . This constant questioning and self-analysis which has become part of our lives has brought us to a better understanding of ourselves. We have had to face our own racism, sexism, homophobia, and do our best to move out of these old frameworks and into new ways of seeing the world . . . The modern philosophy of midwifery is revolutionary.[58]

Learning about themselves was indeed integral to direct-entry midwifery training. The 'learning outcomes' for the chapter entitled 'Understanding world views for midwifery' in the 2006 textbook, for example, included the ability to 'discuss discourses of the self'; and the chapter included Marxist and feminist theories of health, and 'the postmodern self'.[59] Pairman said that she and colleagues watched with delight as more and more of their students left the course with 'confidence' and 'political awareness'.[60]

Farry referred to midwifery's three principles of partnership, continuity of care and informed choice, promising that, 'if we emerge from this course understanding nothing else, these three concepts will be with us until death'. They were, she said, 'like an umbrella extending over the entire course'. Indeed, the topic of 'partnership' occupied almost half of the 600-page 2006 textbook.[61] Pairman reaffirmed in 1999 that partnership 'underpins the philosophy of all pre-registration midwifery education programmes'.[62] The theoretical component of the new courses bothered at least one member of the Nursing Council in the early 1990s who believed it was too extensive, given that students had no prior nurse training.[63]

'Midwifery Knowledge' was taught in each of the three years at Otago Polytechnic, providing students the chance to reflect on information that midwives had previously shared orally.[64] Farry explained that the course also had 'a strong grounding in practical experience', teaching students to be clinically competent health professionals, having spent time in the community and in hospital during their third year. But she also stated that many found the hospital a challenging place: 'Not only because we are expected to apply our practical knowledge, but also because we feel committed to defend all that we have come to believe in as a result of our course.'[65] The hospital setting did not sit comfortably with the midwifery model for these students. One of the four recommended readings for Bronwen Pelvin's chapter in the 2006 textbook, 'Life Skills for Midwifery Practice', was prominent UK homebirth midwife Caroline Flint's *Sensitive Midwifery* (1986), which also featured in the reference list for Pairman and Judith McAra-Couper's chapter on 'Theoretical Frameworks for Midwifery Practice'.[66] Flint's book sought to explain 'how to provide gentle, non-interventionist, non-high technology births', and one reviewer commented that the ideas in *Sensitive Midwifery* reflected 'a rather idealistic and unproblematic approach which is not reality for many'.[67]

In 1996, the College's journal featured an article by two Otago Polytechnic lecturers on the importance of bioscience in midwifery education. While the authors cited a student who worried that learning bioscience would make her nervous about what could go wrong, they believed bioscience had a place in midwifery practice and needed to be more closely integrated with the acquisition of practical experience during the programme. They explained that bioscience at Otago Polytechnic was allocated 'a relatively small proportion of this course's teaching hours (320 over two years)' and was not formally taught in the third year when students spent the largest proportion of their time in clinical environments.[68]

There was no provision for hospital internships or mentoring following graduation, as there was for some other health practitioners. After the first graduates qualified in 1994, some hospitals insisted that they undergo mentoring before they were granted access to the hospital. For instance, in Auckland, the right to attend their clients in hospital was agreed for midwives once they had been mentored for 40 cases – the same as for GPs. As Abel noted, this did not sit well with the College of Midwives. While the latter did not oppose the concept of mentoring, it envisaged a partnership in which the mentor offered support and did not attempt to control practice. Anything else, they explained, would suggest that the midwifery training was inadequate. They complained that what the hospitals wanted was 'an expert/novice relationship based on the hierarchical internship relationship which was a feature of medicine and nursing and not a part of the midwifery model'.[69] Under the LMC system introduced in 1996, hospitals could not restrict access in this way.[70]

In 2001, midwife Dawn Holland contributed an article to the College journal's 'Practice Wisdom' column on mentoring under the midwifery model. She claimed that the knowledge and experience a midwife gained through mentoring would 'empower her and she will move on to the third stage, that of emancipation. Through emancipation she will create a new understanding for herself of the essence of midwifery unconstrained by her previous social context.'[71] Citing American educator Laurent Daloz, she declared, 'Mentors are infused with magic and play a key part in our transformation . . . Mentors give us the magic that allows us to enter the darkness: a talisman to protect us from the evil spells, a gem of wise advice, a map, and sometimes simply courage.'[72]

Pairman said of the 1994 graduates that they were the first midwifery students in New Zealand to be educated to practise independently immediately after graduation.[73] Yet not all chose this path. A survey of the 180 practising direct-entry midwives conducted in 2000 found that only 37.7% were self-employed, whilst 35.6% identified their work type as 'midwifery – core facility' (a secondary or tertiary hospital).[74] Many had not become fully independent-minded midwives after all. However, in 1999, a third-year student at Christchurch Polytechnic went to the other extreme and failed to notify her midwife mentor when a pregnant woman in their care was about to give birth, and attended the birth alone, fortunately without mishap.[75] She had apparently had taken on board the lesson of the midwifery model that childbirth was a normal life event, believing her presence alone was good enough. As Donley had famously told her mothers, 'It's your tea party, I'm just there to pour the tea.'[76]

## Midwifery education, Māori and cultural safety

In 1993 there were 1,547 midwives working throughout the country, but only 24 of them were Māori.[77] One of the arguments in favour of direct-entry training had been that it would attract into midwifery Māori women who would then care for Māori mothers. This did not transpire in the 1990s. Of the 180 direct-entry graduates practising in 2000, 26 (14.4%) defined themselves as Māori, but only four of those worked as Māori health providers.[78] At the 1994 hui at which Nga Maia was established (see p. 155), Waikato Polytechnic agreed to offer a direct-entry midwifery course addressing the needs of Māori women and including Māori birthing practices.[79] Yet, as Hope Tupara, of Ngāi Te Rangihouhiri and Ngāi Tāmanuhiri, a direct-entry graduate from 1994 and a self-employed midwife in Levin, complained in the College's journal in 2001, 'Partnership has not secured a place for Māori within the midwifery education process because we are not equally contributing participants in our own development.' She argued that midwifery education would be enhanced only by positioning a midwifery programme in a Māori wānanga (tertiary college).[80]

One of the core principles of the new direct-entry training courses for all trainees was the concept of cultural safety. Training in cultural safety involved reflecting on one's own cultural identity and how this shaped one's practice in order to more effectively care for an individual or family from another culture.[81] It was the brainchild of Māori nursing educator Irihapeti Ramsden, who had trained as a nurse in the 1960s and began to talk about what she called cultural safety in health services from the 1980s, completing her doctoral thesis on this in 2002.[82] She was a major influence on the midwifery profession as well as nursing. A keynote speaker at College of Midwives' conferences in 1994 and 2002, she was made an honorary member of the College in appreciation of her teachings and advice. In the 1990s the concept of cultural safety was officially incorporated into the New Zealand nursing and midwifery curricula, accounting for 20% of the content of state registration examinations.

Part of the teaching of cultural safety in the midwifery programmes appeared to include instilling an awareness of colonial oppression. In 2001 an AUT midwifery lecturer Anne Barlow wrote an article on the College's review process, including a case study of 'cultural adequacy' based on interviewing six Māori midwives who had undergone review. In her analysis Barlow repeated one midwife's claim that the 1908 [sic] Tohunga Suppression Act forbade burial of the placenta, and outlawed Māori midwives and breastfeeding.[83] This elicited an angry response from Lis Ellison-Loschmann from the Centre for Public Health Research, Massey University Wellington, one of three Māori midwives who met with the College of Midwives in 1994 to discuss Māori representation on the College. Noting that Ramsden had already refuted this allegation, Ellison-Loschmann said she was aware of people teaching in midwifery programmes who had repeated such myths on a number of occasions. It was very disturbing that 'this level of misunderstanding and inaccuracy regarding important legislation . . . [was] being taught to student midwives'.[84]

Barlow replied that she had not undertaken a detailed examination of every piece of legislation affecting New Zealand midwifery, and that she was happy to stand corrected 'on the finer points of this Act'. However, these were hardly finer points; outlawing of Māori midwifery and breastfeeding, and forbidding the burying of placenta would have been significant intrusions into tikanga Māori. In fact, 30 years after the named Act, a Committee of Inquiry into Maternity Services stressed that Māori were 'still confined in the Native fashion with the assistance of their own folk – their relations, or Native "midwives"'; this, it said, was 'effective and, as a rule, applied with reasonable skill and restraint'.[85] Nor was there anything in the brief 1907 Tohunga Suppression Act that could be interpreted as banning breastfeeding and burial of the placenta. But Barlow argued that, regardless of their accuracy, these views were 'widely believed and have influenced midwifery practice for some Māori midwives'.[86] This was surely reason to correct them rather than perpetuate a gross sense of racial injustice.

As part of the celebration of the centenary of the 1904 Midwives Act which had introduced midwifery training, nursing historian Pamela Wood explored myths about midwifery's past in the College's journal. One of these was the belief that early-twentieth-century legislation had prohibited Māori women from breastfeeding their babies. Wood explained that those who perpetuated this myth referred to 'the Native Health Act 1908'. There was no such Act, but she said, 'Sadly, this myth has already become embedded as fact in teaching material, academic theses, research reports and published articles, even within this journal'.[87] Others, equally careless with historical facts, also misrepresented past legislation. For instance, in 2005 Sally Pairman referred to the 1904 Midwives Act, which aimed to reduce infant mortality through improving childbirth services. The Act was passed, she wrote, because: 'It was feared that Māori and other non-white races would outnumber the British settlers and gain advantage in the struggle for resources and power in the new colony.'[88] This is historically inaccurate; whilst there was anti-Asian prejudice at that time, there was no suggestion that Māori would outnumber British settlers.

Māori themselves were not silent in debates on cultural sensitivity. In 2001 Hope Tupara explained how, after being exposed to 'many realities of Māori women in the community', she began to question the accuracy of information she had been taught about Māori during her training. She gave the example of how variously Māori responded when they were asked if they wished to take home their whenua (placenta): reactions ranged from disgust to the making of formal and meticulous arrangements. That some women would decline the practice was evidenced in the account of a Māori woman, Helen Mountain Harte, who had given birth at National Women's Hospital in 1983. She was attended by a Māori doctor, Colin Mantell, who asked her if she wanted to take the whenua home; she politely declined. He persisted, saying he would put it in the freezer until someone came to pick it up, but she again declined. She said that her mother Emere Kaa, an early Māori public health nurse born in 1901 and still alive, 'would have been horrified to have buried the placenta'. Nor, with the exception of one niece, Harte said, did the next generation of her family undertake this practice.[89]

Another example of the wide range of Māori women's experience concerned whānau involvement in the labour and birth process. Tupara pointed out that some Māori women might for personal and situational reasons choose to have no whānau involvement, whilst others might choose to have a large group of family and friends in attendance. She attributed the stereotypes in the midwifery literature to the fact that it was not written by Māori. For instance, she disapproved of Donley's characterisation of what the latter called 'a typical Maori lay midwife'.[90] Citing Māori Studies Professor Mason Durie, Tupara made it clear that Māori women were as diverse as any other population group.[91]

Māori midwifery Master's student Reena Kainamu of Ngāpuhi also cited Durie in pointing out that Māori came from diverse backgrounds. While she believed it was important for health services to collaborate with Māori communities, 'traditional or otherwise', and to be respectful of Māori values and beliefs, she also thought that Māori women were no different from any other women in wanting to have a safe birth.[92]

Teaching in the new midwifery programmes appeared to be politically motivated, whether in relation to colonisation or in opposition to the so-called medical model, an unusual focus for a health professional training programme. The final section of this chapter will focus on the disdain for technology encompassed within the midwifery model more broadly.

## The midwifery model and distrust of modern technology

The midwifery model after 1990 represented a holistic approach to maternity, just as the homebirth movement had before it. The 2006 textbook advised students that, 'because of a greater appreciation of holism displayed by complementary therapists', such as acupuncturists, osteopaths, homeopathists and naturopaths, 'many midwives find working alongside these practitioners very fruitful and mutually satisfying for all involved'.[93] Allied to this holistic approach and a preference for alternative therapies was an ongoing distrust of modern medicine and technology. This section explores that distrust in relation to ultrasound scans, oxytocin, vitamin K and immunisation, all of which had become standard practice within maternity and neonatal care by this time.

Donley continued the campaign against ultrasound in pregnancy which she had launched in the 1980s (see p. 26), at a time when major medical bodies were endorsing it and women were demanding it. In a political commentary in the College's journal in 1990, she warned that those most likely to receive it were 'at the bottom of the socioeconomic heap', implying they were experimental guinea pigs; and she claimed that the manufacturers of this 'very lucrative technology' funded a pressure group who attacked the homebirth movement.[94] Thus she continued to suggest that the use of ultrasound was a capitalist and patriarchal conspiracy, adding that Marsden Wagner, an ardent homebirth advocate, did not support its routine use. The 1990 HBA conference passed a remit endorsing this opposition, and the College of Midwives rejected its routine use a year later.[95]

There was no shortage of literature within the anti-science lobby opposing ultrasound in the 1990s. A 1993 article in the *Yale Journal of Law and Feminism* referred to scientists 'theorising' that ultrasound could cause childhood cancer.[96] In 1994 the HBA reported on overseas studies linking ultrasound to delayed speech development and dyslexia, and in 2001 the Auckland Maternity Services Consumer Council claimed ultrasound scans were linked to fetal brain damage, left-handedness, learning disabilities and epilepsy.[97] In their history of obstetric ultrasound, Nicholson and Fleming pointed out that while it was impossible to prove a negative, ultrasound had been used on millions of fetuses and 'many extensive trawls for adverse effects have yielded no convincing evidence of harm'. They stated:

> The role played by the issue of the safety of ultrasound in the feminist critique of obstetrics would seem to be a symbolic one. Raising the possibility of danger allows the expression of deeper disquiets about the encroachment of technology into the realms of pregnancy and birth.[98]

This certainly held true for Donley, who also warned in 1996 that pregnancy testing including ultrasound could cause midwives to 'slide back into the role of politically unaware and inert doctors' handmaidens'.[99]

Giving oxytocic drugs to mothers and vitamin K to babies were both opposed by the homebirth movement, and this continued under the midwifery model in the 1990s. In her memoirs, Australian obstetrician Caroline de Costa wrote that giving women an oxytocic to contract the uterus and prevent haemorrhaging after birth was 'normal midwifery practice', adding that if women decided to go without because they wanted a natural birth, this was their choice. However, she said, birth attendants were obliged to inform them of the possibility of postpartum haemorrhage (PPH) and the 'natural' consequences of bleeding to death. She also noted that while this discussion was taking place, several women somewhere in the world who had no access to skilled care would be dying of PPH.[100] In the 1990s, Tony Baird commented on the different viewpoints of obstetricians and some midwives on this issue, explaining, 'We've got to spend time now trying to convince a woman who has been told by a midwife that she doesn't need the injection [oxytocin] that she does, and in the meantime she is in danger.'[101] Donley was one of those midwives who told mothers to resist. She said in 1994 that she hardly ever used an oxytocic, preferring a homeopathic or herbal remedy.[102] In 1997 consumer advocate Judi Strid complained that some midwives continued to routinely give interventions that 'should be optional', such as ecbolics for the third stage of labour (such as oxytocin) and vitamin K injections for the baby.[103]

Giving babies vitamin K had been routine in hospitals since the 1940s (see p. 26). The 1992 *HBA Newsletter* reported that almost two-thirds of babies born at home did not receive vitamin K; by 1995 it was still about half.[104] Donley said in 1994 that she had never given a baby vitamin K, preferring herbal alternatives.[105] In 1998 the College of Midwives joined other professional bodies in a consensus statement specifying that: 'It is the responsibility of LMC to discuss Vitamin K prophylaxis and ensure that parents are aware of the recommendation that <u>all babies receive Vitamin K prophylaxis</u>.'[106] Informing parents of the recommendation was not the same as advising it, however, and Donley did not advise it. An account of one antenatal class in 2000 indicates that it continued to be questioned in other quarters too, and a decade later at least one LMC was found not to have administered it – an omission picked up after a disastrous result (see p. 220).[107] New Zealand was not alone; a 2006 article on vitamin K administration in Australia from 1993 to 2017 referred to three neonatal deaths from intracranial haemorrhage that were associated with home delivery and parental refusal of vitamin K.[108]

## The practice of midwifery and the 'midwifery model' in the 1990s

Providing information rather than advice remained core to the midwifery model in relation to immunisation as well. In the 1990s the HBA continued to promote anti-immunisation literature, with its newsletter advertising Hilary Butler's publications, and subscription details for the anti-immunisation Immunisation Awareness Society.[109] It also offered for hire to individuals or groups a video that linked AIDS to immunisation.[110] A 1994 newsletter reprinted the section on immunisation from *A Guide to Healthy Pregnancy: The Auckland Home Birth Association 1993*; the first reference was to the Immunisation Awareness Society.[111] In 1995 editor Brenda Hinton drew attention to the fact that 'a considerable percentage of our members choose not to vaccinate their children'.[112]

The HBA was separate from the College of Midwives, of course, but it had representation on the College's national committee, and Joan Donley was a major link. In 1994, the College published an article by Donley on immunisation written in response to a Public Health Commission immunisation report. Donley began by questioning the nature of informed consent, given that the report labelled the Health Department's *Immunisation Handbook* as factual and anti-immunisation material as opinions or beliefs. She suggested health officials carry out a literature review instead of 'putting a guilt trip on women' who failed to immunise their babies. She argued that women who had not been vaccinated but who had contracted measles carried high levels of antibodies and passed these on to the fetus, affording them lifelong protection. She also claimed serious side-effects of the measles vaccine, introduced in 1969, including ataxia, seizures, aseptic meningitis, hemiparesis, and 'demyelination' affecting a child's neurologic development.[113]

Her article contained 14 references; they were not listed but were available from the author on request, meaning her statements were unverified in the publication.[114] The space at the end of the article was instead used to advertise an international symposium organised by the Immunisation Awareness Society entitled 'The Vaccination Dilemma', to be held in Auckland the following April. The conference was to include talks from 'eminent speakers from around the world on issues such as the safety and effectiveness of vaccines, the role of pharmaceutical companies in research, the relationship between vaccination and cot death, and the international move to compulsory vaccination'.[115]

The next issue of the journal carried a response to Donley's article from Dr Gillian Durham, chief executive of the Public Health Commission. Durham wrote that she hoped Donley's views did not represent the College's position because of the flaws in her arguments. She refuted Donley's claims relating to a recent measles epidemic, the effectiveness of the measles vaccine and side-effects. Above all, in Durham's view:

> It is a matter of grave concern that a midwives' professional organisation is happy to selectively use the medical literature to exaggerate the risks of immunisation, downplay its benefits, and apparently to oppose immunisation which has the endorsement of all major scientific bodies as being one of the most cost-effective means of preventing disease.

She reminded them that midwives played a crucial role in preparing mothers for their newborn children, including their immunisation.[116]

Donley's response in the same issue included another 23 references, as opposed to Durham's nine, again available upon request, which was unusual for the journal.[117] In her piece, Donley cited many small studies, mainly from America, questioning immunisation for rubella and measles, but her main argument was that Durham misunderstood the role of the midwife. She cited Wagner's statement that 'the midwifery model is the social model which sees life as the solution', whilst the 'medical reductionist approach . . . sees life as a problem, full of risks and in almost constant danger'. Whereas medicine aimed for social control, 'the holistic midwifery model includes the social, psychological and spiritual components of technologies'. Donley thus tied anti-immunisation to the midwifery model.

College national coordinator Karen Guilliland also responded to Durham. She explained that, unlike doctors, midwives did not see their role as advisors, but rather as having 'responsibility for providing full information, options and choices for women and families' to encourage them to take responsibility. Yet she made it clear that the College was not convinced by the case for immunisation. In 'the absence of clear unequivocal research', she explained, the College operated in a 'social and wellness model'. Her letter was followed by an editor's note announcing the forthcoming Immunisation Awareness Society conference, which was also included in the 'Coming Events' section of the journal.[118]

Caroline Crawford provided a detailed report of this symposium for the College, noting that the views outlined did not necessarily reflect her own opinions or those of other midwives, and that further study would be needed to make an informed decision. At the symposium, she wrote, immunisation was described as the 'black box' of modern medicine, one which, in general, health professionals did not think (or dare) to question. However, she continued, 15 of the 16 speakers did just that, questioning the efficacy and safety of vaccination; Durham was the exception. Crawford provided a five-page summary of the speakers' objections to immunisation.[119]

The *College of Midwives Journal* also became a platform for the ideas of anti-vaccinationist Erwin Alber, a Swiss-born translator and English teacher, who set up the Vaccination Information Network from his base in Kaeo, Northland. Alber's first letter to the editor, 'Vaccination Information', appeared in 1995, in response to Durham's letter. He exhorted his readers to pay attention to the views of Donley and Viera Scheibner, one of the speakers at the symposium who called vaccination 'the epitome of ignorance and unscientific approach to illness' and the leading cause of cot death. Alber applauded Dr Ulric Williams' book *Hints for Healthy Living*, published 50 years earlier, citing his view that 'modern medicine is the most lunatic system ever devised by man to his own undoing except the financial system, of which it is a part'.[120] A naturopath, Williams had been expelled from the New Zealand Branch of the British Medical Association in the 1930s partly because of his anti-vaccination advocacy.[121]

The same issue of the journal advertised for sale an audiotape on vaccination entitled 'For an Informed Choice'. Speakers included Dr Lisa Lovett (an Australian chiropractor who had written an anti-vaccination book), Dr Eva Snead (an Argentinian-born physician who linked AIDS to vaccines), anthropologist Wendy Lydall (who wrote *Raising a Child Vaccine Free*), and Scheibner. The tape, which could be ordered from the Vaccination Information Network, listed 'some stunning statistics on vaccines and their effects, connections between vaccination, SIDS [sudden infant death syndrome], asthma, AIDS, brain damage and other chronic diseases'.[122]

In April 1996 the journal published another letter from Alber entitled 'Vaccination Awareness' which, among other things, linked vaccination to SIDS and autism.[123] In the same issue, he contributed an article which detailed a German anti-vaccination campaign he had attended with Dr Gerhard Buchwald, medical advisor to the German Parent Association for Support of Vaccine Damaged Children who had spoken at Auckland's Immunisation Awareness Society symposium the previous year. Alber wrote that, if the conclusions of Buchwald and other 'independent researchers' were correct, then 'it may well be the health department policies (*Immunisation 2000*) are the most serious threats to our children's health and well-being, not measles or polio etc.'.[124]

The next issue carried yet another letter from Alber, alongside one from the Department of Nursing and Midwifery, Otago Polytechnic, thanking the journal for passing on the book *Immunisation: Theory vs Practice* by Neil Miller (1996), described as 'another valuable contribution to the debates on vaccination which has been placed in the library where students and practitioners alike can access it'.[125] A midwife from Otago Polytechnic reviewed this book in the same issue. She claimed that Miller did not speak for or against vaccination but aimed to present information so that parents could make an informed choice. However, she added, 'The information he does present is exclusively against vaccination', and that '[s]ome of the language Miller uses is quite emotive'; chapter headings included 'Human Sacrifices', 'Ploys', and 'Genocide'. She concluded, 'If you have never questioned the validity of national vaccination programmes, this may well be a useful book . . .'[126]

In 1999, Alber wrote directly to Guilliland, telling her that independent medical researchers had denounced vaccination as a genocidal practice, a 'huge biological experiment along the lines of biological warfare against civilians (targeting babies and children!)', and a 'particularly nasty form of child abuse and a crime against humanity'. He sent her a copy of a video from well-known American anti-vaccinationist Dr L. Horowitz. He claimed to be disappointed that Guilliland had refuted accusations by Nelson GP Graham Loveridge that some midwives were not promoting immunisation and that some even gave out anti-immunisation information. Alber was further disappointed that Guilliland had told the press that the College actively supported immunisation. He said, 'It is after all midwives' job to deliver babies and not promote controversial pharmaceutical products a growing number of parents and midwives consider damaging and objectionable.' He added, 'I know (and appreciate) that a number of midwives who subscribe to our "anti-immunisation" newsletter pass it (or information in it) to families under their care.'[127]

Despite Alber's extreme stance, Guilliland thanked him for the video, which she said the College was happy to add to its library. She even felt the need to defend her conciliatory response to Loveridge, explaining that she had written in response to doctors' inflammatory comments about midwives in the press. She told Alber, 'As you point out midwives do have a range of opinions and as their professional voice the College is obliged to reflect that position. As with other controversial issues the College takes the view that an <u>informed</u> person has the right to their own decisions in such matters. The College's position therefore gives both sides of the argument.'[128]

The journal continued to publish letters from Alber; in June 2000 Alber called vaccination 'a barbaric and insane practice which could only have been invented by male scientists devoid of the female principle'.[129] The next issue carried a letter applauding his description of the female principle.[130] However, it also elicited an angry response from Elaine Boyd, nurse consultant at the Immunisation Advisory Centre which had been set up at the University of Auckland in 1996 to counter what it considered misleading claims by the anti-vaccination lobby. Boyd urged readers who wanted evidence-based information to contact the Centre. Coralie Zimmer, immunisation coordinator for Northland Health, also wrote criticising Alber and advocated embracing both the female principle and the scientific approach.[131]

College leaders' claimed that they were simply in favour of informed consent and providing information, but a decade of questioning authority, and the support for the anti-vaccination lobby in the *College of Midwives Journal* and elsewhere, did appear to have an influence on midwives' attitudes. For instance, a nurse-midwife at Dargaville Hospital in 1999 commented that, despite the legal requirement that LMCs promote immunisation, only two babies from 20 recent independent midwife-assisted births there were immunised, and this was because they happened to come to the hospital.[132] The 1999 National Health Committee Review also commented on the declining rates of immunisation at six weeks of age, and explained that it had 'heard, from a variety of sources, that some maternity providers [were] not providing objective and adequate information on immunisation to allow informed decision-making by parents'. Worryingly, it reported a North Health's 1996 immunisation coverage survey which found that children who did not commence the immunisation schedule 'on time' were almost 17 times less likely to be immunised at two years. It advocated 'active monitoring of providers on the immunisation information' they were giving to expectant and new parents.[133]

## Conclusion

In the 1990s, under the ongoing influence of Joan Donley, the views of the homebirth movement persisted within the midwifery hierarchy in the College of Midwives. When challenged on their views, the College responded that decisions ultimately rested with the mother. Informed consent formed the main argument in favour of distributing anti-immunisation material to pregnant women, but the opposition to immunisation was based on a broad distrust of what they described as the medical model. Donley tied anti-immunisation to the midwifery model, along with opposition to other forms of technology. The midwifery model also resisted establishing protocols for transfer to specialists and hospitals, based on the argument that these simply reinforced medical control.

The midwifery model did not enjoy the support of all midwives. Many hospital and other midwives who chose to work with doctors in the shared schemes developed in the late 1990s remained sceptical of its tenets and its opposition to the 'medical model'. The 'medical model' and 'midwifery model' were in fact not terms commonly used by doctors and those midwives, but were terms favoured by the College of Midwives leaders and educators themselves; these concepts had emerged from the wider sociological critiques of modern high-tech medicine in the 1970s and had been part of the homebirth package.

The midwifery model, with its anti-science stance, caused anger and frustration amongst some hospital midwives and others who saw midwifery as part of a health service which had as its primary goal a healthy outcome. Chapters 10–12 will explore whether these issues were resolved when, as the new century dawned, midwives as LMCs became the norm. This, too, was when midwives finally got their own professional overseeing body, the Midwifery Council New Zealand, set up in 2004, as midwifery leader Sally Pairman explained at the time, 'to ensure quality and standards [were] maintained'.[134]

# TEN

## *The new century: 'When things go wrong'*

THE 2003 HEALTH PRACTITIONERS Competence Assurance Act provided a framework for the regulation of health practitioners to ensure public safety. While midwives were barely mentioned in the parliamentary debates, *Midwifery: Preparation for Practice* described the Act as 'highly significant for New Zealand midwives' because it established 'what may be the world's first solely midwifery council – a council completely separate from nursing and medicine'. Its establishment 'removed the final barrier to full professional autonomy for midwives'.[1]

The Midwifery Council New Zealand, set up in 2004, took responsibility for ensuring midwives' competency to provide care for women and babies during pregnancy, childbirth and the postpartum period up to six weeks. It developed competencies for entry to the Register of Midwives, detailing the skills, knowledge and attitudes expected of a midwife. The first of these stated that the midwife was to work in partnership with women throughout the maternity experience. The second referred to applying 'comprehensive theoretical and scientific knowledge' and technical skills to ensure effective and safe care. The emphasis was on midwives facilitating the physiological processes of childbirth, which they were to balance with a judicious use of intervention when appropriate. The third competency stated that midwifery was 'a primary health service in that it recognises childbirth as a significant and normal life event. The midwife is therefore responsible for supporting this process through health promotion, education, and information sharing, across all settings.'[2]

These competencies emphasised partnership, and birth as a normal life event, but they also referred to scientific knowledge and technical skills, striving to provide safe midwifery care. This appeared a sensible compromise on the issues which had caused such friction in the 1990s between the midwifery model and the medical model. Marie Burgess, a highly experienced nurse and midwife who specialised in legal-ethical matters for health professionals, described the Health Practitioners Competence Assurance Act itself as 'perhaps the most significant legislation for nurses and midwives since registration began in the early 1900s', in that it introduced new checks and balances such as annual practising certificates and competence review processes. As Burgess explained in 2008, the Act's focus on 'protecting the health and safety of the public by ensuring that mechanisms are in place to monitor the competence and fitness to practise of practitioners, and the disciplinary processes to ensure accountability that it put in place, should ensure that the public is better served than was the case in the past'.[3]

Views on whether this protection was subsequently achieved were, however, divided. A 2012 *New Zealand Herald* article referred to Hamilton coroner Gordon Matenga's 'explosive criticism of the midwifery profession's philosophy and training' which he believed contributed to adverse outcomes.[4] Others, by contrast, continued to see New Zealand as a world leader in midwifery; Sharron Cole, a lay member of the Midwifery Council who subsequently became its chief executive, wrote in the College of Midwives' 2010 history that New Zealand midwives provided 'a primary maternity service that is amongst, if not the best, in the world'.[5]

This chapter explores the grounds for persistent tensions and divergent views. It does so from the perspective of those tasked with investigating adverse outcomes: coroners who examined deaths, and health and disability commissioners who received and adjudicated consumer complaints.

## Coroners' reports 2005–2015

Maternity services received considerable media attention in 2005 when Wellington coroner Garry Evans reported on two neonatal deaths and issued a series of recommendations to the government, as allowed under the Coroner's

Act. When Evans retired in 2015, the *Dominion Post*'s coverage of his work in this role since 1997 referred specifically to this 2005 report, along with another relating to the deaths of a mother and baby during childbirth a decade later. In both reports Evans deemed the deaths preventable. The article referred to the 'unflinching pursuit of knowledge and answers, and the refusal to be cowed by authority' that had defined his term, adding that on the two occasions highlighted he had traded blows with Karen Guilliland of the New Zealand College of Midwives, 'who accused him of overstepping his brief and relying on ill-informed medical opinion'.[6] Outlining his recommendations in 2015, health reporter Donna Chisholm commented, 'For the coroner, there must have been a depressing sense of déjà vu.'[7]

Evans's 2005 findings, reported in the *New Zealand Herald*, concerned the deaths of Saskia Marama Swagerman-Fugle (in 2001) and Cameron Elliot (in 2003), following breech births conducted at home by independent midwives. Evans was highly critical of the midwives involved. He pointed out that midwives were increasingly sole maternity providers and were looking after more high-risk patients experiencing emergencies they might not be prepared for.[8] Karen Guilliland had indeed noted in 2001 that midwives attended not just low-risk screened women but a cross-section of childbearing women.[9] Given their work across the sector, Evans called for an urgent review of midwifery training and greater clinical supervision of graduating midwives. He also called for the reintegration of doctors into maternity services, and for an independent review of maternity and a national audit of birth outcomes. Among his specific recommendations was mandatory vaginal examination in labour. He criticised the midwives' failure to perform such examinations, which, he said, would have diagnosed the breech presentations and alerted them to the need for medical intervention.[10]

According to media reports, the College of Midwives disagreed with Evans, with Chief Executive Karen Guilliland declaring there was 'no evidence to support the coroner's extensive and disruptive recommendations'.[11] Yet a statement by Cynthia (Cindy) Farquhar, chair of a new government committee appointed in 2005, the Perinatal and Maternal Mortality Review Committee (discussed below), suggested that the College appeared to agree with some of Evans's suggestions: 'The College of Midwives have confirmed they do not recommend home birthing for breech presentation and that they recommend vaginal examination during labour, providing there is consent from the woman.'[12]

Nonetheless, there appeared to be ongoing differences attached to the value of vaginal examinations. Dr Gillian White, associate professor of Health Sciences at Massey University, who had previously worked as a domiciliary midwife, said that about 5% of independent midwives never did these examinations, seeing them as an invasion of a woman's body and her privacy. A midwife in the Wellington Home Birth Midwives collective confirmed that some members of the group never did vaginal examinations on these grounds. Around 40% of midwives made the checks only rarely, according to White.[13] A 2009 *New Zealand Listener* article, referring to the Elliot case, reported the College of Midwives' opinion that there was no evidence to support the mandatory use of these examinations. The article's discussion of vaginal examinations in fact called into question one aspect of the midwife–client partnership and informed choice. Amanda Elliot, baby Cameron's mother, told the reporter that it was not until the coroner's hearing a year after her child died that she even knew vaginal examinations could be useful.[14] Women's knowledge could not be assumed.

Nor was there a consensus on breech births. The 2009 *Listener* article reported the College of Midwives' view that the risks involved in caesarean section could outweigh its benefits for breech births.[15] While hospitalisation of breech births did not necessarily mean a caesarean, it was more likely. Homebirth midwife Maggie Banks continued to be wary of hospitalisation of breech births. In 2007 she wrote a follow-up to her 1996 article on performing breech births vaginally at home with an article on 'active' breech birth. Introducing this, the *College of Midwives Journal* editor noted that this was a 'topic for which, I can confidently say, she [Banks] is most famous amongst midwives'. Banks described the midwifery approach to breech birth as opposed to the medical approach; the former, she explained, would 'not wage war on the [women's] bodies and impede their babies' descent'.[16]

Breech homebirths would continue, despite the College's reassurances to Farquhar. While data on homebirths were not collected, meaning the number of breech homebirths remains unknown, the Perinatal and Maternal Mortality Review Committee identified two further deaths from planned breech homebirths between 2007 and 2012.[17]

Evans's 2005 report sparked public commentary. Michael Bassett, Labour's Minister of Health 1984–87, reflected that the balance had swung too far away from the medicalisation of childbirth, and he claimed to be unimpressed by what he described as the College of Midwives' 'extravagant, seemingly contradictory attack on the coroner'. He predicted that the College would bring the same zeal it had shown 20 years previously in lobbying for midwifery autonomy 'to stop an overdue reassessment of maternity services, and any rebalancing required'. In his view, 'When governments allow monopolies to develop, particularly for outdated gender reasons, turf is never surrendered without a fight', but he advised it was time 'to get over such age-old patch warfare'.[18]

A *Kai Tiaki: Nursing New Zealand* article also referred to Evans's 2005 report, and cited Janet Black, a clinical nurse specialist in the neonatal intensive-care unit at Waikato Hospital. Black expressed concern about current midwifery education, explaining, 'The problem is that the new graduates don't know what they don't know.' She worried that new graduates were not trained for hospital work nor taught any nursing skills. Cecile de Bock, a midwife at Taranaki Base Hospital, believed that all new midwifery graduates should spend at least six months in hospital before being allowed to practise independently. She also thought that midwifery education's focus on birth as a normal life event was misplaced, since birth was unpredictable, and that students should be educated from 'normal to abnormal'.[19]

Other coroners weighed into the debates following deaths brought to their attention. Nelson coroner Ian Smith called the death of a baby during a homebirth in Nelson in 2005 an 'avoidable tragedy'. This homebirth took place despite the recommendation from the woman's GP that she give birth in hospital because of her general health condition and because she was aged 40. Smith said more attention to vaginal examination might have provided the impetus for earlier transfer to hospital. The Lead Maternity Carer (LMC) in this case was a first-year practising midwife, accompanied by a third-year student. Another midwife arrived later as back-up and eventually called an ambulance.[20]

Smith also reported in 2010 on a fatal homebirth at Motueka in 2006, under the sole care of midwife Maggie Matthews (also known as Camille Matthews), who had been involved as sole caregiver in a homebirth fatality in 1991.[21] Smith believed that it was not good midwifery practice 'to go it alone' and that back-up midwives should be present at all homebirths – as coroner Dale Hunter had suggested following the 1991 death. Matthews had in fact been suspended from practice by the Midwifery Council in 2007 on the grounds that she posed 'a serious threat to the public'.[22]

Hamilton coroner Gordon Matenga's 2011 report on the death of a baby at Waikato Hospital in October 2009 attracted considerable media attention.

Linda Barlow had been under the care of midwife Jennifer Rowan and was planning to birth at the River Ridge Birthing Centre in Hamilton, a midwifery-owned and -run business that operated a birthing unit.[23] The inquest heard how Rowan had sent Barlow home from the unit owing to lack of space, even though she was having contractions and had been given pethidine. It also heard that, in giving pethidine, Rowan had not followed the unit's guidelines on monitoring the mother's heart rate. The Barlows called Rowan to their home three hours later when Linda Barlow was found to be fully dilated. She returned to River Ridge by ambulance, but when Rowan was unable to hear the baby's pulse, she transferred her to Waikato Hospital. In hospital, Barlow suffered severe complications, leading to an emergency hysterectomy, and ended up on life support and needing 54 units of blood. When she awoke, her husband Robert told her baby Adam had not survived.[24]

Rowan was a newly qualified midwife, 23 years old and just seven months out of training. During her third year of study, she undertook a clinical placement with a community midwife (the new term for independent midwives), Colleen Hugill. After graduating in March 2009, Rowan again worked with Hugill, who became her mentor under the Midwifery First Year of Practice mentoring programme, a scheme introduced in 2007. Hugill withdrew from caring for Linda Barlow when the latter was 36 weeks pregnant, owing to illness. It also emerged during the inquiry that Hugill had been suspended from practice by the Midwifery Council in the month before Adam's death (and was again to be suspended in 2010 and 2011).[25] Rowan had taken over the care of Barlow without telling her that she was a new graduate. Barlow later explained she had wanted an experienced midwife because her first birth had been difficult.

At the inquest into Adam's death, Hugill made it clear that she saw little value in the mentorship programme. She made the point that by law Rowan was 'able to practise anything without a mentor'. She explained to the coroner, 'We are not supervisors, we are there on their request when they feel they need it. People learn better if they do it themselves.' She also said that Rowan had seemed very competent while she worked as a student, explaining that at no time did she say, 'I don't understand.' In reply to Matenga's question to Hugill if anything in the midwives' mentoring programme could be improved, Hugill said that once graduates had completed their training they were 'good enough'. Asked if she would be comfortable with a newly qualified doctor performing open-heart surgery, she replied that she would.[26]

Matenga had also asked North Canterbury midwife Chris Stanbridge, who had 38 years' experience, to review the care Rowan had provided. Stanbridge concluded that Rowan had made 'appropriate and timely decisions' and appeared to have provided a 'reasonable standard of care'.[27] Yet after the coroner's report was completed, Midwifery Council chief executive Sharron Cole regarded the standard of care given less positively. She conceded that the mentoring had not been satisfactory, and explained that this had led to a tightening of rules for mentorship which specified that the graduate could no longer be the practice-partner or mentee of a midwife with whom she had undertaken clinical placement as a student. She also agreed that mentoring should involve experience in different clinical environments, so that mentees would not adopt the methods of those 'not always practising to the highest standards'. She said that the mentoring had 'slipped off-track' in Rowan's case.[28]

Matenga concluded that Adam's death by intrapartum asphyxia (lack of oxygen to the brain during birth) resulted from several factors, including Rowan's failure to recognise Barlow's labour as not normal, and that she did not communicate any urgency verbally or in writing to Waikato Hospital staff during the transfer.[29] He criticised the non-intervention focus of the midwifery profession's philosophy and training generally, considering there to be an 'unacceptable tolerance' of practices outside the 'safe harbour' of referral guidelines. Matenga recommended a review of midwifery education, called for mentoring to be compulsory, and suggested that the role of mentor be enhanced to supervisor.[30] The Midwifery Council told him that it had strengthened midwifery education in 2009, cramming a fourth academic year's work into the three-year programme, with a heavy emphasis on practical placements in the final year, and that it was considering making mentorship compulsory.[31]

Meanwhile, after Matenga had delivered his judgment, Jennifer Rowan changed her name to Campbell and resumed working as a self-employed midwife. The Barlows, when they learned of this, said it was 'alarming' that she should continue to practise without any official record of her involvement in the fatality, and that the Midwifery Council database did not show any conditions for Campbell, even though she had been placed under supervision in 2010. Not only that, she was still under investigation by the Health and Disability Commissioner in 2012; as the Barlows pointed out, she was 'yet to be fully investigated for what the coroner highlighted as a preventable death of a child and also for the severe permanent injuries to the mother'. Cole responded that Campbell had completed the supervision programme. She added that, 'All consumers are free to ask their midwife any questions they wish with respect to her practice, her philosophy, her practice statistics, when she was last reviewed, whether she has had complaints etc.' The Barlows did not consider this to be adequate consumer protection.[32]

Following publicity surrounding Adam Barlow's death, another couple asked Matenga to investigate their baby's death at Waikato Hospital earlier that same year in February 2009. This occurred following transfer from the Waterford Birthing Centre, another midwifery-owned and -run birthing centre in Hamilton.[33] Expert witness Sylvia Rosevear (Fellow of the Royal Australian and New Zealand College of Obstetricians and Gynaecologists since 1992, and of the UK equivalent since 2002) regarded the death as 'potentially preventable'. The baby had died after being starved of oxygen following a prolonged labour. Matenga ruled that the midwife should undergo training on the reading and interpretation of the cardiotocograph (CTG), the external electronic monitoring of the fetal heart rate. The mother told the press she believed that 'the midwifery council need[s] to look at how they do things – like seeking hospital intervention for mums, not staunchly holding off until it's too late'.[34]

Another high-profile case was the death in 2012 of 20-year-old Casey Missy Turama Nathan, a first-time mother, after amniotic fluid entered her bloodstream whilst she was giving birth at a primary maternity unit, Huntly Birthcare. Her baby, Kymani Nathan-Tukiri, died two days later in Waikato Hospital's newborn intensive-care unit. Casey's 19-year-old partner Hayden Tukiri of Tainui was understandably devastated, and the case attracted much media attention.[35] The Press Council did not uphold the College of Midwives' complaint relating to the nature of this reporting.[36]

Jenn Hooper, consumer advocate and founder in 2011 of an activist group called Action to Improve Maternity (see pp. 242–43), alerted coroner Garry Evans to the case, and represented Nathan's whānau at the inquest in February 2014. A reporter noted that Nathan's whānau could be seen crying in the public gallery as the coroner summed up the evidence, and Nathan's uncle told the reporter that he hoped the inquest would lead to change, such as mentoring of new midwives after graduation, 'so that no further members of other families go through this as we have'.[37]

The LMC at Nathan's birth was a midwife who had graduated a year and a half earlier. St John Ambulance staff called to the unit told the inquest they were concerned about the young midwife's apparent lack of experience, with one claiming 'she had no idea what was going on'.[38] Evans asked Auckland midwife Stephanie Vague, an expert witness mandated by the College of Midwives, what support and supervision, if any, a midwife who took up practice as an LMC had after graduating. Vague replied that the responsibility lay with each LMC. She explained that, as a registered midwife, the LMC was accountable for her own practice, and would herself identify any areas where she felt she needed guidance or advice. There was no formal supervision.[39] Evans believed the training and registration of midwives should 'follow the medical and other clinical models'.[40]

Responding to the coroner's suggestion of a hospital internship for newly graduated midwives, the College of Midwives and the Midwifery Council told him this would be 'inappropriate, unsustainable and unnecessary'. They claimed that an internship would lead to de-skilling of the new graduate, just as Donley had suggested back in the 1980s. Evans was puzzled; he could not see how gaining extra experience could mean de-skilling. He replied:

> 'De-skilling' is defined as a reduction in the level of skill required for a job. The natural result of a midwifery internship, as in medicine, would be an 'upskilling' in knowledge and experience through working in a multidisciplinary environment with exposure to the diagnosis, treatment and management of unusual, complex and emergency clinical situations which a midwife may well face in the community, as in this and other cases that have attracted publicity.[41]

In a submission to government, Action to Improve Maternity also commented on the de-skilling argument, wondering whether the 50% of all new midwifery graduates who took up employment as hospital midwives would view themselves as undergoing de-skilling. It claimed, 'Unsurprisingly some core [hospital] midwives have obviously taken exception to this apparently derogatory view of their work by their midwifery leadership.'[42] Obstetrician Tony Baird also argued that Nathan's death strengthened the case for hospital training of midwives. He wrote to the *Listener*:

> The grand assertion about midwifery by Rose Collins (Letters, February 28) that 'We are the envy of the world' is unlikely to

provide comfort to the family of Casey Nathan or help avoid another tragedy. I was a medical expert witness at the Huntly coronial inquiry into the deaths of Casey and her baby Kymani and there is no doubt that the deaths could have been prevented. It's time for midwifery leaders to move beyond complacency to endorse the advice of the coroner about training in hospitals for new graduates.[43]

Sylvia Rosevear was another expert witness at this inquest and maintained that an antenatal ultrasound scan would have picked up warning signs that a transfer was needed. She noted that Nathan had risk factors that should have been recognised, including her youth, irregular attendance at antenatal appointments and maternal smoking.[44]

The online news agency *Stuff* summarised Evans's report in early 2015 under the heading: 'Mum and baby deaths: Coroner slams midwife'. At the inquest, according to Evans, the LMC came across as 'confident, capable, intelligent and articulate', and 'if she had a fault it was an overweening confidence in her own ability'.[45] In the *Listener* Donna Chisholm wrote, 'Over 73 damning pages, coroner Garry Evans laid out the series of shortcomings in the midwives' care that led to what he called Nathan and Kymani's preventable deaths.'[46] Evans advised the Midwifery Council that, among other things, it should ensure more attention was paid to excluding risk factors before proceeding to homebirth or birth in a primary birthing facility, and to providing more advanced training in indicators for the need for transfer.[47] Primary birthing facilities did not have on-site medical specialists, as will be further explored in Chapter 11.

The responses of the Midwifery Council and the College to his report did not impress Evans, who declared their widespread criticisms were not matched by helpful analysis. The Midwifery Council publicly declared that findings in one case should not be used to infer failings in the education and supervision of midwives generally. It explained, 'To do so is particularly concerning to the council as it undermines the trust and confidence of the public in the profession and presents an inaccurate view of what is widely recognised as a world class maternity service.'[48] Home Birth Aotearoa, as the Home Birth Association was now called, issued a media release rejecting the coroner's recommendation to change midwifery training to include hospital internships for new graduates on the basis of findings in this one case: 'Birthing mothers need to have faith in their lead maternity carers in order to feel safe. Expressing doubt that our midwives have been adequately trained – when our maternity system is internationally regarded as of the highest class – does not make mothers feel safe.'[49] Guilliland despaired that tightening referral guidelines for midwives 'further medicalised' normal pregnancy and birth, and lamented, 'A profession which heralds a women-centred approach can feel more and more out of step with the medicalised and fetal-centric world we are increasingly in.'[50]

Hooper, representing Action to Improve Maternity, told journalist Donna Chisholm that the Nathan case reflected failings she consistently found in the 650 cases on her organisation's database of adverse outcomes in birth. These failings included 'normalising' the abnormal, and delays in emergency transfer. She thought the College of Midwives had its priorities wrong, emphasising the childbirth experience rather than the outcome. She explained, 'We don't get pregnant to have a labour and birth', but rather to create a family.[51] Chisholm also interviewed retired National Women's Hospital neonatal paediatrician Ross Howie, who had worked at the hospital since 1963, overseeing major developments in neonatal care.[52] He said that when he viewed the College of Midwives' code of ethics, 'They mention the baby only once, and then casually and in passing. They seem to glorify pregnancy and delivery as an affirmation of woman.' He believed the focus needed to change from 'a celebration of womanhood to a celebration of new life'.[53]

The Nathan case was a springboard for much reflection on maternity services, and yet in some ways little had changed since Coroner Evans's 2005 report, as Chisholm intimated. Guilliland's 2014 lament about a 'medicalised and fetal-centred world' elicited an angry letter to the *Listener* by retired public health physician Margaret Guthrie. In her view, Guilliland had gone too far in glorifying pregnancy and delivery as an affirmation of womanhood. She said that having a well, healthy baby was surely the parents' priority, and concluded that the coroner was right to blame the deaths on current midwifery education and the lack of adequate supervision for new graduates. 'The sooner this is dealt with constructively, the better,' she advised.[54] Deb Pittam and Sue Bree, College of Midwives president and past president respectively, responded: 'Everything midwives do is to try to ensure both a woman and her baby are healthy and happy and, together with their family, in a position to make sure parenthood is started from a positive place.'[55] Coroners' reports suggested that more could be done to ensure that positive place for all.

## The Health and Disability Commissioner and the Code of Health and Disability Services Consumers' Rights

Complaints to the Commissioner for Health and Disability for breaches of patients' rights, a system introduced in 1996, provided another platform for public concerns about birth practices. From 2003, the Commissioner had the option of referring cases of misconduct to a Director of Proceedings, an independent prosecutor who would determine whether the complaint should be referred to the Health Practitioners Disciplinary Tribunal for further investigation, a process that could result in deregistration. If the Commissioner's report concerned midwives, it was also sent to the Midwifery Council for consideration of further action.[56]

The commissioners' reports sometimes complemented the coroners' findings. For instance, Commissioner Ron Paterson reported on the 2005 Nelson death, which coroner Ian Smith had investigated. Paterson found some aspects of the care by the two midwives involved to be substandard, concluding that both breached the Code of Health and Disability Services Consumers' Rights.[57] Anthony Hill, who replaced Paterson as Commissioner for Health and Disability in 2010, reported on Adam Barlow's death in 2014, a case the coroner had previously investigated. Hill found that the midwife had breached the Code in no fewer than eight ways.[58]

In 2011, Hill explained that recurring themes around the 60 complaints received about midwives during the past year included delayed recognition of risk and consequent delayed calls for help, as well as a lack of communication when a multidisciplinary team was involved in the birth. He recommended strengthening postgraduate mentoring and training of midwives.[59] The Midwifery Council's mentoring scheme, introduced in 2007 as an option for newly qualified midwives, consisted of monthly professional development sessions with a mentor. Hill did not think this went far enough. He also called for a culture that encouraged a 'conservative approach in assessing risk and getting help', and better communication among health professionals.[60]

In 2010 Dr Rosemary Godbold, a registered nurse and senior lecturer in Health Care Ethics at the National Centre for Health Care Law and Ethics, AUT, wrote an article for the *College of Midwives Journal* on the Code of Health and Disability Services Consumers' Rights in relation to midwifery. She investigated breaches relating to Right 5 (the right to effective communication), Right 6 (the right to be fully informed), and Right 7 (the right to make an informed choice and give informed consent). Godbold noted that, of the 41 opinions published by Commissioner Paterson relating to complaints about midwifery practice received after 2000, 21 investigated potential breaches of informed consent. She added that the 2008 Midwifery Council report also highlighted the lack of informed consent and communication with clients as two of the themes in the 35 complaints it had received that year about professional misconduct.[61]

Godbold gave the example of a 2006 complaint for which Paterson had determined that a woman having a homebirth for her first baby, and which ended in the baby's death, was not provided with vital information regarding the slow progress of her labour, thus preventing her from being involved in important decisions about her care. Paterson concluded that the midwife had breached Right 6 of Code of Health and Disability Services Consumers' Rights, as well as Standard One of the *New Zealand College of Midwives Handbook for Practice*, which specified that it was 'important that a lead maternity carer fully involve the woman in all aspects of her labour and delivery'.[62]

A key issue Godbold identified was midwives' documentation of discussions relating to the birth process and treatment options. Midwives were required as part of the 2004 Midwifery Council Competencies to keep 'accurate and timely written progress notes and relevant documented evidence of all decisions made and midwifery care offered and provided'.[63] The 2006 midwifery textbook also stressed the importance of documentation. In her chapter, midwifery lecturer Joan Skinner explained that midwives needed to be 'accountable to the public and to the profession within the medico-legal context', and that to protect themselves they needed accurate and complete documentation, providing evidence of care, information given and decision-making processes.[64] Yet Godbold found lapses, referring, for instance, to a case of a stillborn baby where the midwife's documentation was 'so poor that difficulties arose for the Commissioner to establish exactly what occurred' both antenatally and during labour.[65]

The issues raised by Godbold were explored further in a 2013 Law dissertation. Researcher Claire Sweetman assessed 36 Commissioner reports that identified substandard midwifery care since 2002.[66] While she supported a midwifery-led maternity system, Sweetman acknowledged that the midwifery profession had recently found itself under fire in the media and claimed that the commissioners' reports suggested some public concern was justified.[67] She said that the reports showed that the profession was under extreme pressure and that midwives sometimes cut corners to cope with the workload. However, she also believed it likely that graduates were entering practice without the required competence to operate autonomously.[68] She structured her study around central themes in the reports. These included inadequate documentation; lack of informed choice and consent; issues with homebirth; inadequate antenatal care; poor CTG monitoring; poor infant resuscitation; inexperienced midwives; and conflict between doctors and midwives.[69] The following discussion is based on Sweetman's synthesis, backed up by a reading of the health and disability commissioners' evidence and decisions.

Like Godbold, Sweetman noted that issues around inadequate documentation permeated the commissioners' reports on substandard midwifery care. Of the 36 reports she examined, more than 75% expressed concerns about record-keeping. One particularly serious deviation from accepted standards involved a midwife in 2007 who had failed to document the fetal heart rate, the mother's blood loss, the baby's Apgar scores, and even whether the baby was a boy or a girl.[70] The Commissioner concluded in this case that the midwife breached the Code not only in her documentation and failure to communicate with her clients but also by her 'substandard midwifery care' (Right 4).[71] The report noted that the mother and her partner were considerably traumatised by the difficult birth and required counselling. ACC accepted their claim that the baby's hypoxic ischaemic encephalopathy was 'a result of omission of care'.[72]

As in this case, inadequate documentation was often linked with more serious failings, such as failure to provide services of an adequate standard (Right 4) and failure to fully inform the consumer (Right 6). In a 2004 case, Commissioner Ron Paterson found the midwife in breach of Rights 4 and 6 when a baby died after a midwife providing antenatal care failed to respond appropriately to the mother's concerns about reduced fetal movements.[73] In a case investigated in 2010 it was found the midwife's documentation was not of an adequate standard and, more seriously, that she failed 'to recognise, and react in an appropriate fashion' to her client's ongoing symptoms suggestive of pre-eclampsia, leading to an emergency caesarean.[74] In another case in 2010 the midwife's failure to administer a vitamin K injection to a baby resulted in a cerebral haemorrhage which required 'urgent craniotomy and evacuation of a subdural haematoma'.[75] While some midwives had rejected giving vitamin K, since 1998 LMCs were required to discuss vitamin K prophylaxis with parents to ensure they were aware of the recommendation that all babies receive it.

Anthony Hill found no documentation in the midwife's care plan to show that she had discussed this with the woman, and consequently the midwife was found in breach of Rights 4 and 6.[76]

Sweetman commented that homebirth was one of the more controversial choices an expectant mother could make. One of the cases she analysed related to a baby who died in 2000 after a midwife failed to recognise an abnormal and obstructed labour during a homebirth. The case was one of posterior presentation, and the midwife treated her client's failure to progress in the labour 'by encouraging ambulation, by reassurance, surveillance and homeopathy (arnica)'. Eventually the mother was transferred to hospital, but the baby died. The mother disputed that she was told during labour about the slowing of the baby's heartbeat. She claimed that whilst she had wanted a homebirth, she understood the importance of transfer if necessary.[77] Longstanding Invercargill homebirth midwife Terryll Muir provided independent advice to Paterson for this complaint.[78] Among other things, Muir commented on the midwife's failure to administer the standard urine test, and the fact there was no documentation to suggest that the mother had declined this. Muir considered that the midwife's care fell significantly below accepted standards, directly contributing to the baby's death. Paterson reported that he had been told that the midwife 'took the lack of progress . . . to its widest limits'.[79] He concluded that she breached the patient's rights in several ways, including the level of skill she brought to the homebirth, compliance with professional standards relating to hospital transfer, and keeping the mother and family informed.[80]

One of the options following commissioners' findings was to forward them to the appropriate disciplinary body, which happened in this case. The Nursing Council, still the responsible disciplinary authority, upheld the charge of not ensuring adequate communication, and censured the midwife, ordering her to pay 30% of the cost of the hearing. The Council ordered continued name suppression of the midwife, however, since she had since undertaken further professional development and demonstrated a willingness to learn from her mistakes.[81] This midwife had previously been subject to disciplinary charges and had been denied access to the local hospital as a result; Paterson found she had not disclosed this to the client.[82]

In her section on complaints relating to antenatal care, Sweetman referred to a stillbirth in 2006.[83] The mother told Paterson that she had planned a homebirth but did not intend to forsake conventional forms of assessment or refuse medical intervention if needed. She said that the midwife was 'very dismissive of any medical interventions, tending to ridicule them and portray them as heavy-handed and unnecessary'.[84] During the pregnancy, according to the mother, the midwife 'actively discouraged them from taking up testing options and advised that such medical interventions were harmful to the baby'.[85] The mother explained she relied on the midwife's professional judgement, an indication that she did not see herself as an equal partner in the relationship.[86]

This midwife showed no concern as the due delivery date passed, following the textbook advice of 'trusting the childbirth process and trusting women and their bodies'.[87] The mother recalled that at her antenatal class, 'the response of the midwives to the question about what would happen if you were overdue was, "Don't even worry about it . . . Baby's got to come out sometime."' Her midwife went on leave around the time the baby was due, placing the woman in the hands of a colleague who had her own busy caseload. Without providing any clinical records, she told her colleague that she would be needed only if the couple contacted her. According to the Commissioner's notes, the midwife even gave her client instructions on how to deliver the baby herself 'if nobody could reach her in time'.[88] When the midwife returned three weeks later and visited her client, she found no sign of the baby moving. She admitted the woman to a local rural hospital, but, unable to locate a fetal heartbeat, transferred her to a public hospital. An ultrasound scan confirmed the baby had died. Paterson concluded that the midwife had breached Rights 4 and 6 of the Code. This case was passed to the Health Practitioners Disciplinary Tribunal, which found the midwife guilty of professional misconduct, and she was struck off the midwives' register.[89] The system had however, even if inadvertently, encouraged such non-interventionist behaviour.

CTG monitoring was another area explored by Sweetman. She found that the Commissioner continued to receive complaints about undiagnosed fetal distress. She listed seven cases in which, she said, midwives struggled to use CTG equipment effectively. She commented that, as autonomous health professionals, they needed to be able to perform all the tasks required of such a provider. Sweetman gave the example of a newborn baby who died in 2007 after a midwife 'failed to exercise reasonable skill and care' when monitoring the fetal heartbeat via a CTG and failed to refer the case to a secondary-care team. The midwife was found in breach of Right 4 of the Code, and Standard Six of the College's *Handbook for Practice*.[90]

The College's *Handbook* and Midwifery Council's practice requirements, which included being able to assess, monitor and interpret fetal heart patterns 'using a pinard, ultrasound and cardiotocograph equipment', suggested midwifery leaders now accepted this technology.[91] Writing in the College journal's 'Practice Wisdom' column in 2003, Maggie Banks still rejected the use of CTG monitoring.[92] In response, midwife Sian Burgess admitted a sense of unease, explaining that while the significance of fetal movements in labour was still poorly understood, she doubted whether it was wise to replace listening to the heart with detecting the presence of movements as the only determinant of the baby's wellbeing in labour, as Banks had suggested. Burgess explained that not listening to the heartbeat could lay midwives open to charges of negligence for not following commonly accepted practice. Banks retorted, 'I constantly hear of midwives embracing all sorts of interventions, but the rationale is not whether it benefits the woman or baby but rather how it protects the midwife.'[93] A 2011 study, whose authors included Sally Pairman, concluded, 'Fetal heart rate monitoring practices vary according to individual midwife preferences.'[94]

CTG monitoring was recommended by the Royal Australian and New Zealand College of Obstetricians and Gynaecologists when 'there was a high likelihood that the fetus might become hypoxic during labour' – in other words, if the birth was high-risk.[95] But the problem was identifying risk. In 2014, both a coroner and the Health and Disability Commissioner investigated a neonatal death in a case where the midwife had not considered the use of CTG necessary. The mother was attempting a vaginal birth following an earlier caesarean. She insisted that she would not have objected to another caesarean if it was considered necessary, but the midwife caring for her was 'always adamant that a Caesarean would not be needed, and that [her client] needed to change her thinking, as it was all in her head'.[96] The woman was under the impression that her baby would be continually monitored during the labour, and yet the midwife switched off the CTG, against the advice of the hospital obstetrician. The Commissioner's report cited an expert midwife who had advised the coroner that continuous CTG monitoring was indicated, owing to risk factors which included not only the previous caesarean but also maternal smoking and a suspicious CTG on entering the unit. This midwife believed that CTG monitoring 'would have alerted health professionals to the need for earlier intervention, with the probability that death could have been avoided'.[97] The Commissioner listed no fewer than seven ways in which this midwife had failed the mother and her baby and was in breach of the Code, concluding that her care was 'seriously sub-optimal'.[98]

Sweetman also addressed infant resuscitation. She pointed out that this skill was included in the midwife's pre-registration education, and the Midwifery Council required midwives to participate in an annual two-hour refresher. Despite this, she found that the Health and Disability Commissioner received complaints about poor infant resuscitation. An investigation of a case in 2005 revealed delay in establishing effective resuscitation, with the baby sustaining a major brain injury. Another error in this case involved placement of the endotracheal tube in the baby's oesophagus and not the trachea.[99] The Commissioner's report noted that by five months of age, this baby 'exhibited marked limb spasticity, infantile spasms, and limited social awareness, and was thought to be severely visually impaired'.[100]

Paterson accepted the expert midwife's finding that the midwife in question did not exercise reasonable care and skill when attempting to resuscitate the baby, and charged her with breaching Right 4 of the Code. However, the expert witness had qualified her criticism, saying that, 'Peers would view this departure from reasonable care with moderate disapproval.'[101] The parents' response to this statement was utter disbelief, pointing out that the 'actions or inactions of the people we trusted that day have concluded in a truly severe outcome'. Of their daughter they wrote, 'They took her abilities, her personality, and even her smile. Dead or alive, we've lost [her]. They took away the little girl that she was meant to be . . . In replacement they have left us with a lifetime of uncertainty.' Referring to their child's 'extreme health issues, pain, and suffering', her mother wrote:

> At just two years old she has already had a major hip reconstruction. There are many more surgeries to come, no matter how hard we work to avoid them. Due to her extreme scoliosis she must now wear a back brace 23 hours a day. I wanted to be her Mum, but instead I feel like her nurse . . . The midwives did this . . . The consequence to our family has been severe and permanent.[102]

Moving to her next section, Sweetman noted that one of the most heavily publicised aspects of substandard midwifery care related to new graduates, with 'attention-grabbing' headlines asserting that services provided by new midwives were dangerous, and that inexperience was linked to poor-quality care and even death. Although the Midwifery Council firmly denied such claims, she wrote, there was evidence that some new graduates required additional support during their transition into autonomous practice and struggled if this was not available. For example, in two cases reported in 2013 the Commissioner concluded that the midwives involved, both of whom were new graduates, breached the Code with their poor standard of care.[103] The first case, a baby's death in 2010, involved a midwife who graduated in 2009, and whom Commissioner Hill charged with breaching Right 4. He concluded that she communicated poorly with the parents, did not adequately review assessments, did not complete documentation to an acceptable standard, and did not seek medical assistance when indicated.[104]

In the second case, in 2012, the midwife had practised as an independent midwife for nine months, and Hill again found her in breach of Right 4.[105] This case involved a 16-year-old mother who gave birth on the bathroom floor at home, without the midwife present, despite numerous calls having been made to her. The young mother ended up in hospital with a serious infection. Among other things, the midwife had advised her to take evening primrose oil capsules each day for a week from 37 weeks' gestation; she had heard anecdotally that this would bring on labour. The expert midwife at the inquiry disputed that this advice was evidence-based, and said it could even cause harm such as premature rupture of the membranes. Nor was there any reason why the client, a well and healthy woman, would require anything to ripen her cervix or promote labour at 37 weeks' gestation, as she still had three weeks of pregnancy remaining. Hill accepted this assessment and concluded that by prescribing primrose oil the midwife failed to provide services with reasonable care and skill. Hill also charged the midwife with inadequate care of the perineum, which had resulted in the mother being hospitalised, with the infected tissue having to be removed, and her labia and perineum reconstructed.[106] The midwife had called it a 'tiny tear', and laughed when the mother tried to tie her legs together to cope. Hill considered this unkind and unprofessional.[107] Hill recommended the midwife undertake further training and be subject to a College of Midwives review. He referred her to the Director of Proceedings for possible further action, and told the midwife to apologise to her client, to reflect on her failings, and to provide a written report to the Commissioner stating how she had changed her practice.[108] Two years later, this midwife had moved from Blenheim to Northland, and was practising under a different name and with no conditions on her practising certificate.[109]

Under her final overriding theme, Sweetman turned to what she believed was one of the weakest aspects of New Zealand's maternity system: the troubled relationship between some doctors and midwives. She noted that where mothers had high-risk or complicated pregnancies, it was essential for primary- and secondary-service providers to work together, but collaboration was extremely difficult where tension levels were high. Moreover, confusion over roles and responsibilities could lead to gaps in the provision of maternity care, with each party believing the other had the task in hand.[110] She felt that, in light of some graduates entering midwifery practice without the required competence to operate autonomously, these conflicts left midwives even more vulnerable.[111] Like others, she concluded from her investigation that, at a minimum, homebirth care should be strengthened by amending the Maternity Services Notice to require the presence of another midwife, a GP or an obstetrician at the birth, rather than just confirming their availability to attend.[112] This change would affect the safety of more than 2,000 births a year, she said, given that approximately 3.2% of New Zealand women were choosing to birth at home.[113] She noted that two health professionals had to be present at every Western Australian homebirth, ensuring immediate support, consultation, and assistance in emergency situations.[114] Others had shared that concern. The previous year, GP obstetrician Jonathan Wilcox had argued that the move away from having two people present at every homebirth, whether the second be a specialist, GP or midwife, was 'disrespectful of the needs and rights of parents', and 'outright dangerous'.[115] While the government now funded two midwives to attend homebirths, no law or regulation required this.[116]

Sweetman's study highlighted concerns found in health and disability commissioners' reports. Hill told journalist Donna Chisholm that of the 97 complaints received from 2008 to 2010, 21 went to formal investigation and five midwives were found in breach.[117] Guilliland later noted that over the 10-year period to 2015, four or five midwives per annum were found in breach of the Code.[118] Hill explained that it was not the number of complaints that was the issue, but rather the commonality of themes, all of which related to the training of midwives and their philosophies, suggesting systemic issues.

Others also commented on the commissioners' findings. In his study of the tensions between health professions in 2012, law professor Mark Henaghan referred to a 2008 case in which the baby suffered a treatment injury and suspected brain damage. He noted that the midwifery and obstetrics experts had very different viewpoints on the culpability of the midwife. The midwifery expert Chris Stanbridge, who had testified at the high-profile Barlow case and was a member of the Midwifery Council Competence Review Panel, described the midwife's treatment as appropriate. The medical expert, obstetrician and gynaecologist Digby Ngan Kee, said, 'By any first world standard, the care in this case is below what is generally considered acceptable.'[119] The Commissioner also commented that it was 'curious' that the ACC accepted that the midwife's delay in transferring her client from the private birthing unit to hospital (involving an ambulance journey of two and a half hours) amounted to 'poor practice', whilst midwifery advisors described the same care as 'reasonable' and 'close and appropriate'.[120]

Bad outcomes could sometimes lead to police prosecution, as happened in 2006. This followed the death of a baby in 2004 during a first-pregnancy breech delivery in Queen Mary Hospital, Dunedin, following transfer from a maternity unit. The police charged midwife Jennifer Crawshaw with manslaughter, accusing her of allowing an unsafe 'natural' breech birth to go ahead. The midwife's defence rested on informed consent. The midwife delivering the baby did not alert the hospital doctors to the fact that the baby was in a breech position because the mother wanted a natural birth.[121] Crawshaw was acquitted when evidence showed the mother had been well informed about the risks but wanted to go ahead without medical intervention. The Midwifery Council expressed relief at the verdict and the College of Midwives welcomed it, reminding *New Zealand Herald* readers that New Zealand's maternity service was 'world class'.[122]

The High Court trial took place while the Health and Disability Commissioner was investigating the case. Commissioner Ron Paterson doubted whether criminal proceedings were the best way to deal with adverse medical events, as they might hinder regular mechanisms for practitioner accountability. In this case, he reflected on the responsibilities of midwives when mothers acted against medical advice, and the issue of midwives' duty to the unborn child. He also thought the case highlighted tensions between the midwifery and medical approaches to maternity care. While he accepted that the mother had made a choice, he pointed out that she would not have been aware of the tense relationship between primary and secondary maternity-care providers at Queen Mary Hospital, and the practical difficulty of calling in medical staff at the last minute, having earlier excluded them. The midwife had told him of a 'history of stand-up arguments between midwives and obstetricians in the corridors of Queen Mary'. Paterson believed the case highlighted the need for more effective communication between professional groups. Criminal proceedings, in his opinion, did not allow for considerations of such broader systemic problems.[123]

Paterson also drew attention to tensions between LMCs and hospital staff when examining the death of a baby under a midwife LMC at Auckland's North Shore Hospital in 2006. He highlighted what he considered a gap in the access agreement governing use of maternity hospitals by independent midwives, obstetricians and GPs. This agreement prohibited hospitals from checking whether practitioners were 'clinically safe and competent'; nor could hospitals compel practitioners to comply with hospital policies. Paterson noted that the only safety obligation imposed on the practitioner by the access agreement was to ensure the 'cultural safety of the woman'. He maintained that the system put practitioner autonomy ahead of patient safety.[124] Once again, he highlighted systemic problems arising from the consideration of an individual case.

The commissioners' reports also revealed how bad outcomes could have a major impact on providers themselves. In one case, the midwife stopped practising midwifery following the incident. She told the Commissioner that she was reflecting on her role as a health professional in the community with assistance from a clinical psychologist, and that she remained uncertain about returning to midwifery practice.[125] In another case, the midwife was so profoundly affected by the experience that she ceased being a self-employed midwife and took up employment as a hospital midwife.[126]

## Conclusion

A glimpse at these individual cases, whether through the eyes of a coroner or health and disability commissioner, gives a sense of the personal tragedies and the high stakes involved in this area of healthcare. These were life-changing events, and those responsible for investigating them were deeply troubled and sometimes angry about what they saw as avoidable outcomes and were frustrated by the failure of the system to address the shortcomings they repeatedly highlighted. The reports of coroners and commissioners suggested that all was not well within the midwifery model, and challenged the constant refrain from some quarters that New Zealand's maternity services were world-class.

Bad childbirth outcomes also politicised some parents. Following their son's death, and the coroner and commissioner's reports, the Barlows told the press, 'We suffered a shocking lack of basic midwifery care with a lack of humanity on October 25, 2009 by a self employed new graduate LMC midwife in the community.' They challenged the Health Minister and all health professionals, particularly the midwifery sector, 'to accept the findings, to learn from them and put into place a far safer environment for all future mothers, fathers, babies and midwives in New Zealand'.[127] In a rare admission of systemic failure, the College of Midwives joined the Waikato District Health Board and the College of Obstetricians and Gynaecologists in admitting 'the care of Mrs Barlow and the circumstances surrounding the case were tragic and resulted from a failure in the system to provide safe maternity care of mother and baby'.[128] Concerns about systemic failures was not isolated to the discussion of individual cases, however. As will be explored in the next chapter, mounting criticism of the services arose from a wide array of health professionals and consumers as the new century unfolded.

# ELEVEN

## *Maternity system under fire:*
## *The Midwifery Council's first decade*

REPORTS BY CORONERS AND health and disability commissioners elicited sympathy for the families involved in tragedies and adverse maternity events, as well as reflection about what went wrong and how this could be addressed. During the new Midwifery Council's first decade from 2004, when midwifery-led services were increasingly becoming the norm and midwives forming the bulk of LMCs, there arose additional sources of commentary. These included a government-commissioned review; a book by a GP charting changes in maternity services since 1990; consumer submissions to Parliament; and reports by the Health Select Committee, other health professionals and the newly formed Perinatal and Maternal Mortality Review Committee. All attracted considerable media attention, and all were critical of aspects of current maternity services. While midwifery leaders remained confident in their espousal of the midwifery model and in the competence of their midwives, and mostly enjoyed the support of the Ministry of Health, concerns were mounting. This chapter charts those concerns from different quarters and in different settings, including secondary and tertiary hospitals, primary-care units and homebirthing. Mentoring of midwives, levels of training and adherence to directives in the case of immunisation came under scrutiny by those who increasingly claimed the system was broken.

## Calls for audit

In 2006, a *Sunday Star-Times* editorial scolded, 'Fifteen years after the maternity shake-up, health officials cannot say for sure whether it has really made things better or worse, for the simple reason that health bureaucrats never bothered to collect the information needed to make that call.'[1] Others had also drawn attention to the lack of audit. In 2001 obstetrician Neil Pattison called for a national perinatal database to evaluate changes in the system since 1990. He noted repeated calls for such a database, and described the government's failure to act as 'disgraceful' and contrary to World Health Organization guidelines. He acknowledged the existence of some datasets, collected by different government departments, but said they were neither consolidated nor audited and had little clinical input. He contrasted this with Australia and other countries where perinatal epidemiology units independently monitored practices and changes in the provision of healthcare.[2] In 2004 Dr Rosemary Reid from Christchurch Women's Hospital also pointed out that a comprehensive national database to provide information on maternal and perinatal outcomes had long been called for, and suggested New Zealand should adopt a system like the UK triennial maternal mortality reports.[3] Back in 1969 Professor Dennis Bonham had been largely responsible for setting up the Maternal Mortality Review Committee based on the British model, which he chaired until his fall from grace following the 1988 Cartwright Inquiry. His committee did not survive into the new era, with its last report covering 1989–91.[4] As the 1993 commissioned report into maternity services had noted, there was no single information system providing reliable and comprehensive information on the services and the outcomes of those services. As a result, it said, it was 'impossible to undertake an objective evaluation of the effectiveness of services or to investigate issues of access and equity'.[5] Little changed over the following decade.

The 2000 Public Health and Disability Act provided for data collection and analysis, and in 2005 the Ministry of Health finally set up the Perinatal and Maternal Mortality Review Committee (PMMRC), chaired by Cynthia Farquhar, postgraduate professor in Obstetrics and Gynaecology at the University of Auckland since 2002. In its first report in 2007, the committee explained its remit was data collection in order to 'reduce the number of preventable perinatal and maternal deaths'.[6] It also recognised the need to include morbidity, and in particular neonatal encephalopathy resulting from asphyxia during birth.[7] It established a working group on this in 2007 and started collecting data in 2010.[8] From 2011 it reported to the Health Quality & Safety Commission New Zealand, which was set up in 2010 'to support and encourage quality and safety improvements, to identify areas where improvements can take place, and to drive change [in health care]'.[9]

When coroner Garry Evans called for a national audit of maternity services in 2005, Labour's Health Minister Pete Hodgson referred the request to the PMMRC. It responded that New Zealand did not have a centralised perinatal database, and that, while there were some collections, they varied in completeness and quality. The primary purpose of data in the Maternity and Newborn Information System was for service payments, and not to evaluate clinical outcomes. Information collected on stillbirths was incomplete, because most were not assigned a National Health Index (NHI) number at birth. Nor was there any obligation for midwives to submit information on homebirths. Without reliable data, the PMMRC did not recommend a review.[10] In February 2006 Opposition health spokesperson Tony Ryall claimed that Hodgson's failure to institute a review was putting mothers and babies at risk. He asked, 'How many more babies will die before the Government realises that the current system is flawed?'[11]

In 2006, Dr Beverley (Bev) Lawton, founder and director of the Women's Health Research Centre at the Wellington School of Medicine and Health Sciences, also called for an audit.[12] She told Hodgson they urgently needed an independent academic review to ascertain if problems in maternity care were widespread and systemic. Lawton proposed that her centre develop an evidence-based audit template to collect data covering antenatal, intra-partum and postnatal care, explaining that the issues were far more extensive than those covered by existing committee structures such as the PMMRC. Hodgson responded that, on the advice of the Ministry of Health and the PMMRC, he had confidence in New Zealand's high-quality maternity services and would not order an audit.[13] A reporter for *New Zealand Doctor* was not convinced and listed some of the current problems, sourced from a recent Ministry of Health report. These included poorer outcomes for Māori and Pasifika mothers and babies than others, and a high and increasing rate of Asian stillbirths; the reporter also noted that New Zealand ranked twenty-first among OECD countries for infant mortality (falling from around tenth in the 1960s and 1970s) due to relatively high SIDS and perinatal mortality rates.[14]

After the death of another baby, attributed partly to midwives misreading a fetal heart monitor, Ryall again called on Hodgson to institute a review.

Ryall announced that every month there were 'more frightening incidents coming to light, and more professional groups calling for change'. Hodgson responded that a review would only delay improvements currently being developed by professionals.[15]

## The Wellington Area Review 2008

A breech-birth baby's death at Wellington's Kenepuru Hospital's underwater birthing unit in 2008 finally resulted in action. Two midwives had attended the birth, one recently qualified and the other more experienced. The junior midwife failed to diagnose the breech birth despite three examinations, and when she sought help from the senior midwife present during the delivery the latter told her she was 'doing fine'. Nor did they call on any medical support, obstetric or paediatric. The mother, a registered nurse, said the New Zealand College of Midwives should be monitoring graduates: 'Without any experience, they are practising on people's lives. It's not safe.'[16]

Even before the Health and Disability Commissioner reviewed the case, the new Health Minister David Cunliffe announced a review of Wellington maternity services to 'ascertain whether we need to take further steps to ensure public safety and confidence'. This satisfied neither the parents nor Ryall, who asked, 'How many tragedies are there needed before there is action, and not just another report?' The College of Midwives released a statement saying it was unaware of any systemic problems within Wellington's maternity services; it questioned why a government-ordered review was even necessary, claiming there were 'plenty of other ways to investigate what happened'.[17]

The Review of the Quality, Safety and Management of Maternity Services in the Wellington Area was published in October 2008. Chaired by Barbara Crawford, quality and clinical risk manager at the Waikato District Health Board (DHB), reviewers included obstetrics professor Peter Stone and Auckland DHB midwifery leader Anne Yates.[18] The reviewers expressed concern about accountability and the monitoring of standards of maternity services under the current legislative framework. Section 88 of the 2000 Public Health and Disability Act made provision for a notice relating to terms and conditions for payments of service providers, and the 2002 Maternity Services Notice required DHBs to make their facilities available to providers, setting out procedures for referrals and access agreements. The notice was primarily intended to deal with funding and, in the opinion of the reviewers, was useless as a clinical or a quality and safety document, yet it was the only document establishing ground rules for LMC practice in a hospital setting. This shortfall, they wrote, was amplified by the sometimes fraught relationship between LMCs and hospital staff, with no 'common, evidence-based standards for maternity care to which all relevant health professional groups subscribe'.[19] The reviewers pointed to the absence in the notice of any mention of LMC credentials, such as qualification, registration or requirements for continuing professional education, and recommended that the notice include these and make them subject to audit.[20] They also recommended that LMCs' compliance with facility policies and procedures in hospital be audited.[21] They did not believe that the current access agreements under the notice ensured LMC accountability in the hospital setting.

The reviewers also investigated self-employed LMCs outside hospitals. They pointed out that there was no formal requirement to report a serious event either to the Ministry of Health as the funder, or to any agency with oversight of patient safety. While a client death was reported to the coroner and to the newly formed PMMRC, there was no obligation for self-employed LMCs to review, learn from or take actions to prevent recurrence of a serious event that did not result in death. They noted that a self-employed midwife could ask the College of Midwives to conduct a review, but this was not mandatory.[22] In fact, the reviewers objected to the voluntary nature of the College of Midwives' standards review process, and recommended that self-employed midwives be subject to the same requirements as other healthcare providers in New Zealand.[23] The College was unlikely to budge on this, however. As Auckland midwifery lecturer Anne Barlow had explained in 2001 in summarising an evaluation of the process in the Auckland region, removing the voluntary aspect would 'detrimentally alter the nature of the Review'; she said that monitoring credentials, or what she called 'employer controlled evaluation of health services provision', would threaten midwifery autonomy and might not be effective in 'reducing "patient risk"' in any case.[24]

The 2008 reviewers found that some hospital medical and midwifery staff, as well as consumers, were uneasy that first-year midwifery graduates were authorised to deliver babies without formal supervision or mentoring. These graduates were not even required to tell clients they were newly qualified. Some of the reviewers' informants argued that midwives should undergo a compulsory intern year in hospital to learn about abnormal labours and births, how the hospital system worked, and how to access assistance. Just as they had when coroners made this suggestion, the College of Midwives responded that self-employed midwives were better able to learn the differences between normal and abnormal births in the community than in hospital.[25] The College also stated that advances had been made in midwifery education, including, in 2006, expanding the three-year programme from 36 weeks per year to 45 weeks – the first change made since the programmes had started in 1992. In 2007, the College had trialled its Midwifery First Year of Practice programme, giving new graduates the option of a mentor.[26] In their report, the Wellington reviewers did not recommend a compulsory hospital internship but advised that the supervision and mentoring programme should be mandatory during midwives' first year of practice, and should not be over the phone – a suggestion that showed how perfunctory the current set-up was.[27] Ultimately, the reviewers blamed both medical and midwifery leadership for the lack of progress in improving maternity services. They commented on the 'lack of respect, collegiality and collaboration between the obstetric and midwifery colleges that is reflected in some very poor relationships between individual midwives and obstetricians'.[28] There needed to be an attitudinal change. The report mirrored many of the suggestions made by coroners and health and disability commissioners, as discussed in the previous chapter.

While this committee, set up by Labour 'to ensure public safety and confidence', outlined significant deficiencies in the current system and regulatory processes, its report appeared shortly before a general election. Implementation would therefore be in the hands of an incoming National government, with Tony Ryall the new Minister of Health.

## The Baby Business, 2008

Meanwhile, Lynda Exton, a Christchurch GP obstetrician of 25 years' standing, published a trenchant criticism of the midwifery-led childbirth system since 1990. Her main criticism was of government policies that had forced GPs out of maternity services, to the detriment of those services. A press release explained that she had been motivated to write her 'extensively researched book after a disquieting increase in the number of stories she heard from women of near misses, tragedies and unnecessarily complicated pregnancies and births'. It reiterated her conclusion that major changes to this key health service had occurred without adequate monitoring or independent audit.[29]

*New Zealand Doctor* claimed that Exton's colleagues and consumers supported the book, but that she faced criticism from the Ministry of Health and the College of Midwives. It further claimed that to date neither the Ministry nor the College had read the book, but 'remain[ed] at odds with Dr Exton over facts used in promotional material'.[30] The statement they objected to was undoubtedly the claim that New Zealand had one of the highest newborn death rates in the developed world. The Ministry of Health's chief advisor for child and youth health, Dr Pat Tuoy, countered this with a reassurance that the infant mortality rate was a record low, and Karen Guilliland agreed that New Zealand 'compared pretty well internationally for birth outcomes', with the Christchurch *Press* repeating the College of Midwives' view that New Zealand's maternity services were 'among the best in the world'.[31] These assertions were difficult to evaluate in the absence of reliable data. Yet some worrying trends had been revealed in the first PMMRC report published the previous year. It drew attention to an increase in New Zealand's perinatal mortality rate from the years 2000 to 2003, with a much higher increase for Māori than for New Zealanders of European descent.[32]

Two reviews of Exton's book appeared in the *Journal of Primary Health*, one by GP obstetrician William Ferguson and the other by midwife Joan Carll. Clearly the journal strove for balance by inviting these two reviewers, and they offered understandably different perspectives. According to Ferguson, this was 'a modern history book that had to be written', and Exton 'needed a more than usual amount of courage and determination' to do so. In his view, 'All participants in the tortuous saga of New Zealand's maternity services over the last 18 years should be interested, if not required, to read this detailed and extensively referenced account of events.' In contrast, Carll referred to the unfriendly practices at the St Helen's midwifery training hospitals where she herself had trained, all of which had closed by 1990, long before the 1990s reforms. Overlooking Exton's detailed account of policy changes resulting in the GP exodus, Carll simply commented that this needed to happen, asking, 'Hands up those who have been to their GP needing attention only to be left in the waiting room while they dash off to deliver a baby?' She concluded her review with the claim that the challenges for midwives continued to be extreme, but she did not spell out what those challenges were.[33]

## Another 'Unfortunate Experiment'

In 2009 the *New Zealand Listener* reported on a submission by the Royal Australian and New Zealand College of Obstetricians and Gynaecologists to the Australian government's 2009 Maternity Services Review.[34] The submission included a discussion of New Zealand's midwifery-led maternity system, which it described as 'an "unfortunate experiment", responsible for rising baby and maternal death rates, and a disaster that the rest of the world would learn from'. The term 'unfortunate experiment' was well known in the context of events leading to the 1988 Cartwright Inquiry. The College's submission blamed the 1990s New Zealand reforms for the erosion of collaboration and teamwork in maternity care, the exodus of GPs from the sector, a lack of choice for mothers now forced to take whichever midwife was available, and the inability of hospitals to hold independent midwives accountable for safe practice. It also claimed that the reforms had contributed to increased rates of caesarean deliveries and other interventions, when they had promised to do the very opposite.[35] (Caesareans had increased from 11.6% of all births in 1988–89 to 23% by 2005, with a 50% increase between 1996 and 2005.)[36] In its final report, the Australian review pointed to submitters' differing views about the benefits of midwifery-led models.[37] Citing the College's submission, the review raised familiar concerns about midwives' preparedness for 'advanced practice', and suggested the need for additional qualifications and experience. The review also commented that improving harmony within the maternity workforce was crucial to achieving maternity reform.[38]

The College of Midwives dismissed the obstetricians and gynaecologists' submission as 'patch protection and scaremongering by Australian specialists keen to keep their stranglehold on the sector as it considered reforms similar to ours'.[39] Karen Guilliland and Sally Pairman reported in their 2010 history of the College that New Zealand had achieved a 'unique maternity service, based on a relationship model of midwife and woman as equal decision-makers and supported by legislation'. They claimed that it was still the only country in the world to have achieved such a model.[40] However, they also believed that in New Zealand, as in Australia, midwifery autonomy was 'regularly challenged', since some people did not think a woman-dominant profession could be trusted to provide a safe service without medical supervision.[41] Authors of a 2012 Australian College of Midwives publication agreed with this assessment, referencing Guilliland and even Sandra Coney's 1988 book on the

Cartwright Inquiry to argue that, despite recent wide-ranging developments, New Zealand's maternity system was 'constantly under threat from political forces which seek to return it to medical control'.[42]

However, the Royal Australian and New Zealand College of Obstetricians and Gynaecologists' submission was not written by Australian specialists concerned about patch protection, as the College of Midwives suggested. The *Listener* explained that it was compiled by a New Zealand committee, and its chair, Auckland obstetrician Gillian Gibson, stood by every word of it.[43] In 2009, commenting on two stillbirths resulting from midwives failing to pick up signs of distress from heart-monitoring equipment, Gibson reiterated the Wellington Area Review's plea for standardised guidelines when self-employed midwives accompanied their clients to hospital.[44] The *Listener* article, itself entitled 'Another unfortunate experiment', repeated the claim that: 'In what some say is an extraordinary omission by the Health Ministry, it launched New Zealand into some of the most dramatic public health reforms ever seen, without following that up with data to show if it works.'[45]

This article and Exton's book also inspired Lannes Johnson, a GP obstetrician who had attended about 3,000 births over 30 years, to contribute an article to *New Zealand Doctor* entitled 'Experimenting with maternity services'. He revisited the history of the reforms and the social and political factors that had led to what he called the 'awful decisions' made during the 1980s and 1990s, arguing they were ideologically and politically driven. He still wondered why so many of the medical colleges and GP leaders were ignored, and why the 'small voice of pregnant women was lost in the hubris'. He asked, 'What have been the consequences, do we even know?'[46]

## Petitioning Parliament and the select committee 2009–2010

It was not only health professionals who raised issues. In 2009, a maternity action group called 'The Good Fight' was set up, comprising consumers along with health professionals. Founding member Shannon Beynon told the press how she had lost her two-day-old daughter Emma at Christchurch Women's Hospital in 1996 after complications from a prolonged labour. She said that the coroner had ruled that Emma would have lived had she and her mother been transferred from the primary birthing centre to hospital earlier, and that midwives had a 'professional responsibility to refer to others when they reached the limit of their expertise'.[47] Another founding member, Jenn Hooper, was motivated to speak out after her daughter Charley was born with severe cerebral palsy following apparently inadequate monitoring by two midwives and a bungled resuscitation at her birth in a Morrinsville birthing unit in 2005, which also nearly killed Hooper.[48] Her baby, she told a reporter in 2014, was left 'brain damaged, blind, tetraplegic, not knowing who I am'.[49]

In June 2009 Hooper presented to Parliament a 121-page submission on behalf of The Good Fight, backed by a petition with 1,500 signatures. It exhorted the government to change New Zealand's maternity system to enhance the safety and protection of all mothers and babies.[50] Recommendations revolved around monitoring and ensuring accountability of providers, but the first called for 'a complete change in the philosophy behind New Zealand's maternity providers to move the emphasis away from "a normal life experience" towards "a safe and satisfying birth experience"'. The submission drew attention to certain funding incentives the petitioners did not believe encouraged best practice, such as giving bonuses to LMCs who booked their client at a private birthing facility or non-tertiary hospital, and a bonus to midwives whose clients were not admitted to hospital. It asked for an independent review of the changes to the maternity system over the past two decades by a panel of international experts 'with no vested interest in the outcome'. The petitioners urged the establishment of an accessible perinatal database, together with standardised, evidence-based documentation and monitoring of pregnancy, labour and birth, along with a review of the training and funding of all LMCs, and better safety nets to pre-empt and deal with emergency situations.[51]

Health Minister Tony Ryall met with the group in 2009, assuring them that several matters they raised were in hand.[52] He also referred their submission to a Health Select Committee headed by National MP and obstetrician Paul Hutchison, which published a 20-page report in 2010, recommending that the government take the petition seriously.[53] The select committee thanked the petitioners 'for the enormous effort, thought, and courage' they put into presenting their petition and the stories behind it, and agreed that serious work was needed to improve New Zealand's maternity services.[54] The committee's recommendations included enhanced postgraduate monitoring and supervision of providers before they entered independent practice; for midwives this should be for at least a year. It also recommended continuous peer review, audit, and educational updates for practitioners.[55]

In 2010 *New Zealand Doctor* announced another online petition to the Minister of Health. The 528 signatories included consumers and senior hospital midwives, who expressed concern about the performance of new midwifery graduates and also requested a two-year internship in a tertiary hospital.[56] The petition was reportedly prompted by more parents coming forward whose babies had died or been compromised through midwifery inexperience.[57] The Waikato Hospital midwives who signed the petition said they had previously gone to the press about poor practice in a local birthing centre (where two midwives had mixed up drugs), rather than approaching the College of Midwives, because of the manner in which the College had responded to complaints including their own.[58] In response to the petition, chair of the Midwifery Council Sally Pairman said there was no evidence to suggest that new midwifery graduates needed to undertake a hospital internship. She said they had increased the training hours in 2006 not because new graduates lacked 'competence' but because they lacked 'confidence'.[59]

## 'Failure to Deliver', 2011

In 2011 the PMMRC presented its first report to the new Health Quality & Safety Commission, based on 2009 data. In her introduction, Cynthia Farquhar reported their finding that 14% of all perinatal deaths and 33% of maternal deaths were potentially avoidable. The report analysed contributory factors. It found those most frequently cited were 'lack of policies, protocols, guidelines, inadequate education and training, and poor organisational arrangements of staff'. Assessing contributory factors under the heading 'Personnel', it concluded the most common were the failure to follow recommended best practice, lack of knowledge and skills, and failure to recognise the complexity or seriousness of a condition. Dr Vicki Culling, who compiled the section on 'Issues for parents, families and whanau', commented that reading about this lack of policies, inadequate training and communication, and failure to follow best practice, would be 'heart-wrenching for many parents'.[60]

The following month the Auckland-based magazine *North & South* picked up on the concerns expressed in the report and also that mortality in itself did not give the whole picture. Journalist Donna Chisholm repeated the claim that, despite this 'most profound change in the make-up of our maternity workforce', no one knew the impact this had had on the health of mothers and babies, because 'despite decades of urging and official recommendations', data were still only being collected on deaths and not on harm.

Chisholm interviewed well-known figures in the debates around childbirth services, including former perinatal physiologist and the prime minister's chief scientific advisor Sir Peter Gluckman, Cynthia Farquhar, Lynda Exton and Jenn Hooper. All expressed disquiet about the current system. Gluckman thought the reforms should have been piloted before being rolled out nationally. Farquhar told Chisholm that she strongly supported graduate midwives spending their first year under supervision in hospital to get more exposure to complications of pregnancy and birth than they might experience in training. Exton spoke of her concern that since 1990 the maternity system had been premised on a philosophy of birth as a normal life event rather than aiming for a healthy outcome. Hooper said of the current midwifery rubric, 'Being an expert in normal birth is like being a meteorologist who specialises in fine weather.'

From her interviews, Chisholm identified training and mentoring of midwives as the most pressing issue. She reported that even some midwives questioned whether their training equipped them well enough for independent practice, at least in the early months, and cited midwife Jennifer Rowan's comment that her practice had 'changed heaps' since 2009 and that she did not believe her training had been robust enough.[61] Tony Ryall referred to the 'persistent calls' for graduate midwives to spend a supervised year in hospital, but said that on the advice of the Midwifery Council he preferred to strengthen the current system rather than opt for the more expensive hospital internship.[62]

In contrast to the views of doctors Gluckman, Farquhar and Exton, Karen Guilliland told Chisholm that she found the debate over the quality of midwives 'frustratingly, tediously circular and anti-feminist'. Of the repeated calls for a supervised, in-hospital postgraduate year for midwives, she said the only people suggesting it were doctors and lawyers. She believed it was based on gender and the failure to see that a woman's profession could be highly competent. She told Chisholm that the 'establishment of law, medicine and politics is deeply entrenched in thinking that a women's profession really needs help', and insisted, 'A few other people need help and it's not us.'[63]

## Consumers and Action to Improve Maternity, 2011

Guilliland's suggestion that doctors and lawyers were alone in criticising the midwifery-led system was incorrect. Consumers were mobilising. Jenn Hooper expanded the lobby group The Good Fight into a charitable trust called Action to Improve Maternity (AIM) in 2011, and its database grew rapidly to encompass about 500 families whose children had died or been damaged at birth; by 2013, that number totalled 650.[64]

This was a very different consumer group from those which had supported the College of Midwives upon its foundation. Two Australian midwives writing in 2012 about New Zealand's unique midwifery system of maternity care enthused that the 1990 reforms had resulted from partnerships between midwives' organisations and groups representing childbearing women, and that this 'continues to be important today'.[65] This was in line with the statement in the 2006 midwifery textbook that: 'The continued involvement of women (consumers) in the policy formation and processes of the College ensures that midwives uphold the needs and wishes of women.'[66] But which women?

As discussed in previous chapters, the consumers who had supported the College in 1990 were closely involved in the homebirth movement in alliance with homebirth midwives, and came to the movement with a strong feminist orientation. But to some extent feminism itself had changed over the decades, as had attitudes to the natural childbirth movement. In her study of American childbirth history, Jacqueline Wolf referred to a new generation of feminists who were demanding the choice of caesarean birth. '[E]pidural anesthesia and elective caesarean section,' she explained, 'had come to represent the essence of female empowerment in relation to birth.'[67] This was echoed in a 2011 article on childbirth in the Netherlands that relayed how feminists there were calling for women's right to pain relief, in particular epidurals, and were questioning the ideology of natural delivery and midwives' insistence that it was good for women to deal with pain without pharmacological support.[68]

Elective caesareans were also on the rise in New Zealand, although they still constituted a minority of all births. In 2009, National Women's Hospital noted 14.6% of all births were elective caesareans but these included those planned for medical reasons as well as by maternal request.[69] Women choosing this option often felt judged for doing so.[70] In Australia, obstetrician Caroline de Costa, a self-proclaimed feminist, believed that women had the right to demand a caesarean without being criticised as 'too posh to push', with the safety and wellbeing of the woman and her child being paramount.[71]

There was no consumer group in New Zealand demanding the right to caesarean birth. The consumer group AIM believed, however, that some people took the natural childbirth philosophy too far. AIM paid close attention to the PMMRC reports and publicised its findings, including the fact that the 2013 report showed that between 2006 and 2011, '35 per cent of maternal deaths were identified as being potentially avoidable'.[72] Jenn Hooper was delighted when the PMMRC expanded its remit to include morbidity as well as mortality, including outcomes like her daughter's cerebral palsy.[73] She believed that the long-term costs to the country of these outcomes should make the government pay attention. She noted that the tax-funded compensation system, ACC, had recently put the treatment cost for each birth-related brain injury at $54 million per child. Reporting that 149 babies had been born with brain damage in 2010–11, with inadequate resuscitation listed as the cause in 15% of those cases, she maintained this was a considerable public burden.[74]

Hooper set up a website to gather information and to act as a contact point for AIM, whose network included not just affected families, but also doctors, midwives, paediatricians, nurses and other health professionals concerned about the current system.[75] She insisted in 2013 that they were not 'uninformed and obsessive lobbyists with a long held agenda to undermine midwives in New Zealand', as 'certain lobbyists' had been described in a recent College of Midwives media release and which Hooper assumed referred to AIM.[76] Indeed, in 2015 retired public health physician Margaret Guthrie wrote that she was 'deeply grateful to Hooper who, despite her numerous tragedies, has emerged to become such a knowledgeable [and] humane . . . advocate for safe maternity care'.[77] GP obstetrician Pippa MacKay also complimented Hooper as 'a tenacious and articulate advocate for mothers and their babies' to whom they should all be listening. She added, 'Many doctors involved in obstetrics and neonatal paediatrics have tried to bring the same failures of midwifery care to public notice in the past, but always get tarred with the brush of "self-interest".' Challenging this view, she defined herself as a mother of three daughters, a sister, aunt and patient advocate, whose interest and concern had always been much wider than that of her profession. She referred to 'medicine's apprenticeship model' which supported learning and experience, and felt that midwifery would 'do well to embrace it a little more'. She described Guilliland and the College's dismissal of any criticism as 'arrogant and out of touch'.[78]

## Primary birthing units, homebirth and transfers

Much of the concern relating to maternity services revolved around the philosophy and skill levels of LMC midwives, particularly when they practised outside the hospital setting – in private homes or primary birthing units. Jenn Hooper told Donna Chisholm in 2016 that, of the 650 families AIM had represented, 95% of concerned mothers (like herself) had planned to birth in a birthing unit or at home; Lynda Exton had calculated it at around 90%.[79] This was at a time when only 3% to 4% of births occurred at home and around 10% in primary birthing units, as later calculated by the PMMRC for the period 2016–2020.[80]

In 2012 Hooper led another submission to Parliament demanding, among other things, the strengthening of referral guidelines for transfer from home and primary-care units to base hospitals.[81] Transfer from primary birthing units to hospital (either one of the six tertiary or 19 secondary hospitals in the country) was also one of the features of many of the cases that ended up before coroners and/or health and disability commissioners.

Primary units were regarded as an alternative to homebirth, and were run by midwives, with no on-site obstetric presence. By the early twenty-first century, there were about 60 primary maternity units in New Zealand. Māori women were twice as likely to give birth in primary units than non-Māori women, with a 2010 study calculating that 16.9% of Māori births and 8.8% of non-Māori births occurred in the units. The reason for this higher Māori occupancy probably related to location, with most of the units situated in rural areas or provincial towns.[82]

The opening of a birthing centre in Bethlehem near Tauranga in 2014 by Prime Minister John Key afforded the opportunity for a journalist to investigate broader issues around these primary-care facilities. The centre offered free (public-funded) births; for an additional cost, clients were entitled to stay longer than the statutory three days, and have various upgrades, which managing director Roy Younge explained was a good business model. Like other such units, the Bethlehem unit was intentionally low-tech; there were no specialists, obstetricians or GPs on site, but they shared the building with a chiropractor, an acupuncturist and a physiotherapist.[83] Therapies on offer at the unit included 'HypnoBirthing', which was described as the 'art of birthing in a way that allows her [the mother] to summon her natural birthing instincts and to birth her baby in safety and with ease'.[84]

One mother who was planning to birth at the centre using HypnoTherapy told the journalist that her two-page birthing plan did not consider transfer to hospital. Hooper told the journalist that birthing centres did not generally publicise their transfer rates or give realistic timelines for emergency transfers. But one study the following year found that fewer than half of the women who planned to birth in a primary unit did so, and that the average emergency transfer time was 58 minutes.[85] The Bethlehem Birthing Centre itself took part in a practice transfer scenario with Tauranga Hospital before opening; it took 40 minutes. This could make a difference to the outcome, but transfer was more problematic for more remote rural units. A 2006 study recorded average transfer times in rural areas of around 90 minutes, but they ranged from 29 minutes to 1,440 minutes (24 hours).[86] A 2008 survey of rural primary maternity-care facilities found that the waiting time for ambulance services in some areas could be three to four hours. Many areas were reliant on an urban ambulance coming out to the rural area, then returning to the city with the woman and midwife. It found rural ambulances were mostly staffed by volunteers, generally a single driver, leaving the midwife alone in the back to manage any emergencies.[87] This was a long way from the flying squad concept employed in Britain as part of its homebirth services.

The College of Obstetricians and Gynaecologists was supportive of low-technology stand-alone primary childbirth units, provided they were sited 'wherever possible' within or immediately adjacent to a 24-hour hospital facility.[88] In the Netherlands, birthing centres run by midwives generally met these criteria.[89] Even for homebirths, a Dutch midwife had to be able to reach the home of any woman booked for a homebirth within 15 minutes, and emergency care had to be not more than 15 minutes away by ambulance. In 2008 it was reported in that country that 49% of those having their first babies and 17% of those having their second or subsequent babies were transferred during labour.[90] Birthing units in other countries also commonly had ready access to secondary facilities. In the mid-1990s Australian homebirth midwife Maggie Lecky-Thompson had complained that none of the nine birthing centres in New South Wales were free-standing; all had varying degrees of obstetrician and/or GP involvement.[91]

The journalist reporting on the Bethlehem Centre also interviewed the Health Quality & Safety Commission chair Alan Merry, professor of anaesthesiology at the University of Auckland. Merry had made his views known in his foreword to the recent PMMRC report, where he commented that there was 'clearly still work to be done to improve safety of our maternity services'.[92] The executive summary of that report had noted that 'labouring in an isolated location and the need for a long transfer for secondary or tertiary care when required' was a significant contributory factor to preventable perinatal deaths.[93] A later PMMRC report would recommend improvements in transfer availability and support to deal with neonatal encephalopathy in particular.[94] Given that the PMMRC found that over 13% of neonatal encephalopathy cases in 2010–2012 occurred at home or in primary facilities without specialist facilities, this was no minor consideration.[95]

When homebirths had been discussed by the Maternity Services Committee back in the 1970s, and comparisons made with homebirth experience in the Netherlands, one of the issues raised was the long distance New Zealanders had to travel to hospital. There were few studies in New Zealand on the outcome of homebirths. Despite pointing out that the country's homebirth rate (2.5%) was the second highest in the world after the Netherlands, a 2015 international review included only one reference to a study of homebirth in New Zealand which did not focus on issues of safety.[96] A reason for this absence could have been the lack of data. A 2015 Auckland DHB strategic plan for maternity services noted that neither the boards nor the Ministry of Health collected statistics on homebirths.[97] This absence of studies on outcomes of planned home births contrasted with Australia where such research continued to be conducted.[98]

In the second decade of the twenty-first century, low-tech birthing as practised in the primary units continued to enjoy official support. The Auckland DHB's 2015 10-year maternity strategic plan, for example, included the aim to: 'Support and increase primary birthing options for women which will encourage women to give birth out of hospital.'[99] However, evidence accumulated by the consumer group AIM, alongside the findings of coroners and health and disability commissioners and the PMMRC, suggested that the maternity-led care which formed the basis of practice in these locations was at times concerning.

## Immunisation in the early twenty-first century

While the midwifery-led maternity system continued to enjoy government support, with the Ministry of Health often leaping to its defence when it was under fire, there was one area where independent or self-employed midwives practising as LMCs did not win the Ministry's backing, albeit with the critics coming from the latter's public health rather than its maternity sector.

Part of the contract for the LMC system from 2002 was that LMCs were required to provide mothers with Ministry of Health information on immunisation.[100] In the 1990s the College of Midwives had seen its role as providing parents with information on both sides of the immunisation debate. In 2002, Director of Public Health Collin Tukuitonga was shocked to find that some midwives were not promoting immunisation and were even directing parents to anti-immunisation material. He considered this inappropriate for state employees: 'People who are receiving state subsidies ought to be providing what the state says is good practice.' Natalie Desmond from the Immunisation Advisory Centre which had been set up at the University of Auckland in 1996 explained that, in the interests of informed consent, it was currently standard practice for many LMCs to pass on anti-immunisation material produced by the Immunisation Awareness Society (IAS) when they gave parents the Ministry pamphlet. She herself considered this unethical since the IAS pamphlet was 'based on anecdotes and pseudoscience' and 'extraordinarily emotive'. She added, 'It's not just a few fringe LMCs – it's mainstream LMCs.'[101]

In June 2002 the *New Zealand Herald* reported Tukuitonga's claim, based on information he had received from GPs and hospital paediatricians, that midwives were distributing anti-immunisation material to expectant mothers. It also reported the claim by Dr Nikki Turner, a GP and director of the Immunisation Advisory Centre, that midwives were spreading misinformation: 'At first we thought it was just a few isolated cases, but we then realised through our networks it was quite widespread.' She described the IAS pamphlet as scaremongering and wildly inaccurate, and pointed out that, as nearly 90% of mothers made up their minds on the issue antenatally, midwives as LMCs carried a significant responsibility.[102]

Tukuitonga ordered LMCs 'to cease handing out the Immunisation Awareness Society's anti-immunisation pamphlets', a move endorsed by the Immunisation Advisory Centre.[103] This resulted in letters sent directly to

Tukuitonga from the IAS, consumer advocates and midwives. Erin Hudson and Sue Claridge of the IAS, copying in the College of Midwives and Women's Health Action, told Tukuitonga that the IAS was not anti-immunisation but pro-choice. They maintained that all the information in their brochures was 'backed up by solid references, much of it from peer reviewed medical journals'.[104] Long-time homebirth advocate Lynda Williams told Tukuitonga it was 'inappropriate and unacceptable for the Ministry of Health to be trying to suppress or blacklist other organisations or other sources of information in this way'.[105] Midwife Sian Burgess expressed concern about Tukuitonga's 'deriding' of midwives for not promoting immunisation. She told him that midwives were very concerned about immunisation but chose to contribute to babies' immune status by focusing on breastfeeding, which would enhance the babies' immunity, along with good nutrition, good baby care, lack of stress and lack of poverty, 'all issues that engage the midwifery profession'. She added that midwives were committed to the Code of Patient Rights and ensuring that parents receive full information that enables them to make an informed choice regarding all aspects of their care and vaccination choices.[106]

Later that year, Sue Claridge wrote an article for the magazine *Education Effects*, in which she was described as the mother of two very healthy unvaccinated children, aged three and one, editor of IAS's monthly newsletter *WAVES* (Warnings about Vaccine Expectations), and author of a forthcoming book for IAS on vaccination.[107] Her nine-page article was titled 'Making INFORMED Decisions about Vaccinating your Child'.[108] Claridge claimed that Tukuitonga made 'thinly veiled threats against the job security of midwives who disseminated information on vaccination that was not sanctioned by the Ministry of Health'. She stated categorically that unvaccinated children were generally healthier than vaccinated children.[109] *Education Effects* subsequently published letters from Helen Petousis-Harris from the Immunisation Advisory Centre, and Simon Clendon, both highly critical of Claridge. Clendon declared he hoped the magazine did not mean to endorse the latter's article by printing it.[110]

*Education Effects* had been set up in 1989 as the mouthpiece of Childbirth Educators New Zealand. The close association between the childbirth educators who ran many of the antenatal classes and the homebirth movement was discussed in Chapter 2. The College of Midwives continued that association, with its journal advertising courses for childbirth educators who would 'assist women to make informed choices throughout their pregnancy, during childbirth and in the weeks following'.[111] In 2009, a mother and medical graduate penned an account of her antenatal class in *O&G Magazine*, reporting her concern that 'rather than being advocated for, immunisation was presented very neutrally as an option that parents may wish to pursue'.[112] Turner also said she knew of antenatal classes where anti-immunisation information was handed out in the interests of informed choice, but she worried that, without accompanying explanation, this would effectively give equal weight to evidence-based and non-evidence-based information.[113]

When asked by *New Zealand Doctor* in 2010 about the obligation on LMCs to provide Ministry of Health information on immunisation, the College of Midwives affirmed that these requirements meant that a midwife's personal beliefs were irrelevant, and that very few midwives were opposed to immunisation in any case. 'The trouble is,' said Amanda Cameron of *New Zealand Doctor*, 'the anecdotes keep piling up.' Cameron consulted Sue Baines, who coordinated Northland DHB's National Immunisation Register. Baines told her that 'a handful of self-employed midwives working in the area refuse to provide information about immunisation in their antenatal education classes, don't report home births to the NIR [National Immunisation Register], and, anecdotally, direct mums-to-be and new mothers to anti-immunisation websites'. Cameron decided to randomly call a Northland midwife, who 'did nothing to dispel these allegations'. The midwife told her it was the woman's choice, but then directed Cameron to the IAS. The midwife also told her that the Ministry of Health website 'always makes you afraid of all the diseases' and was 'sponsored by big drug companies that want to push [vaccines]'.[114]

The Nurses' Organisation claimed to know of a minority of health practitioners who did not support immunisation or give parents the recommended information. It called for consistent training in immunisation for health practitioners and childbirth educators, and advised that attendance at two-yearly immunisation training courses should be 'compulsory for all health professionals involved in immunisation, especially educators and LMCs'.[115] In 2011 a Health Select Committee headed by Paul Hutchison and tasked with improving immunisation rates also called for increased training for LMCs. The committee recommended that contracts for LMCs be strengthened to recognise the obligation of healthcare professionals to promote only evidence-based medicine.[116]

In 2013 disquiet was expressed about practising midwives who were not immunised against influenza. Apparently, only 37% of midwives employed by

DHBs had accepted free flu vaccinations in the previous year, the lowest of all health providers. The uptake in some areas was as low as 22%. The *Herald* interviewed an independent midwife of 40 years' standing who complained that all the information was pro-vaccination, inhibiting an informed decision. She explained that she believed in bolstering immunity through a healthy diet, exercise, and covering mouths when sneezing.[117]

## Conclusion

Despite the 2003 Health Practitioners Competence Assurance Act, the Midwifery Council's Competencies for Entry to the Register of Midwives from 2004, and Section 88 of the 2000 Public Health and Disability Act setting out guidelines, there appeared to be ongoing concerns from some quarters – notably other health professionals and consumers – about the quality of maternity care. While immunisation was one such concern, others related to training and mentoring of new midwives, protocols for transfers from home and primary-care units to secondary and tertiary care, and auditing and accountability of LMCs in different settings. These were by no means new concerns, and many had been raised by coroners and health and disability commissioners in relation to individual cases they investigated. This chapter has shown commentary coming from a much wider range of sources, although with equally little impact on practice or policy.

Meanwhile, the PMMRC was gathering information for the first time since the changes to the maternity system in 1990, revealing some worrying trends. By 2017 it noted that there had been no statistically significant change in the maternal mortality ratio in New Zealand since data started to be collected in 2006, and that maternal mortality continued to be significantly higher than that in the UK.[118] In 2015 New Zealand ranked seventeenth in an international table of the lifelong risk of dying in maternity.[119] The neonatal death rate had not changed materially in New Zealand from 2007 to 2015, whilst there had been significant reductions in the UK, Australia and Scandinavia.[120] Was New Zealand keeping up with international trends? During the second decade of the twenty-first century these outcomes would be subjected to more rigorous academic scrutiny, systems failures would be addressed by the PMMRC and others, and the results would once again be hotly debated.

# TWELVE

## *Research into maternity outcomes during the 2010s*

THE SECOND DECADE OF the twenty-first century finally saw the emergence of academic research into New Zealand's maternity services, including across different population groups. This chapter examines this research, and responses from the New Zealand College of Midwives, along with the Midwifery Council and the Ministry of Health, who had oversight of the services. Those conducting the studies and other commentators described the College's reaction to that research as defensive and unconstructive. For its part, the College regarded any concerns arising from the research as scaremongering, refused to take the findings seriously, and continued to express pride in New Zealand's unique midwifery-led childbirth system. Divergent views, if anything, appeared to become even more entrenched and irreconcilable. Similar divisions were being exposed in some parts of England around this time, although there the Royal College of Midwives appeared to take on board the concerns revealed following investigations, providing a possible model for its New Zealand counterpart.

## Bev Lawton's research and responses

Professor Bev Lawton from the Wellington Women's Health Research Centre is a longstanding advocate for women's health, and has had ongoing concerns about the maternity system and poor auditing. In 2010 she and her co-researchers reviewed 29 cases from 2005 to 2007 of severe acute maternal morbidity or 'near misses' at Wellington Hospital's intensive-care unit. Their study concluded that 10 of these, or 35%, were preventable, including all five of the septicaemia cases. Worryingly, three of the 10 women concerned were Māori (50% of the Māori in the total audit) and four were Pasifika (67% of the Pasifika women in the total audit). While this was a small sample, they considered it indicative, and called for a national system to record and review maternal morbidity. Their findings identified several contributory factors: 'Failure to diagnose infection, failure to follow up abnormal results, failure to recognise high risk status, delay in recognition of abnormal vital signs, delay in referral to experts, lack of knowledge, inadequate treatment and poor documentation.'[1]

Another study published by Lawton and colleagues in 2013 suggested that rising caesarean rates (up from 15.69% in 1996 to 23.5% in 2010) could be related to delayed referrals to specialists by midwives. As autonomous practitioners, LMC midwives had to take the initiative in requesting help from an obstetrician. The study concluded that failure to recognise the need for obstetric intervention could lead to a delay in the active management of labour and deterioration in maternal and fetal health, requiring urgent surgical intervention via caesarean delivery.[2]

In a 2014 paper, Lawton and her co-researchers pointed to the importance of reducing preventable severe maternal morbidity not only for the woman but also because of the potential effects on her baby. In line with their 2010 study, they found that 38.8% of adverse delivery outcomes for women with severe maternal morbidity were potentially preventable (38 out of the 98 analysed), and a further 36 (36.7%) women could have received better care. They concluded that 'the most frequent preventable factors were clinician related: delay or failure in diagnosis or recognition of high-risk status (51%); and delay or inappropriate treatment (70%)'.[3] Their research led to setting up of a system to evaluate severe maternal morbidity by district health boards, starting in 2015.[4]

However, it was a much larger study, published in 2015, which brought Lawton into direct conflict with the College of Midwives over midwifery-led maternity care. In November 2015, *New Zealand Doctor* announced that Lawton was calling on the government to review maternity training and consider supervision rules for new midwives. Lawton urged mandatory clinical supervision in hospital for newly graduated midwives for up to two years, followed by a supervised year in the community for independent midwives. The two-year study had found strong evidence that levels of midwifery experience were associated with baby mortality.[5]

Published online in the *International Journal of Gynecology and Obstetrics* on 13 October 2015, the article reported research conducted by New Zealand researchers and colleagues at the University of Illinois, USA. They used Ministry of Health data to match the years of experience of midwives to the life/death outcomes of 234,215 babies born in New Zealand from January 2005 to December 2009. Nurse-midwives oversaw 150,172 of those births and direct-entry midwives 84,043. Of the latter, 10,573 were cared for by midwives in their first year out of training. The researchers found that perinatal mortality rates did not differ by experience in the nurse-midwife group, but the 86 baby deaths involving direct-entry midwives with less than one year's experience was 33% higher than among those cared for by those midwives with five to nine years' post-registration experience.[6] Lawton told the press that this involved 21 more deaths over the five-year period for the direct-entry midwives than would be expected from more experienced midwives (practising five to nine years). She said that the higher rate among first-year graduates was statistically and clinically significant, as was the lower rate as midwives gained more experience.[7]

Action for Maternity (AIM) spokesperson Jenn Hooper applauded the study as confirming AIM's impressions. The College of Midwives, however, did not accept the findings. Chief Executive Karen Guilliland claimed the researchers' data was flawed, as it assumed that the midwife who was initially registered to work with the woman was the same one who attended the birth, which was often not the case when the woman transferred to hospital. She also said the data covering 2005–09 was out of date, and that deaths had declined from 2009 to the present, when the number of LMCs with midwife-only training had markedly increased and the number of doctors providing LMC care had decreased (the latter comment was hardly relevant, as the research was not about doctor LMCs). Guilliland concluded, 'Clearly the presence of highly educated midwives has improved the birth outcomes for babies. This is in contrast to the misguided claims made by Dr Lawton's study.'[8]

The issue attracted considerable media attention: 'Researcher faces backlash from midwives', Radio New Zealand reported.[9] The day after the research was published, College of Midwives' advisor Lesley Dixon declared that the research was out of date and scaremongering. Hooper, on the other hand, repeated that the study supported what some families had been saying about graduate midwives, and Lawton called for an urgent review of New Zealand's maternity training system.[10]

One of the study's authors, Stacie Geller, professor of Obstetrics and Gynecology at the Centre for Research on Women and Gender, University of Illinois, spoke of how careful they had been in their data collection and methodology, and in drawing conclusions. She was shocked by the College of Midwives' reaction, saying this was 'an academic disagreement that should have been handled in an academic professional [manner], instead it has been highly unprofessional'. She noted that Lawton had 'really been personally attacked', adding, 'I'm astounded by this.'[11] University of Otago Pro-Vice-Chancellor of Health Sciences Professor Peter Crampton was also appalled, claiming never to have seen such a strong reaction to research. The response, he said, had been 'very intense, very rapid and focused on her [Lawton] as a person and her professionally more than it would be customary in this situation'. He insisted that the attacks on Lawton must stop, and discussions moved 'from the intensely personal' to policy issues, 'in which there is legitimate public interest'.[12]

Hooper told Radio New Zealand that Lawton's findings provided evidence of the need for a hospital-based internship.[13] The College of Midwives and the Midwifery Council declined a Radio New Zealand interview but issued a statement that: 'Women can have confidence in knowing our midwifery-led maternity system is one of the safest if not the safest maternity services in the world.' They added that a compulsory midwifery hospital internship had been rejected as unnecessary and would add no value to the quality of maternity care. Lawton was not convinced, and pointed to Australia, where three years working in a hospital were required before government-funded midwives practised independently; she considered this 'very sensible'.[14]

Lawton said that the idea that new midwives could benefit from more experience was 'not rocket science', and she was disappointed the College had taken it as personal criticism. She explained, 'We want zero mistakes, zero avoidable deaths, that's what we should be aiming for here.' While acknowledging New Zealand had a good midwifery system, she believed more supervision of new midwives could bring further improvements. She estimated that in 2015 there might be about 1,500 pregnant women whose LMC was an independent midwife with less than one year's experience post-graduation, so the issue was not insignificant.[15]

Within four weeks of the research appearing online Guilliland, on behalf of the College, had lodged a complaint about the research findings with the Medical Council, which Lawton thought 'must be the first time anybody's made a complaint about public health research to the council'.[16] The Medical Council eventually rejected the complaint, but in the meantime Guilliland and colleagues had published a rebuttal of the research in the College of Midwives' journal, and in a letter to the *International Journal of Gynecology and Obstetrics*, which invited Lawton to respond.

In their rebuttal, Guilliland and her co-authors argued there were inaccuracies in the register information used to classify midwives, as some from overseas would be registered as first-year midwives, whilst others, although registered, did not enter practice for some time and would not be included in the first-year category. This misclassification, they argued, would lead to erroneous conclusions. Lawton responded that, if anything, such miscalculation could blur the real effects of inexperience of the first-year group, with more experienced midwives from overseas possibly inadvertently improving outcome statistics for the group.[17]

Guilliland and colleagues also claimed that the findings from 2005–09 could not be generalised to 2015. They explained, 'The historical dataset was taken from a period that bears little resemblance to the present system', referring to the increase in midwife LMCs. However, this increase was from around 80% of LMCs in 2009 to over 90% by 2015; the real change in providers had already occurred. There was no fundamental systemic change between 2009 and 2015 to support the assertion that there was little resemblance between the two periods. Guilliland and colleagues also delivered an inherent criticism of independent academic research, claiming that: 'To achieve robust, high quality research there is a need to involve midwives as one of the key maternity health professionals on any multidisciplinary research group exploring women's health and maternity care.' For added emphasis, this statement was repeated in a text box.[18]

The College of Midwives asked Health Minister Jonathan Coleman to initiate a separate study of first-year midwifery graduates.[19] In October 2016 the College announced that the Ministry of Health believed a more robust methodology than Lawton's was needed, together with more recent data, and had commissioned a new study led by Auckland District Health Board epidemiologist Dr Lynn Sadler.[20] Lawton agreed that access to more recent data not available to her team would be useful.[21] Contributors to the paper included the chair of the Midwifery Council Dr Judith McAra-Couper and the College of Midwives president Deb Pittam, who 'provided advice on the protocol, the analysis and interpretation of the findings', revealing the Ministry had heeded the advice to include midwives in academic research teams on maternity.[22]

The paper, published in the *British Medical Journal Open*, in 2018, covered the period 2008 to 2014. The authors found that there was indeed a significant reduction in the incidence of perinatal mortality among those under the care of midwives beyond the first year compared with those within the first year, affirming Lawton's findings. However, they pointed out that first-year-of-practice midwives cared for more women whose babies had a higher risk of perinatal mortality, including Māori, Pasifika, Indian, those under the age of 20, smokers, women living in socio-economic deprivation, and those with high body mass index, hypertension, type 2 diabetes, and antepartum haemorrhage. After adjusting for these risk factors, they concluded that the risk of perinatal mortality for those under the care of new midwives was not significantly higher than for those cared for by midwives beyond their first year.[23]

The paper criticised Lawton's paper for not 'adjusting for potential confounders in the association between midwifery experience and outcomes'. It also expressed concern that Lawton's paper 'eroded some of the community's trust in the unique midwifery model of care in place in NZ since 1990', suggesting why they believed a corrective necessary: 'The current study is important internationally as NZ has a unique maternity model of care . . . and is a model for the development of midwifery models worldwide.'[24] They had a reputation to maintain.

The College of Midwives welcomed the Sadler paper, which they said showed that outcomes for pregnant women registered with a graduate midwife were just as good as those registered with more experienced midwives.[25] Lawton and some of her colleagues were not convinced, finding the conclusion of the paper – that the increase in perinatal deaths was not a 'real' increase but due to first-year midwives looking after a riskier population – in itself concerning.[26] This also begs the question as to why these new graduates were looking after high-risk clients. Perhaps part of the answer lay in the finding of the 1999 National Health Committee review of maternity services that:

> Women who have adverse risk factors due to medical, mental or obstetric complications, often had very limited choices. The NHC heard about providers who would not register as a LMC for women whose care was likely to be more complex and costly. This was also the case where there was a threat of lost income due to the high probability that care during labour and birth would have to be transferred to another provider.[27]

In other words, experienced midwives could be more selective about who they took on. Deputy chair of the New Zealand Medical Association, GP obstetrician Don Simmers, had also noted in 2006 that, 'LMC midwives have been reluctant to take on women with medical problems who will inevitably require base hospital delivery.'[28]

Yet another study found less choice of carers amongst those most at risk of poor pregnancy outcomes. In 2015 public health researcher Karen Bartholomew, Professor Susan Morton and others published a paper on choice in the LMC system. Morton led the University of Auckland's 'Growing up in New Zealand' longitudinal study, and this article was based on a survey of over 6,500 women from the study who were pregnant in 2009 and 2010. They found that 145 women (2.2%) did not engage an LMC for maternity care, and that 694 women (or 12%) did not have a choice of providers (the 1999 Health Committee review had noted that a third of the women surveyed were unable to secure the LMC of their choice).[29] Bartholomew's study found that women not engaging an LMC, and those not experiencing choice, were more likely to be of non-European ethnicity, younger, or living in more deprived areas. They concluded that choice of LMC was 'unequally distributed in the NZ maternity population', and that those women missing out on an optimal service were also most at risk of poor pregnancy outcomes and potentially most in need of care, just as the 1999 review had found.[30]

The Perinatal and Maternal Mortality Review Committee would also later make the point that Māori, Pasifika and Indian mothers who were among those most likely to experience adverse outcomes in pregnancy were also 'less likely to have registered, or been able to register, with an LMC in the first trimester of pregnancy'.[31] The College of Midwives too intimated this in their initial response to Lawton's article. It stated that first-year midwives were still building up their caseloads, so had more room to take women later in their pregnancy who were more likely to have risk factors for perinatal mortality.[32] The system was inherently unfair.

Meanwhile Hooper led a submission to Parliament in 2015, drawing on Lawton's research and advocating a year's hospital internship for midwives. In its response, the Ministry of Health revealed that it had rejected the concept of a hospital internship on the advice of the College of Midwives, who argued it would compromise midwives' ability to deliver high-quality community-based midwifery care. Hooper's submission also suggested upgrading mentoring in the Midwifery First Year of Practice programme. It criticised the documentation around the Midwifery Council's mentoring programme, which stressed support for new independent midwives rather than measuring outcomes or benefits of the programme for the women and babies they cared for.[33]

The midwifery mentoring programme was made compulsory in 2015, but it consisted of educational opportunities such as lectures, along with a one- to two-hour session usually once a month with a trained midwifery mentor, and no direct supervision. Hooper and AIM did not consider this enough, and in 2019 sent another submission, declaring, 'Beyond statistics and facts and figures are real families and real people providing care, all of whom have to live with tragic results when they occur', adding that this was even more tragic when the outcomes were preventable. The submission noted that 'it was customary [in Britain] for newly qualified midwives not to work as community midwives for at least two years after graduation and to have completed a range of preceptorship competencies prior to entering community practice'. Urging more direct supervision, they stated, 'Maternity is not, in our view, the place for postgraduate "experiential learning" as it stands currently. That equates to something like gambling, but with someone else's chips.'[34]

In response to the 2019 submission, the College of Midwives referred to the expansion of midwifery training to a four-year programme, and pointed out that their profession was different from those of nurses and doctors, and more akin to the work of pharmacists, physiotherapists and allied health professions, who could also work in a hospital or community setting after graduation.[35] This was an odd comparison to make, and counter to previous assertions that midwives' work was equivalent to doctors', a point Guilliland had made in 1999 when she said that midwives had 'equal status' to doctors and obstetricians (as discussed on pp. 145–46); and midwives' equivalence to GPs had been accepted by the 1993 tribunal (see p. 159). When Dr Allan Sutherland had compared midwives to physiotherapists in the 1990s, he made the point that midwives were presented with very different challenges from physiotherapists, since childbirth could be a life-or-death matter. Nor was the College's comparison of midwife training to pharmacy training totally accurate, since the four-year pharmacy programme was followed by a year-long pre-registration training after graduation, administered by the Pharmaceutical Society of New Zealand under the supervision of a registered pharmacist.

Others were also reflecting on the midwives' level of training before practising in the community. An award-winning *University of Auckland Law Review* paper from 2017 asked, 'Should Midwives be Held to a Different Standard of Care, Given New Zealand's Unique Autonomous Midwife-led Framework?' Author Cherry Ngan argued that, with the exodus of GPs from maternity services, 'One could argue that midwives should be held to the same standard of care as GPOs [General Practitioner Obstetricians], as midwives play the role that GPOs did before the reforms.' The current framework, she wrote, assumed LMC midwives to be 'quasi-doctors solely responsible for detecting concerns and taking the correct action'. At the same time, she argued that imposing the same standard would be 'hugely unfair on midwives due to their lower education and training standards'. To explain this, she set out the training for GPOs, including admission to medical school, undertaking a six-year degree, spending at least two years working in a hospital, completing the three-year General Practice Education Programme to specialise in general practice, and obtaining the one-year full-time (or four-year part-time) Postgraduate Diploma in Obstetrics and Medical Gynaecology, amounting to 12 years. By contrast, a midwife undertook a three-year degree before she could practise autonomously, with minimal training in abnormal birth.[36]

Whilst she believed it was unfair to expect midwives to be as highly trained as GPOs, Ngan felt that midwifery educational requirements should be raised. She pointed out that the first few years of any doctor's professional life involved working in a hospital under the supervision of more experienced practitioners, and midwives should be required to do the same before 'making autonomous decisions'. This would not raise the midwife's standard of care to equal a GPO, she said, but it would 'reduce the gap'.[37]

Lawton herself led a submission to the Health Select Committee in 2019 with nine other signatories (three obstetricians, a neonatologist, two statisticians, and three research fellows at the Centre for Women's Health Research). Noting that both the Lawton and Sadler studies showed increased perinatal deaths associated with care by first-year midwives compared to more experienced midwives, they postulated that the lack of support and mandated supervision of early-career midwives added to their stress, and placed women and children at increased risk of harm and mortality. They pointed out that Māori continued to be disproportionately impacted by such disparities. They explained that doctors had two years' intensive supervision as house surgeons, in a model that supported practice development and collegial teamwork with more experienced practitioners, and thought this would be a helpful model for midwifery clinical practice. They also argued that this aspect of the maternity system could be easily addressed. They concluded, 'These are babies and women that are suffering preventable harm. We cannot in all conscience not submit this evidence to the committee even though several of us have had considerable stress from our previous foray into these system issues.'[38]

Meanwhile Lawton and others at the Centre for Women's Health Research, and in Illinois, published another paper in 2018 on severe maternal morbidity, blaming provider inadequacies in almost all cases (93.4%). Once again, the most common problems identified were inappropriate or delayed diagnosis, failure to recognise 'high-risk' patients, and inappropriate or delayed treatment.[39]

## Ellie Wernham's study and responses

In 2016 midwife Ellie Wernham led a multi-authored retrospective cohort study comparing midwifery-led and medical-led care, and the relationship to adverse fetal and neonatal outcomes in New Zealand. The results were published in *PLOS Medicine*, a high-ranked peer-reviewed open-access journal.[40] The comparison of midwifery-led and medical-led maternity care had become a hot topic internationally, especially after a 2010 study published in the *British Medical Journal* covering nearly 40,000 women who were pregnant during 2007–08 in the Netherlands. This study had found that infants of 'low-risk' women whose labour began under the supervision of a midwife were 2.33 times more likely to die during delivery than infants of 'high-risk' women whose labour began under the supervision of an obstetrician. Concluding that 'the Dutch system of risk selection in relation to perinatal death at term is not as effective as was once thought', the researchers called for a critical evaluation of the Netherlands obstetric care system.[41]

An article in *O&G Magazine* the following year, entitled 'Trouble in Paradise', pointed out that homebirth in the Netherlands, despite its international reputation, had recently been criticised as the 'main culprit for the relatively high Dutch perinatal mortality rate, one of the highest in Europe'. The debate, the author noted, had become highly polarised, with finger-pointing and mutual recrimination between midwives and obstetricians, with both groups publishing articles in their respective professional journals to bolster their views.[42] Articles did indeed appear in midwifery and nursing journals countering the 2010 *British Medical Journal* study. One 2015 study from Amsterdam, published in *Midwifery*, found no difference in outcomes between midwifery and obstetric-led care.[43] A systematic review published in the *Journal of Advanced Nursing* in 2012 concluded there was no evidence of negative impacts for mothers and infants receiving midwifery-led care rather than medical-led care.[44] There was no reference to the New Zealand model in that systematic review, despite its unique midwifery-led system, probably because of the lack of available studies to draw on. As Wernham and her colleagues noted, 'Despite a radical change in the way maternity care was delivered [from 1990], there has never been a full and proper evaluation to ensure the maternity system in New Zealand is safe.'[45]

Ellie Wernham had trained as a midwife and qualified in 2007. She later explained that, although she could have practised independently on graduation, she chose to work in hospital for a year, supervised by hospital midwives. She believed that any new graduate would feel underprepared to work independently when the stakes were so high. After her year in hospital, she took up a post in a clinic, working with midwives, GPs, social workers and other health workers, where she said she felt supported; she had chosen to work in a low-income area where the community's healthcare needs were high. In 2012 she enrolled for a Diploma in Public Health at the University of Otago Wellington. Professor of Public Health Diana Sarfati supervised her Master's thesis, which formed the basis of the article.[46] Co-authors of the article included Jason Gurney, Lis Ellison-Loschmann and James Stanley. Gurney and Ellison-Loschmann were both involved in Māori health research, and Stanley was a biostatistician and later one of the signatories of Lawton's 2019 petition.

The study covered 244,047 births between January 2008 and December 2012. Of these, 91.5% registered with a midwife as LMC and 8.5% with a medical LMC. While midwives managed the vast majority, the number in the medical group – 20,662 – was statistically large enough to draw comparisons. The study found that, after adjusting for likely confounding factors, medical-led births were associated with substantially lower odds for certain issues when compared with midwifery-led births. These were: an Apgar score of less than 7 at five minutes after birth (48% lower odds), birth-related asphyxia (55% lower odds), and the more severe neonatal encephalopathy that could cause brain damage (39% lower odds).[47] The authors concluded there was 'an unexplained excess of adverse events in midwife-led deliveries in New Zealand where midwives practice autonomously'. They believed the findings were concerning and demonstrated a need for further research that specifically investigated the reasons for the apparent excess of adverse outcomes in midwifery-led care.[48]

The authors stated that their findings should be interpreted in the context of New Zealand's internationally comparable birth outcomes, but cautioned that this did 'not preclude the possibility that avoidable adverse outcomes are occurring, potentially both in New Zealand and in other countries'.[49] They also advised that the findings should be viewed in the context of research that supported the many benefits of midwifery-led care, such as greater patient satisfaction and lower intervention rates.[50] A recent international systematic review had argued midwifery care with its many benefits was just as safe as medically led care.[51] This review was subsequently invoked to question Wernham's findings.[52] However, in their article Wernham and colleagues addressed this study and questioned whether it was relevant to New Zealand. They argued that the midwifery-led care included in the review was carried out by a small number of midwives (in most cases 10 or fewer), which made it difficult to generalise findings to a population-based setting with autonomous midwives. They noted 'a paucity of systemic evaluation that formally investigates safety-related outcomes in relationship to midwife-led care within an entire maternity service'. They also believed the review was not relevant to New Zealand, where midwives were more autonomous than in the countries where even in midwifery-led births there was some medical input.[53] A decade earlier, an Australian article had pointed to difficulties in interpreting data from an international systematic review of birth centres that argued in favour of midwifery-led services, noting that, among other variables, 'Some birth centre models had the routine involvement of medical practitioners while others did not.'[54]

Wernham later explained that when their striking findings of the different outcomes between doctor-led and midwifery-led care became apparent, she and Sarfati were mindful of what had happened after the release of Lawton's research, so they approached the Ministry of Health and the College of Midwives to explain the results and discuss how to use them constructively.[55] This was a forlorn hope; the College was not going to be happy with their findings. A later *Stuff* investigation revealed Wernham and Sarfati met with the Ministry and the College of Midwives a year before the article was published, giving them time to address the issues. Using records obtained under the Official Information Act, reporter Michelle Duff found evidence that the latter went into damage control, dismissing the research rather than constructively engaging with it. These documents included notes from a College National Committee meeting that described the research as flawed, and the comment: 'Watch for publications – College and MOH prepared to address the concerning issues of this poor research.' Guilliland accused the researchers of 'scaremongering, bias and naivety', and the Ministry's chief advisor for child and youth health Pat Tuohy assured her that the study would 'soon be consigned to the back pages'.[56]

One of the criticisms of the study was that it focused on the maternity carer at the time of registration and not at the time of birth – a criticism aimed at Lawton's earlier study. Wernham and her colleagues, however, thought the LMC should take responsibility for the outcome. Sarfati explained, 'For example if a problem occurs and it's missed and it's missed and it's missed, and then someone delivers the baby who is in a bad way, it wouldn't be fair to say that was the fault of the person who delivered the baby.'[57] Obstetricians had long complained of having to pick up the pieces.[58]

The College of Midwives also argued that the study showed 'inequality between private and public care and was not a reflection on midwives'.[59] Guilliland commented that women under the care of midwives were 'more likely to be rural and remote, Māori, Pasifika, younger, smoke, obese, sicker and book late with a carer . . . well-known risk factors that cause the adverse outcomes described'. These women, she said, were being compared with those 'who live in big cities (mainly Auckland) and who can pay thousands of dollars and afford to have a private obstetrician'.[60] A system that ostensibly required private (and expensive) care for a better outcome was not a good one. If true, this was a serious indictment of the post-1990 structure in a country that had prided itself on free maternity care since 1939, changes in which the College itself had taken a lead. In any case, epidemiologist Charlotte Paul, who reviewed the paper, pointed out that the study design accounted for factors like smoking, age, ethnicity, deprivation and weight, and that the results remained sound.[61]

Wernham's research was the subject of a feature article in the *New Zealand Listener*, which blazoned a series of statements on its cover: 'Alarming Maternity Research: Birth: Where the Revolution Went Wrong: The dangers of midwives in charge'. Writer Donna Chisholm affirmed in the opening paragraph that 'no one is throwing the reform baby out with this lot of bathwater', but added, 'our maternity system could be doing better – some say much better.'[62] Chisholm interviewed a range of experts about the new research findings, in addition to Ellie Wernham and Diana Sarfati. These included three obstetricians and three senior midwives, along with others such as Bev Lawton, Jenn Hooper and Lynda Exton.

As the senior academic involved in the research, Sarfati told Chisholm that, while no epidemiological study based on routine data would ever be perfect, they had been 'extremely careful in their approach' and the international experts who had reviewed the research all found the study robust and the results concerning.[63] Wernham reflected on what had prompted her research. She described how, in her hospital year following midwifery training, she saw far more complications and births that went wrong than she had in training. She explained:

> It was mentioned during training that one of the things that might occur if we worked in a hospital was that we'd be more set in a medicalised model of birth. The midwifery philosophy has always focused on the normal, and that care should be provided in a primary care setting. My personal experience and belief around the first new graduate year are that in order to really understand that something is normal, you have to have a good understanding of what is not normal.[64]

In response to a claim by the College of Midwives that the issue lay with the shortage of obstetricians to whom midwives could refer clients, Hooper said that AIM had helped more than 700 families and not one had complained about a delay in medical intervention in hospital after a midwife flagged an issue. She said, 'Instead, there has been lack of transfer, of recognising the severity of issues, a lack of communication and communicating the sense of urgency, specifically by independent, self-employed midwives. There are families that these numbers represent, families who have been avoidably hurt, a lot of them permanently.'[65] Lawton was of the view that, although Wernham's research did not examine reasons for the disparity in adverse outcomes, when added to her own findings there was strong evidence of some 'clinical performance issues'. She said the findings did not surprise her, and added, 'I think it is time for some action, some swift action.'[66]

Following publication of Chisholm's article, College of Midwives president Deb Pittam laid a complaint on behalf of the College to the Press Council. She complained of breaches of three of the Press Councils' principles, two of which related to the reporter, and the third to the headlines and captions. She argued that the latter did not accurately and fairly convey the substance of the article, the study it was based on, or maternity care in this country. She believed the same applied to the cover picture of a 'hippie genre' couple carrying a banner reading 'DELIVER US FROM DOCTORS'. She also maintained that Chisholm did not allow midwifery leaders an opportunity to respond to other interviewees' opinions, that the reporting was inaccurate, with inflammatory language, and that Chisholm did not identify personal views as opinion. [67]

As an example, Pittam referred to comments reported in the article by Ken Clark, past president of the Royal Australian and New Zealand College of Obstetricians and Gynaecologists and current chair of the national DHB Chief Medical Officers' Group. Claiming that his comments were untrue, Pittam said that Chisholm did nothing to discredit these 'false claims' but reinforced them by quoting them. Clark had stated that a shortage of obstetrical assistance in hospitals (obstetricians, house officers and registrars) had never been brought to his attention in his role on the DHB, and he added that he would 'need real evidence' of such a shortage. It was also his opinion that while the new research did not suggest the 1990s reforms were a mistake, he believed the system would be better if GPs had remained part of it, either as lead carers or just as a part of the care. He said, 'We missed a trick, frankly . . . If we could relive history, and we were smart, we would have done it so we had the best in all senses – midwifery-led care, but still with strong involvement of GPs and obstetricians in public and private.'[68] This viewpoint was by no means unique.

If Pittam had looked at *New Zealand Doctor*, for example, she would have seen this widely canvassed amongst doctors over the previous two decades. Responding to the complaint, *Listener* editor Pamela Stirling noted that the *Listener*'s reporting of Wernham's research was like that of other media, and the article did not express the author's opinion but 'only factual information and the opinion of people interviewed'.[69]

In its response to the complaint, the Press Council determined, 'In relation to principle 1 (accuracy, fairness, and balance) the Council's view is that the article canvasses a wide range of views and is balanced and accurate.' However, it upheld the complaint relating to the cover headlines and captions. It said these conveyed 'a much more negative view of midwives, the level of risks posed by midwifery-led care and the changes to maternity care in the 1990s' than did the article itself, the views it canvassed, or the research on which it was based. The hippie couple and their placard exacerbated this.[70]

In her response Stirling had defended the headline 'Where the revolution went wrong', arguing that it 'fairly reflected a key element of the article – a political decision in the mid-1990s to transfer control of delivery from doctors to midwives and whether this had resulted in the optimum outcomes'.[71] She could have gone further; the hippie couple and their placard, 'DELIVER US FROM DOCTORS', was a fair reflection of the movement which had fuelled the 1990 Nurses Amendment Act. The *Listener*'s response to the Press Council also included a letter from Peter Crampton who had spoken out following criticisms of Lawton's research. He thought that the article fairly and accurately represented the study – apart from the error acknowledged by the *Listener* that it employed the term 'midwife' rather than 'LMC' in some instances.[72]

Among the letters published in the *Listener* following the article was one from Deb Pittam, who repeated her claims that the article was 'unbalanced, inadequately researched and gave undue weight to a study that had major limitations'. She ended her letter with the statement that New Zealand's maternity system was admired internationally and that 'overall we are achieving the best outcomes ever for mothers and babies'.[73] Retired neonatal paediatrician Ross Howie was not so sure, maintaining that preventability was more important than crude figures, and that, 'When I last heard, some 19% of deaths were regarded as preventable'; he did not believe this signalled a safe system. He also thought safety standards had declined since 1990.[74]

In response to Pittam's letter, Stirling said that she stood by the coverage of the research and the surrounding issues:

> We believe New Zealand women have a right to informed consent
> and it is the role of the media to draw attention to important
> evidence-based research in a compelling and accessible manner.
> Our coverage was fair and balanced and in no way sensationalist.
> We chose not, for example, to include the report by the Health
> and Disability Commissioner – released in the same week our
> article was published – that is highly critical of a midwife's care of
> a woman whose child was born dead after the baby's heart stopped
> during labour. We did not state the system is 'broken' but rather,
> suggested that it has shortcomings, as it assuredly has.[75]

Michelle Duff's subsequent *Stuff* article noted that Wernham's paper was the first study to take an overarching look at the safety of babies within the system that had evolved since 1990. She described how, on the day the research was published in 2016, the Ministry of Health's maternity advisor Bronwen Pelvin announced that the Ministry's National Maternity Monitoring Group, of which she was an ex-officio member, would consider the research and the next steps.

The Monitoring Group, according to Duff, recommended the Ministry develop a 'co-ordinated maternity research programme that recognises the need for improvements within an already high-quality … system'. When Duff contacted the Ministry two years later, she discovered nothing had happened; instead, the Ministry directed her to the Sadler study as 'covering off questions raised by the research'. That paper had been published in response to Lawton's article and not Wernham's. The Ministry told her:

> We support the findings of Sadler … that is, that graduate
> midwives in New Zealand provide safe care when comparing their
> performance with more experienced midwives. The message is
> that pregnant women in New Zealand can have confidence in our
> midwives. When compared internationally, New Zealand women
> receive excellent care.

Wernham's colleague Diana Sarfati spoke with Duff about the personal toll the response to their work had taken: 'It was so draining and exhausting and seemed to have so little effect, and it was so stressful personally. It had a big impact on Ellie and me for quite a long time, and despite all our efforts it had no impact at all.' Duff also interviewed Peter Crampton who, she noted, had

had oversight of hundreds of studies in more than four decades in academia. He told her, just as he had remarked following Lawton's research, 'I've never seen anything quite like it. The extent to which [the researchers] felt beaten up and traumatised by the experience was way outside of the normal.' In his view, the response was 'more about the management of a contentious issue than a policy engagement with important findings'.[76]

In its 2019 response to AIM's submission, the College repeated the claims that robust data demonstrated that midwifery graduates did not have poorer outcomes in their first year of practice, and that maternity care in New Zealand was safe and met women's needs. The College acknowledged the work of AIM in supporting women and their families following an adverse outcome, but noted that AIM represented 800 women/families, which was only 0.13% of the 614,735 women who gave birth from 2008 to 2017.[77] Such a response could be seen as tantamount to rejecting a demand to upgrade a particularly hazardous stretch of road where fatal accidents had occurred on the basis that thousands of cars passed over it each year without ill-effect. Or, as the presenters of a paper to the European Congress of Perinatal Medicine in 2012 expressed it, it was equivalent to relegating those who experienced adverse events to the category of 'collateral damage', an assignation they considered unethical, no matter how small the number.[78]

## The Perinatal and Maternal Mortality Review Committee

The Perinatal and Maternal Mortality Review Committee (PMMRC), the official monitor of outcomes in maternity services, also took a very different stance from the College when the latter dismissed AIM's members as representing a small minority of childbearing women. Rather, the PMMRC declared in its 2021 annual report that, 'Every loss of life is mourned and acknowledged', and that its vision was to work 'across the system towards zero preventable deaths or harm for all mothers and babies, families and whānau'. In his introduction to this report, chair John Tait said that the information presented did not begin 'to demonstrate the lifelong heartache experienced following each one of the deaths included'.[79] PMMRC member and Māori mother Lisa Paraku, who was tasked with commenting on the report on behalf of bereaved parents, families and whānau, had considered its findings in 2018 to be 'alarming'.[80] The PMMRC itself expressed frustration in 2021, commenting that 'year after year' its reports showed continuing inequity and no significant progress towards reducing mortality and morbidity for Māori, Pasifika and Indian families and those living in areas of high deprivation in particular.[81] In his foreword to the 2022 report, the chair of the Health Quality & Safety Commission Dr Dale Bramley (Ngāpuhi), a public health specialist and National Director of Improvement and Innovation for the new national health authority Te Whatu Ora – Health New Zealand, wrote:

> As with previous reports from the PMMRC, the content has been difficult to read, and we appreciate how much harder it is, and has been, for families and whānau who personally endure the loss of a loved one. We owe it to them to listen and learn – and to improve.

He continued: 'The whole Commission Board wishes to emphasise the clear lack of improvement over the years highlighted within this report and the ongoing serious systemic issues demonstrated. Many of these deaths are preventable.'[82]

The 2021 report noted that there had been no reduction in neonatal (the first 28 days of life) mortality for the period 2009–18 overall, and it drew attention to the higher rates amongst certain ethnic groups, mothers under the age of 20, and those living in areas of high deprivation.[83] This finding had become depressingly familiar to the committee since its first report in 2007.[84] From 2010 the committee had included neonatal encephalopathy in its remit, and in 2017 it noted no significant improvement in rates since then, with Māori, Pasifika and Indian mothers at increased risk compared to other population groups.[85] In 2022 it again stated, 'Neonatal encephalopathy rates remain static with no significant improvement.'[86]

In 2018 the committee identified 25% of babies' deaths (79 in total) as potentially avoidable.[87] Because pre-term birth was the leading cause of neonatal death, and Māori babies were over-represented, it cautioned, 'Care for these babies needs to occur in one of Aotearoa/New Zealand's six tertiary neonatal centres.'[88] Yet their mothers were the very ones most likely to give birth in hospitals or birthing units with no neonatal intensive-care unit.[89] Others had drawn attention to the fact that Māori women and women living in New Zealand's most deprived areas often relied on primary units in both rural and urban settings.[90] These low-technology units generally did not have easy access to specialist services. The PMMRC also found that statistically

Māori, Pasifika and Indian babies were significantly less likely to have an attempt at resuscitation than babies from other ethnic groups.[91]

On maternal mortality, the 2021 report drew attention to the two major causes of maternal death: suicide and amniotic fluid embolism. Disturbingly, the 2017 report had noted that maternal death from amniotic fluid embolism was four times higher and maternal death from suicide seven times higher than in the UK.[92] Addressing deaths from amniotic fluid embolism, the 2021 report cited a recent study (including New Zealand data) which identified that 'having an obstetrician and/or anaesthetist present at the time of the event and the use of interventions to correct blood clotting abnormalities' was associated with lower mortality.[93] Investigating deaths from suicide, the report noted that not only was this the leading cause of maternal death in New Zealand but there were also 'alarmingly higher rates of maternal suicide' among Māori – 18 of 30 suicides between 2006 and 2018 – making Māori 3.35 times more likely to die by suicide than New Zealand European women.[94] The midwifery-led partnership model had not met the needs of these women, and the reports stressed the need for 'culturally appropriate maternal screening tools and treatment'.[95] When suicide had been identified as the leading cause of maternal death in 2012, PMMRC chair Cindy Farquhar told the press that there needed to be 'better co-ordination between existing services in the primary and specialist sectors and processes for sharing information between providers'.[96] Nonetheless, the issue continued to fly under the radar until drawn to public attention by a 2022 report by the Helen Clark Foundation which attracted a short burst of media attention.[97] The 2022 PMMRC report once again drew attention to the disproportionate number of Māori women affected by suicide.[98]

Each PMMRC report included recommendations. Disturbingly, in 2021 the committee reported that only half of the 120 recommendations it had made since 2007 had been fully implemented.[99] Among those was that DHBs provide 'free interdisciplinary fetal surveillance education for all clinicians involved in intrapartum care on a triennial basis' at no cost to LMCs. It explained that the aim was to strengthen supervision and support 'to promote professional judgement, interdisciplinary conversations and reflective practice'.[100] Discussing maternal mortality, the committee noted another recommendation not yet fully implemented: that all clinicians involved in the care of pregnant women should 'undertake regular multidisciplinary training in management of obstetric emergencies and resuscitation'. It maintained that women with serious pre-existing medical conditions required a 'multidisciplinary management plan for the pregnancy, birth and postpartum period' which should be communicated to 'all relevant caregivers'.[101] These recommendations were repeated in the section on 'Recommendations not yet fully implemented' in 2022.[102] Over its many reports, the PMMRC stressed multidisciplinary collaboration and medical training for all caregivers, as had many health professionals since 1990.

One possible obstacle to implementing the PMMRC's recommendations on multidisciplinarity could be that they were mediated through the Ministry of Health's National Maternity Monitoring Group from 2012. The group's 2017 annual report explained, 'Where the PMMRC recommends specific action by maternity system stakeholders, the National Maternity Monitoring Group will advise the Ministry on an appropriate response to these recommendations', and it further noted that decisions within the group were by consensus.[103] The monitoring group was chaired by obstetrician John Tait, and included Judith McAra-Couper (Midwifery Council chair) as vice-chair, College of Midwives president Deb Pittam, and Bronwen Pelvin, ex-officio in her capacity as the Ministry of Health's principal maternity advisor.

Indications are that these senior midwives did not rate multidisciplinarity in a hospital setting. As explained in Chapter 3, Bronwen Pelvin had played a key role in lobbying for midwives' autonomy in the late 1980s when she practised as a homebirth midwife at the Riverside Community, Lower Moutere, in Nelson Tasman. Despite now overseeing maternity services across the sector, a position she held from 2008, her views appear not to have changed. In her address to the 2015 homebirth conference at the Riverside Community, for example, she reflected that many of the challenges she had faced before 1990 were mirrored by the challenges midwives still faced, which included 'difficult medical professionals' and 'hostile working environments'.[104]

Other midwifery leaders continued to be wary of collaborating with medical professionals. In 2017, an article in the College journal by McAra-Couper, among others, pointed to the 'empowerment' of midwives in partnership with women in the community as a 'unique foundational feature of New Zealand maternity care', and to their 'disempowerment' if they worked in hospital. There were ongoing philosophical barriers inhibiting multidisciplinarity in a medical setting.[105] These philosophical barriers were also evident in McAra-Couper's 2007 PhD thesis and her subsequent publications critiquing the role of technology in modern childbirth.[106] Journalist Michele Duff had noted little activity on the part of the Monitoring Group or the Ministry of Health following Wernham's research findings, despite assurances.

If Karen Guilliland's comment at the thirtieth anniversary of the 1990 Nurses Amendment Act is anything to go by, the College of Midwives was never going to take seriously academic research which showed flaws in the maternity services. She claimed that there was endless research showing the safety and efficacy of midwifery care, but added, 'We could research 'til the cows come home, it's not about evidence, it's about ideology.'[107] Academic research – or evidence – was dismissed by her as having no real value. This did little to help the PMMRC in its plea for research into 'possible causes for the increase in perinatal-related death of babies born to Pacific women, Māori women, women under the age of 20 and over the age of 40, and women who live in areas of high socioeconomic deprivation . . . in order to develop appropriate strategies to reduce these possibly preventable deaths'. It had made this recommendation in 2010 but repeated it in the section of 'recommendations not yet fully implemented' in 2022.[108]

## Learning from others: The Morecambe Bay, Ockenden and other inquiries in the UK

Failure to work as a team was at the forefront of criticisms in inquiries into maternity care at certain hospitals in the UK around this time. In 2015, maternity and neonatal services at the University Hospitals of Morecambe Bay NHS Foundation Trust were subject to a review chaired by gynaecological oncologist Bill Kirkup, following the revelation of 'a distressing chain of events' at the maternity unit at Furness General Hospital.[109] The reviewers found 20 instances of significant failures of care at the hospital, associated with three maternal deaths and 16 baby deaths, after events were brought to light by bereaved families.[110] The review concluded that clinical competence at Furness General Hospital was substandard, with deficient skills and knowledge, and poor staff relations (with a 'them and us' culture). They noted that midwifery care there was strongly influenced by a small number of dominant individuals whose over-zealous pursuit of natural childbirth led at times to inappropriate and unsafe care:

> Whilst natural childbirth is a beneficial and worthwhile objective in women at low risk of obstetric complications, we heard that

midwives took over the risk assessment process without in many cases discussing intended care with obstetricians, and we found repeated instances of women inappropriately classified as being at low risk and managed incorrectly.[111]

A national Maternity Transformation Programme was set up following this inquiry, stressing multidisciplinary teamwork through the establishment of 'Local Maternity Systems'. These were intended to bring together those involved in maternity care, including midwives, obstetricians, service users, neonatal staff, managers, commissioners, public health, educators, perinatal mental health providers and GPs, to achieve better results in maternity care.[112]

In 2017, Shrewsbury and Telford Hospital NHS Trust became the subject of an inquiry following complaints by bereaved parents about potentially avoidable birth outcomes. Initially 23 cases were investigated, but the number quickly ballooned to 1,486 families affected during the first two decades of the twenty-first century (with 170 prior to 2000). According to the inquiry's chair, midwife Donna Ockenden, the size and scale of the review was unprecedented in the history of the National Health Service.[113] When Ellie Wernham et al. cautioned in 2016 that the apparent international comparability of New Zealand's maternal and neonatal outcomes did 'not preclude the possibility that avoidable adverse outcomes are occurring, potentially both in New Zealand and in other countries', they could have been presaging the findings of Britain's 2022 Ockenden report.[114]

The Ockenden review committee investigated maternal deaths, maternal morbidity, stillbirths, neonatal deaths and brain injuries, and found significant shortcomings in services. Of 12 maternal deaths they investigated, they concluded that none had received care in line with best practice at that time. They had 'major concerns' about the maternity care in a quarter of the stillbirth cases they reviewed. The final report stated, 'Many hundreds of families who received maternity care at the trust have told us of experiencing life-changing tragedies that have caused untold pain and distress.'[115]

Like the Morecambe inquiry, the Ockenden review found a lack of 'multidisciplinary communication and collaboration and/or senior clinical supervision, both of which are key to providing safe care'.[116] It also found a failure to follow national clinical guidelines, whether for the monitoring of fetal heart rate, maternal blood pressure, management of gestational diabetes or resuscitation. This failure, combined with delays in referrals and failure to work collaboratively across disciplines, resulted in many poor outcomes for mothers or their babies, including death. Like the Morecambe inquiry, the Ockenden review found an unhelpful culture of 'them and us' between the midwifery and obstetrics staff.[117] Its recommendations included the need for 'multi-professional training' and 'the suspension of midwifery continuity of carer model until – and unless – safe staffing is shown to be present'.[118]

In May 2022 Donna Ockenden was again called upon to lead a review, this time into baby deaths at the Nottingham University Hospitals NHS Trust. *The Times* reported, 'More than 450 families have now come forward to take part in the review.'[119] Commenting on the alternative therapies used at the facility (specifically aromatherapy), obstetrician Jayne Terry claimed that 'a dogmatic pursuit of natural birth can have serious consequences'; and a patient safety campaigner declared, 'It is clear the ideological push to "de-medicalise" maternity care has gone too far.'[120]

Dr Bill Kirkup also led another review in October 2022, into East Kent Maternity Services. This review found a serious lapse in care in more than half of the 202 cases investigated from 2009 to 2020 at two local hospitals (with 45 of the 65 baby deaths, or 69%, considered preventable). The review identified 'gross failures of teamworking', which it attributed partly to different philosophies among staff, with midwives positioning themselves as 'defenders of women against . . . [obstetricians'] over-medicalised models of care'.[121] The Ockenden review had stressed that quality care required teamwork, with each sector contributing unique skills; Kirkup's East Kent review also recommended that different sectors should train together to learn how to work 'in a mutually supportive way'.[122]

Following the Ockenden report in March 2022, the *Sunday Times* reported that the Royal College of Midwives had apologised for its normal birth campaign's role in contributing to poor care in that region and accepted that elements of its campaign were not evidence-based. 'It is now calling for renewed focus on improved culture and investment in safe staffing.'[123] In September 2022, the College of Midwives announced a new working group to lead the Maternity Transformation Programme, overseen by the Royal College of Midwives along with various medical colleges.[124]

Constructive dialogue and action plans involving multidisciplinarity appear to have emerged from these various damning reviews. Such multidisciplinary training and collaboration was repeatedly rejected by the New Zealand College of Midwives as undermining midwifery autonomy. As Sally Pairman commented in 2020, only as 'a truly autonomous profession can we make a real difference to mothers and babies and their families', in this way prioritising autonomy over multidisciplinary teamwork.[125]

## Conclusion

The establishment of the Midwifery Council to oversee professional standards in 2004 had not calmed troubled waters within New Zealand's maternity services. The Council along with the College of Midwives, whilst supported by the Ministry of Health, came under fire from other health professionals, coroners, health and disability commissioners, consumers, journalists and academic researchers. The principal complaint was that midwives should have more training in a medical environment and more interaction with medical providers outside of emergencies. This was strenuously opposed by those who subscribed to the midwifery model and were intent on normalising birth, as they had been since the early days of the homebirth movement. Others were of the view that the philosophy of low-intervention community-based midwifery did not meet the needs of high-risk groups, and that this was made more urgent by the apparent increasing co-morbidities since the 1990s both in New Zealand and internationally, leading to more high-risk births. They believed that changing the mindsets of those in charge was needed.

In 2020 an article entitled 'Professor Bev Lawton fighting for change in New Zealand's "flawed" maternity care system' pointed out that at the Te Tātai Haouroa o Hine Centre for Women's Health at Victoria University, led by Lawton, the current focus was Māori women's health, particularly in maternity services. Lawton, of Ngāti Porou descent herself, noted that the Māori perinatal mortality rate was double that for Pākehā and commented, 'If you get it right for Māori, you get it right for everyone.' Referring to the overall static perinatal mortality rates (no change in 11 years), she said that there was 'harm occurring' in a maternity system she described as flawed, and declared, 'It's not as safe as it should be and we need to change that.' For change to occur, she advised, 'We need to think as a team.'[126]

# CONCLUSION

## 'NZ – the best place to give birth?'

IN JUNE 2021 CHRISTCHURCH journalist Sally Blundell began her article 'NZ – the best place to give birth?' with the reflection by Karen Guilliland, long-serving New Zealand College of Midwives' chief executive until her retirement in 2018, that she was 'always surprised at how famous New Zealand midwifery is everywhere else … except in New Zealand'.[1] This overseas renown is perhaps not surprising; the New Zealand model sounds idyllic. Each woman can choose a Lead Maternity Carer to look after her, mostly free of charge, from early pregnancy through childbirth to six weeks postpartum. As a Ministry of Health-commissioned report explained in 2012, she would usually choose a midwife, who would be her partner throughout, helping her to make informed decisions in a truly woman-centred model of maternity care: 'In this model each woman and her midwife are partners, working together to ensure that the woman has care that best meets her individual needs.'[2] As Guilliland had previously noted, the partnership model was a uniquely New Zealand concept.[3] Two Australian midwives had admired New Zealand in 2013 as having 'arguably one of the most woman-centred national maternity systems in the world'.[4]

So why, then, was it not famous in New Zealand? Idyllic as it sounds, the midwifery-led system contains unresolved issues that can be grouped around four themes: accessibility, philosophy, training, and accountability.

These were well illustrated in the circumstances around the death in 2019 of the first baby of a young Māori woman who lived in a rural area, which was investigated by the Deputy Commissioner of Health and Disability Rose Wall and reported just two months after Guilliland's interview.[5] The concerns expressed in Wall's report were unfortunately not peculiar to this case, and they can also be directly related to the maternity reforms from 1990 and the midwifery model of care that has formed the subject matter of this book.

## Accessibility

Accessibility was a clear issue in the case investigated by Wall. The chosen midwife, who had cared for other whānau, lived outside the district, about an hour's drive from the woman's home. As a result, the midwife specified that visits were to be at the clinic and 'primary consultations' made over the phone; even in labour, the midwife assessed her client over the phone.[6] The midwife did not ask to see her in person, which meant she was unaware that in the final weeks of pregnancy the woman developed oedema, headaches, and elevated blood pressure — symptoms of a pregnancy complication called pre-eclampsia. The midwife did no blood test or urine analysis which would have picked up the problem. As discussed in Chapter 8, women living in rural areas were particularly vulnerable in the midwifery-led maternity model introduced in the 1990s. Independent (also known as community, self-employed or caseload) midwives tended not to set up practices there, as there was not enough work to sustain them; instead, they worked from a distance. This meant that in many cases there were no postnatal checks. But it could also be an issue in pregnancy: in this case, prenatal testing would have detected pre-eclampsia. The midwife in this case admitted that 'distance was a barrier'.[7] Moreover, midwives often struggled to keep up with demand. Discussing the midwifery shortage in 2021, Guilliland said, 'Most midwives nowadays will work for about six years because the work is unsustainable. There's a lot of burnout.'[8]

GPs and obstetricians, who had pressed for multidisciplinary team-based practices, had predicted this since the 1990s. The 1990 Nurses Amendment Act had given midwives parity with general practitioner obstetricians in maternity services, and the LMC system introduced in 1996 made maternity care untenable for most GPs. Many of them continued to regard maternity as an important part of their practices, hence their involvement in the late 1990s and early 2000s in schemes which operated outside the LMC system, offering shared care by doctors and midwives. These schemes appeared to be very successful, and many midwives liked working in them. Consumers liked them too. With the backing of the New Zealand College of Midwives, however, the government shut them down in favour of a sole-midwifery system. Demands for midwife/GP teams in rural areas, which had special needs, fell on deaf ears. Combining midwifery with other aspects of nursing care of the woman and her family was also rejected in favour of stand-alone midwifery, as midwives sought to distance their profession from nursing. The result for midwives was, as Blundell noted in 2021, 'burnout from working seven days a week and a lot more hours than expected from a full-time role'. Midwives had literally been left holding the baby, and this system was not viable. It certainly failed the young Māori woman whom Wall was investigating.

## Philosophy

The second theme, highlighted by this case, was the philosophy that underpinned the midwifery-led system. The midwife had worked with the woman's whānau for previous births and explained that she 'had no doubt that they also believed everything to be normal for [Ms B]'.[9] This raises an important issue. Why do we need health professionals at all if other household members could be relied upon to assess the situation? In this case they clearly could not.

The College of Midwives' philosophy that birth should be regarded as a normal life event can be traced directly to the homebirth movement of the 1970s that had been core to the College's founding in 1989. Indeed, the College's perspective can only be explained by reviewing the homebirth movement and an ideology rooted in non-interventionist or 'natural' childbirth. The midwife in the 2021 investigation reflected, 'My actions were not proactive enough and I have considered the desire for her to homebirth may have clouded my judgement and caused my inaction.'[10] As discussed in this book, these concerns were not new. Dr Allan Sutherland had suggested in 1995 that the non-interventionist attitudes of some homebirth advocates had 'clouded their judgement' (see pp. 184–85). Homebirth doctor William Ferguson told Health Minister Annette King in 2000 that the primary focus of a maternity service should never be normal births but rather the prevention and management of complications, morbidity and mortality (see p. 173). Jenn

Hooper, spokesperson for the consumer group AIM, believed the College of Midwives' childbirth philosophy needed to change from an emphasis on 'normal birth' to a 'safe and satisfying birth experience' (see p. 239).

Addressing a complaint two years before Wall's report, Health and Disability Commissioner Anthony Hill had commented that partnership was 'at the very heart of midwifery in New Zealand'.[11] The philosophy around partnership had its roots in the homebirth movement, which encouraged women to take control and to be the decision-makers in the birth process in the belief that this would enhance their capability as mothers. The philosophy underpinned approaches to immunisation as well, with the College of Midwives in the 1990s staunchly claiming that its role was not to advise but rather to give both sides of the debate on whether to immunise. Hill's comment on partnership came in relation to a case in which he determined there had been a breach of informed consent – or 'partnership'. The midwife in question had given the mother saline instead of the requested pethidine for pain relief (stipulated in her birth plan) for a difficult posterior-presentation birth without informing her of the substitution. Hill described the midwife's conduct as 'disgraceful', 'paternalist', breaching the right of informed consent, lacking integrity, and undermining any real partnership.[12]

Yet, the very concept of partnership was itself fraught with inconsistencies, as discussed in Chapter 9. Karen Guilliland had explained in relation to immunisation that under the partnership model midwives were not to be advisors but were to provide information to allow women to make up their own minds and take responsibility. But elsewhere midwifery leaders showed a lack of real partnership. For instance, Sally Pairman reminded midwives that they might have to 'persuade' women of the safety of homebirth; another senior midwife, Maggie Banks, explained that, even within the partnership model, midwives should not acquiesce to all demands women made, but rather 'honour their innate promise' to be as non-interventionist as possible.

The partnership model was not part of the equation for the young Māori woman whose situation the Commissioner investigated in 2021. She told the latter that she booked the midwife because of her 'expertise and experience'.[13] Discussing her antenatal care, she explained that she had not found all the midwife's questions clear; nor did she fully understand the condition of pre-eclampsia.[14] Equal knowledge and understanding could not be assumed. The philosophy which saw birth as a normal life event, with women and midwives as equal partners, did not serve this woman well.

## Training

Training was the third theme emphasised by the 2021 case, with Wall concluding that the midwife's training was insufficient in the areas of record-keeping and diagnostic skills.[15] Rosemary Godbold's 2010 article in the College of Midwives' journal on consumers' rights and Claire Sweetman's 2013 law dissertation had identified midwives' documentation of discussions about the birth process and treatment options as a key concern, often indicative of a casual attitude to the birth process and a reliance on letting nature take its course, something midwives were taught in the new 'direct-entry' midwifery training programmes of the 1990s.

Legislated for under the 1990 Act and introduced from 1992, direct-entry midwifery training (that is, without prior nurse training) allowed midwives, unlike other health professionals, to practise independently after three and later four years' training, with no hospital internships. This caused consternation among health and disability commissioners as well as coroners, consumers, health professionals and academic researchers, who believed midwives should have the same educational requirements as other health professionals. Their concerns fell on deaf ears, with the College of Midwives even arguing that hospital experience would be counterproductive to independent practice. The new training programmes embraced a holistic/social model – also known as 'the midwifery model' – with the express purpose of steering students away from the so-called medical or technocratic model, as discussed in Chapter 9.

The extent to which the new courses, with no mandatory hospital internships, prepared graduates for adverse events was hotly debated. The original intent of the 1990 Act seemed to be that midwives would be caregivers for 'low-risk' pregnant women. Yet, as Karen Guilliland and Sally Pairman later pointed out, the legislation did not require midwifery practice to be restricted to so-called normal childbirth. The assumption that midwives would confine their practices to normal pregnancies – and that they would be able to define a normal pregnancy – was based on trust. Ministry of Health officials at the time the Bill was introduced into Parliament had urged that safety measures such as back-up services be included in the legislation and were wary of the introduction of direct-entry midwifery training. Health Minister Helen Clark ignored their advice in favour of that of homebirth midwife Joan Donley. As Clark's officials forewarned, without legislative restrictions, independent midwives extended their practices beyond low-risk pregnant women, leading some investigators to question whether their training was robust enough.

The studies by Bev Lawton and Lyn Sadler in 2016 and 2018 respectively, and addressed in Chapter 12, found that newly graduated midwives often cared for pregnant women with major underlying health issues, sometimes with sub-optimal outcomes. Lawton and others unsuccessfully lobbied the government for more education for midwives and for hospital internships, arguing that training and post-registration mentoring left much to be desired. This was particularly problematic when midwives worked alone in the community or in midwifery-run birthing centres. When Rose Wall investigated another baby death in 2021, she found that the LMC had failed to interpret an ultrasound scan correctly and to recognise the complexity of the clinical picture. She concluded that this LMC had not identified that the woman was no longer in the low-risk category and therefore unsuitable to birth at a primary birthing unit. The LMC was found to have breached Right 4 of the Code (failure to provide services of an adequate standard) and was instructed to undertake further education.[16]

In the case of the young Māori woman with pre-eclampsia, Wall also found the midwife's education to be inadequate and recommended that she undertake further instruction on pre-eclampsia in pregnancy, documentation and the Growth Assessment Protocol.[17] The implication was that her training had not served her well. Nor was this an isolated concern. As discussed in Chapter 12, the Perinatal and Maternal Mortality Review Committee tasked with charting avoidable deaths and making recommendations for improvements repeatedly recommended three-yearly 'free interdisciplinary fetal surveillance education' for all LMCs – a measure which still had not been implemented by 2021 (see p. 270).

## Accountability

The final theme relevant to this study and highlighted by Wall's 2021 report into the death of the young Māori woman's baby was accountability. Apart from recommending further training, Wall asked the midwife to write an apology to the woman and her whānau.[18] The midwife did so, writing of her 'deepest aroha for [Ms B], her partner, and her whānau for the loss of [the baby]. A precious daughter, mokopuna, cousin, and niece.'[19] Was this aroha enough compensation for a dead baby? The no-fault ACC system that had been in place since the 1970s meant that New Zealand's unique midwifery-led maternity service was predicated on a structure which did not allow lawsuits. This made independent practice a much more viable option in New Zealand than in Australia, for example, as noted in Chapter 7.

Consumers did have the option of having complaints heard by the Health and Disability Commissioner from 1996. Commissioners could demand that the health professional apologise to the complainant, request additional education and, if the complaint was considered serious enough, could refer the case to further disciplinary bodies: the Nursing Council prior to 2004, and thereafter the Health Practitioners Disciplinary Tribunal and the Midwifery Council. Yet even the Commissioner's involvement as a channel of redress for parents had been criticised by Joan Donley in 1998 for its failure to honour the partnership model of care and for being too punitive; in one case that same year Karen Guilliland described the Nursing Council's ruling as 'exceptionally harsh' and 'punitive', and – strangely – as 'likely to have serious consequences for women's health and status in society' (see p. 189).

Accountability was further addressed in a 2022 article about the state of maternity services in New Zealand in the magazine *North & South*. Jenn Hooper (who had been awarded the New Zealand Order of Merit in 2019 for her work with AIM) claimed that the system had 'no real accountability'. She pointed out, 'We train our midwives less and trust our midwives more than in any other developed country.' Her suggestion that midwives should be employed by DHBs rather than remain independent was rebuffed by the chief executive of the College of Midwives Alison Eddy, who favoured the midwifery-led model of care with pathways for referral support.[20] Presumably, the College saw Hooper's suggestion as a ruse for medical control, just as the Domiciliary Midwives Society had in the 1980s when it vehemently opposed transferring homebirth midwives' contracts from the Health Department to hospital boards because this would mean midwives losing their autonomy. The very meaning of 'autonomy' was defined by two contributors to the 2006 midwifery textbook, Sally Pairman and Judith McAra-Couper, when they explained that autonomy involved 'a specific philosophy and body of knowledge, together with the ability to practise without reference to another discipline' (see p. 135). Independence of practice was fiercely protected by these midwifery leaders who were building their professional identity with their own overseeing body, the Midwifery Council, from 2004.

The College of Midwives envisaged disciplinary processes primarily as a learning tool for the midwife. As discussed in Chapter 10 (see p. 213), the parents in one tragic case in 2010 were appalled to discover two years later that the self-employed midwife was practising with no official record of her involvement in the fatality and whilst still being investigated by the Health and Disability Commissioner. The Midwifery Council, then the overseeing body, informed them that she had completed her supervision. Another midwife who had been severely criticised by a coroner for a homebirth death in 1991 continued to practise for the next 15 years until she was suspended in 2007 following another death in a case where she was a sole practitioner (see pp. 140, 211). There appeared to be little accountability in a system that stressed partnership between a midwife and her client; they were equally responsible for the outcome. As we saw in chapter 7, midwife Bronwen Pelvin explained in 1992, 'Tragedies *do* occur at birth and less than perfect babies *are* born', and she believed the complaints procedure should be about increasing understanding of these events and not about apportioning blame (see pp. 147–48). This was little consolation to the parents of dead or damaged babies.

In the 2021 case, as in so many others, the outcome of the investigation by the Health and Disability Commissioner was a letter of apology and a requirement to undertake further training. The Midwifery Council carried out a competence review of the midwife and determined that she was 'competent across the midwifery scope of practice'.[21]

## 'New Zealand – the best place to give birth'

When the young Māori woman who lost her baby in 2019 was invited to respond to Rose Wall's findings in 2021, she wrote of the impact of what had happened. She hoped that no one else would ever have to experience what she and her whānau had, and that 'all the measures are taken to ensure the health and safety of mother, baby and whānau are upheld and respected in the future'.[22]

This had become a familiar refrain, from the Board of Health's Maternity Services Committee in the 1970s to submissions to Parliament by major consumer groups such as the National Council of Women in 1990 and AIM from 2011. When planned homebirth was first advocated by a small minority of midwives and alternative lifestylers in the 1970s, the Maternity Services

Committee did not attempt to shut it down but to incorporate it safely within New Zealand's maternity system. However, the ideological movement which informed homebirth eschewed any association with hospitals and modern medical technology. It is perhaps surprising that the movement managed to persuade the government in 1990 that this was what women wanted. In fact, most women did not choose homebirth, and homebirth did not take off as some had anticipated (with the most recent calculations being 3.9% of all births in the period 2016–2020).[23] Despite its failure to flourish, the precepts of the movement were incorporated into the New Zealand College of Midwives and its educational bodies which oversaw and guided independent or caseload midwifery after 1990.

The College of Midwives claimed that it was rooted in feminism. But this was a 1970s brand of radical feminism which had an aversion to medical technology and science on the grounds that these upheld patriarchy. Feminism itself changed over the decades, with women increasingly arguing for the right to choose intervention in childbirth and no longer wedded to the tenets of so-called natural childbirth. The College found itself under fire from multiple sources, including consumers, other health professionals and academic researchers. Many voices were raised in protest, but even the government's Perinatal and Maternal Mortality Review Committee has not been able to facilitate a more multidisciplinary approach to maternity services. This history has shown that there have been many people since the reforms of the 1990s who would disagree with the College of Midwives' 2015 assessment that New Zealand's unique midwifery-led maternity system is 'one of the safest, if not the safest maternity services in the world', or the College's chief executive's view in 2010 that New Zealand midwives provided 'a primary maternity service that is amongst, if not the best, in the world'.[24]

# NOTES

## INTRODUCTION

1. Martin Johnston and Natalie Akoorie, 'Babies' deaths reignite maternity row', *Weekend Herald*, 23 June 2012, p. A22, https://www.nzherald.co.nz/nz/babies-deaths-reignite-maternity-row/GDROFD7RHGC4ZGXUIHS6AULMCY/ These deaths were of Adam Barlow (2009) and Kymani Nathan-Tukiri (2012) along with Kymani's mother, Casey Missy Turama Nathan (see Chapter 10).
2. On Donley, see Linda Bryder, 'Donley, Joan Elsa', *Dictionary of New Zealand Biography*, 2018, *Te Ara – the Encyclopedia of New Zealand*, https://teara.govt.nz/en/biographies/6d2/donley-joan-elsa (accessed 24 August 2021).
3. This expression was first used by Donley in her article 'Political Comment: Autonomy for Midwives', *New Zealand College of Midwives Journal* (*NZCOMJ*), vol. 3, November 1990, p. 7. It became common in, for example, Sally Pairman, 'Welcome to Conference', *NZCOMJ*, vol. 15, October 1996, p. 5, and most recently: Alison Eddy, webinar: 'Emancipating Midwifery – Reflecting on 30 years of midwifery autonomy', 3 September 2020, hosted by Alison Eddy, Chief Executive, New Zealand College of Midwives, https://www.midwife.org.nz/news/webinar-emancipating-midwifery-reflecting-on-30-years-of-midwifery-autonomy/ (accessed 10 March 2023).
4. Lynda Exton, *The Baby Business: What's Happened to Maternity Care in New Zealand?*, Craig Potton Publishing, Nelson, 2008.
5. Karen Guilliland and Sally Pairman, *Women's Business: The Story of the New Zealand College of Midwives, 1986–2010*, New Zealand College of Midwives, Christchurch, 2010.
6. Sally Blundell, 'NZ – the best place to give birth?', *Newsroom*, 3 June 2021, https://www.newsroom.co.nz/page/nz-the-best-place-to-give-birth
7. Ollie Neas, 'Risky business', *North & South*, May 2022, p. 53–55.

## CHAPTER 1: *Homebirth 1970s-style*

1. See Philippa Mein Smith, *Maternity in Dispute: New Zealand, 1920–1939*, Historical Publications Branch, Department of Internal Affairs, Government Printer, Wellington, 1986.
2. Janet Greenlees and Linda Bryder (eds), *Western Maternity and Medicine, 1880–1990*, Pickering & Chatto, London, 2013; in particular see chapters by Linda Bryder and Alison Nuttall.

3   Report of Committee of Inquiry into Maternity Services, *Appendices to the Journals of the House of Representatives (AJHR)*, H31A, 1938, p. 76.
4   Linda Bryder, *The Rise and Fall of National Women's Hospital*, Auckland University Press, Auckland, 2014, p. 21.
5   Irvine Loudon, 'Childbirth', in Irvine Loudon (ed.), *Western Medicine: An Illustrated History*, Oxford University Press, Oxford, 1997, p. 219; see also Irvine Loudon, *Death in Childbirth: An International Study of Maternal Care and Maternal Mortality, 1800–1950*, Oxford University Press, Oxford, 1992.
6   Bryder, *The Rise and Fall*, p. 118.
7   Ibid., p. 104.
8   Ibid., p. 82; Department of Health, *A Review of Hospital and Related Services in New Zealand*, Department of Health, Wellington, 1969, p. 50.
9   Bryder, *The Rise and Fall*, p. 10.
10  Gabrielle Bourke, 'Illuminating the Dark Hour: Auckland's St Helens Hospital, 1906–1990', MA thesis, University of Auckland, 2006, pp. 100, 117.
11  Information paper for meeting of Maternity Services Committee of the Board of Health, 27, 28 March 1979, R20459385, 1978–81, Box 5, Record 29-21, Archives New Zealand Wellington (ANZW); Helen Brown, 'When birth becomes an "occasion" at home', *New Zealand Woman's Weekly*, 7 August 1978, p. 5; Lyn McLean, 'Home Birth in New Zealand', *New Zealand Nursing Journal: Kai Tiaki*, vol. 73, 7, July 1980, p. 7.
12  Information paper, 1979; Maternity Services Committee, *Mother and Baby at Home: The Early Days: A Report of the Board of Health Maternity Services Committee*, Board of Health Report Series 30, Wellington, 1982, p. 10.
13  *Home Birth Association (HBA) Auckland Newsletter*, 35, March 1987, p. N15; ibid., 43, June 1989, pp. N19–20.
14  Ibid., p. 5.
15  Jennie Nicol, 'A Choice of Birthing: Part 1: Homebirth and Domiciliary Midwifery', Department of Health, Wellington, November 1987, p. 6, https://www.moh.govt.nz/notebook/nbbooks.nsf/0/6D092B4E4F967CBC4C2565D7000DD6A4/$file/Choice-of-birthing.pdf (accessed 10 September 2022).
16  Terry Craig and Michael Mills, *Care and Control: The Role of Institutions in New Zealand*, Social Monitoring Group Report 2, June 1987 (convened by Peggy Koopman-Boyden), Wellington, New Zealand Planning Council, p. 6, https://www.mcguinnessinstitute.org/wp-content/uploads/2016/11/NZPC-June-1987-Care-and-Control-The-Role-of-Institutions-in-New-Zealand-FULL.pdf (accessed 10 September 2022).
17  *HBA Auckland Newsletter*, 43, June 1989, p. N19; see also Sally Abel and Robin Kearns, 'Birth Places: A Geographical Perspective on Planned Home Birth in New Zealand', *Social Science and Medicine*, vol. 33, 7, 1991, pp. 825–37, doi: 10.1016/0277-9536(91)90387-r (They noted Māori women in 1987–88 made up just 2.7% of homebirths.)
18  Nicol, 'A Choice of Birthing', p. 3.

19  'Non-smoker for our children's sake: Reply by Bonham', *Auckland Star*, 15 October 1980; Public Health Commission, *Our Health, Our Future; Hauora Pakari, Koiora Roa: The State of Public Health in New Zealand*, Public Health Commission, Wellington, 1993, pp. 66–67.
20  'No smoking – and watch your diet', *New Zealand Woman's Weekly*, 30 October 1978, p. 30; 'Midwife is one of the family', *North Shore Times*, 10 April 1979, p. 15.
21  *HBA Auckland Newsletter*, 43, June 1989, p. N19.
22  McLean, 'Home Birth in New Zealand', p. 7.
23  Brown, 'When birth becomes an "occasion" at home', p. 5.
24  *HBA National Newsletter*, 2, October 1980, p. 11.
25  Maggie Banks, 'Out on a Limb: The Personal Mandate to Practise Midwifery by Midwives of the Domiciliary Midwives Society of New Zealand (Incorporated), 1974–1986', PhD thesis, Victoria University of Wellington, 2007, p. 80.
26  'What Kind of People Choose a Home Birth?', *HBA National Newsletter*, 7, November 1982, p. 10.
27  *HBA Auckland Newsletter*, 43, June 1989, p. N19.
28  *HBA National Newsletter*, 7, November 1982, p. 10.
29  Brown, 'When birth becomes an "occasion" at home', p. 4.
30  *HBA National Newsletter*, 6, July 1982, p. 1.
31  Celine Kearney, 'Delivering on Low Pay', *Broadsheet*, 140, 1986, p. 6.
32  *HBA National Newsletter*, 7, November 1982, p. 11.
33  *HBA Auckland Newsletter*, 43, June 1989, p. N19.
34  Joan Donley, *Herstory of N.Z. Home Birth Association*, New Zealand Home Birth Association, Auckland, 1992, p. 4.
35  Pauline Ray, 'Whose body is it? Whose baby is it?', *New Zealand Listener*, 15 March 1980, p. 22.
36  *HBA Auckland Newsletter*, 45, December 1989, p. L5.
37  Kearney, 'Delivering on Low Pay', p. 6.
38  Transcript of interview of Joan Donley by Sally Abel, 6 July 1994, p. 17, Joan Donley Papers 1933-2003, MSS & Archives 2007/15, 1638, Manuscripts and Archives, University of Auckland Library (JDP).
39  *HBA National Newsletter*, 1, July 1980, p. 7.
40  Robert Mannion, 'The great home birth debate hots up again', *Dominion Sunday Times*, 23 December 1990, p. 9; Maria Crotty, Andrew T. Ramsay, Rosemary Smart and Annabelle Chan, 'Planned Homebirths in South Australia 1976–1987', *Medical Journal of Australia*, vol. 153, 1990, p. 666.
41  McLean, 'Home Birth in New Zealand', p. 7.
42  *HBA National Newsletter*, 2, 2, June 1984, p. 15.
43  Ohu Advisory Committee, *Ohu: Alternative Life Style Communities*, Department of Lands and Survey, Wellington, 1975.
44  Information paper, Maternity Services Committee, 1979, p. 8.
45  *Mother and Baby at Home*, p. 27.
46  Banks, 'Out on a Limb', p. 73.

47   Ibid., p. 75.
48   *HBA Auckland Newsletter*, 28, July 1985, p. 12.
49   'Steadfast advocate for new mums and babies', *Press*, 9 June 2012, https://www.pressreader.com/new-zealand/the-press/20120609/282260957527810
50   Banks, 'Out on a Limb', p. 181.
51   Ibid., p. 72.
52   *HBA Auckland Newsletter*, 41, October 1988–January 1989, p. 10; Bronwen Pelvin, 'On the Edge: Midwifery and the Art of Knowing', *New Zealand College of Midwives Journal (NZCOMJ)*, vol. 15, October 1996, p. 14.
53   Lynn Rain, *Community: The Story of Riverside 1941–1991*, Riverside Community, Lower Moutere, 1991, pp. 81, 89, 92, 116. Pelvin noted her address as 'Riverside Community, Upper Moutere', *Domiciliary Midwives Society (DMS) Newsletter*, April 1989, p. 1.
54   Rain, *Community*, p. 116.
55   Report from Editor Heather Waugh, *DMS Newsletter*, March 1985, p. 3.
56   Rain, *Community*, pp. 118–20.
57   *HBA Newsletter*, 2, October 1980, p. 16; 'Future Events', *New Zealand College of Midwives Newsletter*, 3, 3, February 1991.
58   Joan Donley, Report of meeting of DMS, 28 March 1982, in *HBA National Newsletter*, 6, July 1982, p. 11.
59   Lynley McFarland, in Halina Ogonowska-Coates, *Born: Midwives and Women Celebrate 100 Years*, New Zealand College of Midwives, Christchurch, 2004, p. 18.
60   Samantha Skiff, 'Machine-minders and Handmaidens? Hospital Midwives and Childbirth in New Zealand, 1950–1990', MA thesis, University of Auckland, 2014, p. 80.
61   C. S. Harison, Obstetric Advisor, Thames Hospital Board, Submission to Maternity Services Committee, Domiciliary Midwifery, 11 June 1980, R20459385, ANZW.
62   Report from Nelson, *HBA National Newsletter*, May 1983, p. 9.
63   'Rock music festivals Page 3 – Nambassa', https://nzhistory.govt.nz/culture/rock-music-festivals/nambassa (accessed 10 September 2022).
64   'Cultural guests' at Nambassa listed in: https://en.wikipedia.org/wiki/Nambassa#:~:text=Nambassa%20was%20a%20series%20of,and%20an%20environmentally%20friendly%20lifestyle
65   'Homebirth at Nambassa', *HBA National Newsletter*, 3, January 1981, p. 4; *HBA Auckland Newsletter*, 11, May 1981, p. 3; Gaskin's qualification was a Master of Arts in English from the Northern Illinois University: Ina May Gaskin, *Spiritual Midwifery*, The Book Publishing Co., The Farm, Summertown, Tennessee, rev. edn,1978 p. 19.
66   Wendy Kline, *Coming Home: How Midwives Changed Birth*, Oxford University Press, New York, 2019, pp. 73, 79.
67   Ibid., p. 87; see also Wendy Kline, 'Communicating a New Consciousness: Countercultural Print and the Home Birth Movement in the 1970s', *Bulletin of the History of Medicine*, vol. 89, 3, 2015, pp. 543–48.

68  Kline, *Coming Home*, pp. 86–87.
69  Paula A. Michaels, *Lamaze: An International History*, Oxford University Press, Oxford, 2014, pp. 115–16.
70  Gaskin, *Spiritual Midwifery*, pp. 14, 283, 285.
71  Jean Patterson, 'Book Review: Ina May Gaskin, *Guide to Childbirth*, 2003', *NZCOMJ*, vol. 31, October 2004, p. 27.
72  Jane Ellen Esther Stojanovic, 'Placental Birth: A History', PhD thesis, Massey University, 2012, p. 7.
73  Banks, 'Out on a Limb', pp. 73, 75, 185.
74  Harison, Submission to Maternity Services Committee, 1980, R20459385, ANZW.
75  'Book List: Special edition – Happy birthday! Changing attitudes to birth, bonding & babies', *Centrepoint Magazine*, 12, March/April 1983, p. 33.
76  Bronwen Pelvin, 'Life Skills for Midwifery Practice', in Sally Pairman, Jan Pincombe, Carol Thorogood and Sally Tracy (eds), *Midwifery: Preparation for Practice*, Churchill Livingstone Elsevier, Marrickville NSW, 2006, p. 234; Sally Pairman and Judith McAra-Couper, 'Theoretical Frameworks for Midwifery Practice', in Pairman et al. (eds), *Midwifery: Preparation for Practice*, p. 255.
77  *HBA Auckland Newsletter*, 32, June 1986, p. 6; 'Report from Christchurch', ibid., 45, December 1989, p. 8.
78  Helen Brew, 'Viewpoints in Antenatal Education. The Parents' Viewpoint', speech at National Women's Hospital 1958, pp. 3, 12, cited in Bryder, *The Rise and Fall*, p. 62.
79  Frances Parkin, 'Giving birth back to mothers', *New Zealand Listener*, 16 April 1977, p. 18; Jillian Wittmer, 'Place of Birth: A Longitudinal Study Comparing Delivery Outcome, Maternal Attitudes and Coping', MA thesis, University of Auckland, 1981, p. 5.
80  Brown, 'When birth becomes an "occasion" at home', p. 3; 'Producer plans $1.5m series on childbirth', *Auckland Star*, 15 February 1979; see also Bryder, *The Rise and Fall*, pp. 173, 195.
81  Brenda Hinton, *HBA Auckland Newsletter*, 43, June 1989, p. 1.
82  Ivan Illich, *Medical Nemesis: The Expropriation of Health*, Calder & Boyars, London, 1975.
83  Donley, *Herstory*, p. 3.
84  Kitty Wishart, 'The Birth of Kate', *Broadsheet*, 35, December 1975, pp. 16–19. See also Sandra Coney, 'Taking Childbirth Back', ibid., 49, May 1977, pp. 22–23, 25.
85  *HBA National Newsletter*, 2, October 1980, p. 5.
86  Brown, 'When birth becomes an "occasion" at home', p. 5. Davis was one of the most prominent American health-food writers; her books sold more than 10 million copies before she died in 1974.
87  Catherine Carstairs, 'The Granola High: Eating Differently in the Late 1960s and 1970s', in Franca Iacovetta, Valerie J. Korinek and Marlene Epp (eds),

*Edible Histories, Cultural Politics: Towards a Canadian Food History*, University of Toronto Press, Toronto, 2012, p. 318, cites Adelle Davis, *Let's Have Healthy Children*, New American Library, New York, 1972, p. 92.
88  F. D. (Flora Davidson), 'Q for Quackery', *Health*, September 1960, np.
89  *HBA National Newsletter*, 2, 2, June 1984, p. 28.
90  Brown, 'When birth becomes an "occasion" at home', p. 5; Coney, 'Taking Childbirth Back', p. 23; McLean, 'Home Birth in New Zealand', p. 7.
91  Michele Simpson, 'Raspberry Leaf: Panacea for Pregnancy and Labour or Problem?', *O&G Magazine*, vol. 12, 4, Summer 2020, p. 55.
92  Donley to Maggie Lecky-Thompson, 10 November 1995, MSS & Archives 2007/15 Series 1, Sub-Series 1/2, File 7/2/C/1, JDP.
93  *HBA National Newsletter*, 7, November 1982, p. 3.
94  Julie Leibrich, Janet Hickling and George Pitt, *In Search of Well-being: Exploratory Research into Complementary Therapies*, Health Services Research and Development Unit, Department of Health, Wellington, 1987, p. 137.
95  McLean, 'Home Birth in New Zealand', p. 8; Classified Ads: International Home Birth Week Seminar, *Broadsheet*, 104, November 1982, p. 56.
96  Editorial, *HBA Auckland Newsletter*, 34, December 1986, p. 2A.
97  *HBA Auckland Newsletter*, 37, 1987, pp. 4, 5.
98  Leibrich et al., *In Search of Well-being*, p. 134.
99  *DMS Newsletter*, 2, March 1985, p. 2.
100 *HBA National Newsletter*, 3, January 1981, p. 2; *DMS Newsletter*, 1, 1984, p. 2; Leibrich et al., *In Search of Well-being*, p. 16; *DMS Newsletter*, 4, July 1987, Part 1, pp. 6–11; ibid., 5, March 1988, Part 2, pp. 7–14.
101 Home Birth Aotearoa, 'We Follow Midwifery Students: Lian Pansino', September 2014, in *Home Birth Matters*, 1, 3, Spring 2014, p. 86, https://homebirth.org.nz/magazine/wp-content/uploads/2014/09/Home-Birth-Matters-Spring-Issue-PDF.pdf (accessed 6 January 2023).
102 *Northern News*, 20 April 1989, in Wise Woman Archives Trust Inc. (WWAT), http://wwat.nz/wp-content/uploads/1989-4.pdf (accessed 10 March 2023).
103 Pamela Stirling, 'Hard labour', *New Zealand Listener*, 12 March 1990, p. 11.
104 Ibid.
105 *HBA Auckland Newsletter*, 45, December 1989, p. 8.
106 Ibid., 46, Autumn 1990, p. 9.
107 Alice Coyle, 'Six Years of Independent Midwifery in London: Presented for the NZCOM Conference', *NZCOMJ*, vol. 7, December 1992, p. 22.
108 Leibrich et al., *In Search of Well-being*, p. 131.
109 Donley Q and A, 29 July 1985, p. 2, Appendum to *DMS Newsletter*, 2, March 1985.
110 Yvonne Morgan, 'Letter to the editor: Induction via Acupuncture', *NZCOMJ*, vol. 3, November 1990, p. 6.
111 *HBA Auckland Newsletter*, 36, June 1987, p. 9.
112 Vanya Hogg, 'Acupuncture mothers find childbirth easier', *Auckland Star*, 31 October 1979.

113 T. E. Kjellstrom, 'Home Birth – A Viable Alternative?' A fifth year Community Health Project carried out by 10 students under supervision of Dr T. E. Kjellstrom, Department of Community Health, School of Medicine, University of Auckland, 1982, p. 13, MSS & Archives 2007/15, 1638, JDP.

114 Leibrich et al., *In Search of Well-being*, p. 66. Later, a four- to five-year approved Bachelor degree programme with a major in acupuncture was recommended by the Australian and Chinese Medical Association; see John Schibeci (collator), 'Non-pharmacological Pain Management in Childbirth', *O&G Magazine*, vol. 11, 4, Summer 2009, p. 26.

115 Leibrich et al., *In Search of Well-being*, p. 66.

116 Hogg, 'Acupuncture mothers find childbirth easier'.

117 Harison, Submission to Maternity Services Committee, 1980, R20459385, ANZW.

118 Penelope and David Robie, 'A warm and loving welcome', *New Zealand Listener*, 15 January 1977, p. 19.

119 'Birth: Back to basics', *New Zealand Listener*, 30 April 1983, pp. 20–21.

120 'Rose: Our first baby', *Centrepoint Magazine*, 12, March/April 1983, p. 34; Don McKenzie, 'A family affair', ibid., p. 9.

121 Rhonda Evans, 'Having a choice about birthing', ibid., p. 4; Sue Mendelssohn, 'Western women have many problem-inducing body tensions', ibid., p. 7; 'Waveney's story', ibid., p. 16; Book list, ibid., p. 33.

122 Barbara Hasslacher, 'Birth at Home', *New Zealand Nursing Journal: Kai Tiaki*, April 1988, p. 25.

123 *Save the Midwives Newsletter*, December 1984, p. 8.

124 Sally Pairman, in Ogonowska-Coates, *Born*, p. 62; her visit was also mentioned in *Save the Midwives Newsletter*, 5, 1984, p. 8.

125 Leibrich et al., *In Search of Well-being*, p. 131.

126 Robyn Maude and Shea Caplice, 'Using Water for Labour and Birth', in Pairman et al. (eds), *Midwifery: Preparation for Practice*, p. 431; 'Waterbirth in New Zealand: Herstory and Politics', *Birthspirit Midwifery Journal*, vol. 1, 2009, pp. 13–19, rev. 3 March 2014, https://www.birthspirit.co.nz/waterbirth-new-zealand-history-politics/ (accessed 10 September 2022); *New Zealand Herald*, 18 January 1982; *HBA National Newsletter*, 7, November 1982, p. 5.

127 Report by Henriette Kemp, *HBA National Newsletter*, Special Conference edition, May 1983, p. 6; also reported in *New Zealand Herald*, 3 August 1982.

128 *HBA National Newsletter*, 2, 2, June 1984, pp. 17–19.

129 Pauline Ray, 'Whose body is it? Whose baby is it?', *New Zealand Listener*, 1980, pp. 15, 20–24.

130 *HBA National Newsletter*, 2, 2, June 1984, p. 17; Shelley Ashcroft, 'Modern Women or Tree-hugging Hippies? A Foucauldian Discourse Analysis of the New Zealand Media's Representation of Waterbirth', Master of Health Science Midwifery, Auckland University of Technology, 2007, p. 53; Charkovsky did not always have a favourable media coverage; his methods were compared to child abuse by a midwife in 1988: Deseret News, https://www.deseret.

com/1996/2/9/19224104/russian-father-of-sea-births-faces-charges (accessed 10 March 2023).
131 *DMS Newsletter*, 3, July 1986, p. 8.
132 Ashcroft, 'Modern Women', p. 52.
133 *HBA Auckland Newsletter*, 44, September 1989, pp. N6, 13.
134 Maude and Caplice, in Pairman et al. (eds), Midwifery: Preparation for Practice p. 443; J. Balaskas, *The Water Birth Book*, Unwin Hyman, London, 2004.
135 Malcolm Nicolson and John E. E. Fleming, *Imaging and Imagining the Fetus: The Development of Obstetric Ultrasound*, Johns Hopkins University Press, Baltimore, 2013.
136 *HBA National Newsletter*, March 1984, p. 36.
137 Department of Health, *Your Pregnancy, To Haputanga me to Whakawhanautanga*, Department of Health, Wellington, 1985, Code 4146, pp. 26, 36, https://www.moh.govt.nz/notebook/nbbooks.nsf/0/50BA5494E2C12B5F4C2565D70018BC95/$file/your-pregnancy.pdf (accessed 10 September 2022); *HBA Auckland Newsletter*, 30, November 1985, pp. 6–7; *HBA National Newsletter*, 32, June 1986, p. 3.
138 Transcript of interview of Donley by Abel, p. 7, JDP.
139 *HBA Auckland Newsletter*, 45, December 1989, pp. L4–5.
140 'Scans . . . How safe for babies?', *New Zealand Woman's Weekly*, 9 October 1989, p. 18.
141 Bryder, *The Rise and Fall*, pp. 130–33.
142 'Home Birth – a Viable Alternative?', pp. 13–14.
143 Dennis G. Bonham, 'Maternal and Child Health', in Douglas. P. Kennedy (ed.), *Health in the 1970s: A Collection of Informed Opinions*, N. M. Peryer, Christchurch, 1970, pp. 28–29.
144 Linda Bryder, *A Voice for Mothers: The Plunket Society and Infant Welfare 1907–2000*, Auckland University Press, Auckland, 2003, pp. 219–22.
145 See, for example, *HBA Auckland Newsletter*. 32, June 1986, p. 3; 33, September 1986, p. 3; 37, September 1987, p. 2; 41, October 1988–January 1989, p. 26; 44, September 1989; 47, Winter 1990, p. 17.
146 Ben Schrader, 'Magazines and Periodicals – Specialist and lifestyle magazines: 1890s to 2010s', *Te Ara – the Encyclopedia of New Zealand*, http://www.TeAra.govt.nz/en/magazines-and-periodicals/page-5 (accessed 31 October 2021).
147 "Giving it her best shot", *More*, October 1987, pp. 117–20.
148 *HBA Auckland Newsletter*, 41, October 1988–January 1989, p. 23.
149 Ibid., 45, December 1989, Report from Christchurch, p. 9; ibid., Mac McDonald, 'Immunisation – yes or no?', pp. 12–14.
150 Ritchie was described as a homeopathic doctor in the Christchurch *Press*, 2 August 1997, included in *HBA Auckland Newsletter*, 68, Spring 1997, p. 46; International Medical Council on Vaccination, 'A Collection of Comments by Doctors on the Myths and Dangers of Vaccination-immunization', http://www.blatantpropaganda.org/propaganda/articles/vaccination_doctors.html (accessed 12 March 2023).

151 Nicola Legat, 'Measles on Elm Street: The argument against immunisation', *Metro*, December 1991, p. 102.
152 Ibid., p. 103.

## CHAPTER 2: 'Everyone should do it': Why choose homebirth?

1. Jenny Wheeler, 'Home or hospital birth? The case for both . . .', *New Zealand Woman's Weekly*, 30 October 1978, p. 30.
2. See Linda Bryder, *The Rise and Fall of National Women's Hospital*, Auckland University Press, Auckland, 2014, p. 61.
3. Helen Brown, 'When birth becomes an "occasion" at home', *New Zealand Woman's Weekly*, 7 August 1978, p. 4.
4. Wheeler, 'Home or hospital birth?', p. 30; see also Bryder, *The Rise and Fall*, p. 197; 'Auckland champion of home births dies', obituary, *Auckland Star*, 5 October 1982.
5. Joan Donley, 'Conference 1982', *Home Birth Association (HBA) National Newsletter*, 6, July 1982, p. 2.
6. T. E. Kjellstrom, 'Home Birth – A Viable Alternative?' A fifth year Community Health Project carried out by 10 students under supervision of Dr T. E. Kjellstrom, Department of Community Health, School of Medicine, University of Auckland, 1982, p. 23, Joan Donley Papers 1933-2003, MSS & Archives 2007/15, 1638, Manuscripts and Archives, University of Auckland Library (JDP).
7. Ibid., p. 24.
8. John Stevenson, *Melbourne Age*, 3 July 1984, reported in *HBA National Newsletter*, 2, 3, September 1984, p. 14.
9. See Bryder, *The Rise and Fall*, p. 195.
10. Julie Leibrich, Janet Hickling and George Pitt, *In Search of Well-being: Exploratory Research into Complementary Therapies*, Health Services Research and Development Unit, Department of Health, Wellington, 1987, p. 136.
11. Penelope and David Robie, 'A warm and loving welcome', *New Zealand Listener*, 15 January 1977, p. 18.
12. Jillian Wittmer, 'Place of Birth: A Longitudinal Study Comparing Delivery Outcome, Maternal Attitudes and Coping', MA thesis, University of Auckland, 1981, p. 29.
13. *HBA National Newsletter*, 1, July 1980, p. 8.
14. Ibid., 2, June 1984, pp. 13–14; Joseph Chilton Pearce, *The Crack in the Cosmic Egg: Challenging Constructs of Mind and Reality*, Julian Press, New York, 1971, reprinted 1988, and *Magical Child: Rediscovering Nature's Plan for Our Children*, Dutton, New York, 1977.
15. Bryder, *The Rise and Fall*, p. 61.
16. *HBA Auckland Newsletter*, 46, Autumn 1990, p. 3; Birth and Being Conference, Australian Birth Foundation and the Childbirth Education Association of Victoria, in Wise Woman Archives Trust Inc. (WWAT), http://wwat.nz/wp-content/uploads/20072-2-022.pdf (accessed 10 March 2023).

*Notes*

17  Kjellstrom, 'Home Birth – A Viable Alternative?', pp. 3–4.
18  *HBA Auckland Newsletter*, 34, December 1986, pp. 3A–4A.
19  Ibid., 35, March 1987, p. 19.
20  'Lynda's Story', in Karen Guilliland and Sally Pairman, *Women's Business: The Story of the New Zealand College of Midwives, 1986–2010*, New Zealand College of Midwives, Christchurch, 2010, p. 179.
21  Pamela Stirling, 'Hard labour', *New Zealand Listener*, 12 March 1990, p. 15.
22  Ibid., p. 15.
23  Marilyn Garson, 'Mother and baby bond best in home birth', *Northern News*, 20 April 1989.
24  *Auckland Star*, 9 July 1980.
25  Stirling, 'Hard labour', p. 15; see also Diana Nash, 'Foreword' to Joan Donley, *Save the Midwife*, New Women's Press, Auckland, 1986, p. 8.
26  Working Group on Safe Options for Low Risk Pregnancy, sixth draft, October 1989, p. 8, in WWAT, http://wwat.nz/wp-content/uploads/20073-91-005.pdf (accessed 10 March 2023).
27  Maya Howat (Hicks Bay), Letter to the editor, 'Home births', *New Zealand Listener*, 15 October 1983, p. 11.
28  Mrs D. Windelborn (Katikati), ibid., 12 November 1983, p. 8.
29  Wittmer, '*Place of Birth*', p. 121.
30  Ibid., p. 123.
31  *HBA Auckland Newsletter*, 35, March 1987, p. 8.
32  Ibid., 34, December 1986, p. 2; ibid., 36, June 1987, p. 1. See also Joan Donley, *Herstory of N.Z. Home Birth Association*, New Zealand Home Birth Association, Auckland, 1992, p. 4.
33  'Glynette's story', in Guilliland and Pairman, *Women's Business*, p. 202.
34  Alastair Shaw, 'Telling the Truth about People's China', PhD thesis, Victoria University of Wellington, 2010, p. 114; Joan Donley, Workshop on Women and Health, Auckland University, March 1978, MSS & Archives 2007/15, Series 1, Sub-Series 2, 2007/15, file 2/4/c/1, JDP.
35  Joan Donley, 'Having the Baby at Home', *Broadsheet*, 132, September 1985, p. 17.
36  Joan Donley, Letter to the editor, 'For healthier babies', *Auckland Star*, 16 February 1983, reproduced in Donley, *Herstory*, p. 27.
37  *HBA National Newsletter*, 2, October 1980, p. 6.
38  Sandra Coney, *The Unfortunate Experiment: The Full Story Behind the Inquiry into Cervical Cancer Treatment*, Penguin, Auckland, 1988, p. 16.
39  Donley, *Herstory*, p. 3 (there are some discrepancies in spelling in different published sources: Deryn or Derryn and Macfarlane or MacFarlane).
40  Barbara Macfarlane (secretary), Letter to the editor, *Auckland Star*, 16 October 1980 (in *New Zealand Listener*, 15 March 1980, p. 24 the journalist called her the president).
41  Boston Women's Health Book Collective, *Women and Their Bodies*, New England Free Press, Boston, 1970, reprinted and revised as *Our Bodies Ourselves* with editions in 1971, 1976, 1984, 1985, 1995, 1998, 2005.

42   Sarah Calvert, 'Knowledge is Power: Reasons for the Women's Health Movement', *Broadsheet*, 80, June 1980, pp. 26–30.
43   *HBA National Newsletter*, 1, July 1980, p. 2.
44   Donley, *Herstory*, p. 11.
45   Linda Daly-Peoples, 'The Politics of Childbirth', *Broadsheet*, 48, April 1977, p. 21.
46   Ibid., p. 24.
47   'Getting By: Marilyn Garson Looks at Life for Women in the Hokianga', *Broadsheet*, 182, October 1990, pp. 18–19.
48   Sandra Coney, 'Alienated Labour – Foetal Monitoring', *Broadsheet*, 69, May 1979, pp. 16–17, 38–39.
49   Phillida Bunkle, *Second Opinion: The Politics of Women's Health in New Zealand*, Oxford University Press, Auckland, 1988, pp. viii–ix (emphasis in the original).
50   Vanya Hogg, 'I put babies first, says doctor', *Auckland Star*, 4 October 1978, p. 23.
51   Cited in Donley, *Herstory*, p. 14.
52   Editorial, *Save the Midwives Newsletter*, 5, January 1985, p. 2.
53   Christine Bird, 'Using Womens Health Groups', *Broadsheet*, 137, March 1986, pp. 19–21.
54   Judi Strid, 'Midwifery in Revolt', ibid., 153, November 1987, p. 16.
55   HBA Auckland Branch, Submission to Maternity Services Committee, 23 September 1979, R20459385, 1978081, 5, 29-21, 53139, Archives New Zealand Wellington (ANZW).
56   Donley, 'Having the Baby at Home', p. 47.
57   Lyn McLean, Wellington, Submission to Maternity Services Committee, 23 June 1980, R20459385, ANZW.
58   Strid, 'Midwifery in Revolt', p. 15; Judi Strid, 'A Consumer Viewpoint', *New Zealand College of Midwives Journal* (NZCOMJ), vol. 5, October 1991, p. 5.
59   Joan Donley, 'Professionalism: The Importance of Consumer Control Over Childbirth', *NZCOMJ*, vol. 1, September 1989, p. 6; this had been previously reported by Sandra Coney, 'Health: Take the Power from the Docs', *Broadsheet*, 170, July/August 1989, p. 24.
60   Baird to Guilliland, 6 January 1990, MSS & Archives 2007/2 NZCOM Auckland Region 1985-2002, R300388602, Item 5, Special Collections, University of Auckland Library (NZCOM AR Papers).
61   M. A. H. Baird, 'Letter to the New Zealand College of Midwives and Apology', *NZCOMJ*, vol. 2, March 1990, p. 5.
62   COM National Committee Meeting, 5 May 1990, Item 5, NZCOM AR Papers.
63   *HBA Auckland Newsletter*, 43, June 1989, p. N8; Thea Roodra, 'New Choices in Childbirth', *Health*, 40, 9, Spring 1989, p. 3; Ruth Joy Surtees, 'Midwifery as Feminist Praxis in Aotearoa/New Zealand', PhD thesis, University of Canterbury, 2003, p. 35.
64   Joan Donley, 'Women in Partnership', *Broadsheet*, 182, October 1990, p. 7.
65   Joan Donley, 'Political Comment: Protocols?', *NZCOMJ*, vol. 7, December 1992, p. 11; Joan Donley, '"What Does the New Zealand College of Midwives Do For Me?" A response to the New Zealand Nurses Association', ibid., 19,

November 1998, p. 20; Joan Donley, 'Independent Midwifery in New Zealand', in Tricia Murphy-Black (ed.), *Issues in Midwifery*, Churchill Livingstone, Edinburgh, 1995, p. 79.

66   *HBA National Newsletter*, 3, January 1981, p. 2; repeated in Karen Guilliland, 'Maintaining the Links: A History of the Formation of the NZCOM', *NZCOMJ*, vol. 1, September 1989, p. 14.
67   *HBA National Newsletter*, 3, January 1981, p. 2.
68   Jean Donnison, *Midwives and Medical Men: A History of Inter-professional Rivalry and Women's Rights*, Schocken Books, London, 1977, reprinted as *Midwives and Medical Men: A History of the Struggle for the Control of Childbirth*, Historical Publications, London, 1988.
69   *HBA National Newsletter*, 2, 3, September 1984, p. 16.
70   Wendy Kline, *Coming Home: How Midwives Changed Birth*, Oxford University Press, New York, 2019, p. 95.
71   Ibid., pp. 95–96.
72   *Domiciliary Midwives Society (DMS) Newsletter*, 3, July 1986, p. 12.
73   *HBA National Newsletter*, 2, 2, June 1984, pp. 12, 25; Judy Cochrane, 'Diony Young: A Profile', *International Journal of Childbirth Education*, vol. 5, 4, 30 November 1990, pp. 19–20, https://www.proquest.com/openview/46cab465ccfaade75b756270bf919c3f/1?pq-origsite=gscholar&cbl=32235https://www.ourbodiesourselves.org/publications/our-bodies-ourselves-2011/contributors/diony-young/ (accessed 8 September 2022).
74   Sharon [sic] Cole, 'Antenatal Education: Why Childbirth Educators?', *NZCOMJ*, vol. 5, October 1991, p. 21.
75   Donley, *Herstory*, p. 49; Carolyn Young, 'The Honouring of Joan Donley, OBE', *NZCOMJ*, vol. 2, March 1990, pp. 10–11.
76   *Save the Midwives Association Newsletter*, December 1984, p. 8; *HBA Auckland Newsletter*, 35, March 1987, p. 19; 'Lynda's Story', in Guilliland and Pairman, *Women's Business*, p. 181.
77   'Press Release: ICEA: International Appointment for Dunedin Woman', *NZCOMJ*, vol. 2, March 1990, p. 20.
78   Jenny Drew, 'Teacher to Teacher', *International Journal of Childhood Education*, August 1990, p. 41.
79   Donley, *Herstory*, p. 62; *HBA National Newsletter*, 4, August 1981, p. 15; Donley report, 1988 Homebirth Australia Conference, Hobart, in WWAT, http://wwat.nz/wp-content/uploads/20001-22-006b.pdf (accessed 10 March 2023).
80   Donley, Sixth National Homebirth Australia Conference, Report, 5–8 April 1985, in WWAT, http://wwat.nz/wp-content/uploads/20001-22-009.pdf (accessed 10 March 2023).
81   *HBA Auckland Newsletter*, 36, June 1987, p. 19.
82   Ibid., 37, September 1987, p. 23.
83   Ibid., 39, March 1988, p. 9.
84   Sian Burgess, 'Report from the First International Home Birth Conference', *HBA Auckland Newsletter*, 37, November 1987, pp. 22–23 [both September 1987

and November 1987 are listed as no. 37]. Recordings of speeches can be found in WWAT 2005/1, http://wwat.nz/sian-burgess-papers-relating-to-domiciliary-midwifery-and-home-birth-1983-1992-wwat-20051/ (accessed 10 March 2023).
85  *Auckland HBA Newsletter*, 37, November 1987, p. 23.
86  Lyn Bell, 'Sheila Kitzinger: Childbirth and women's choice', *Woman's Day*, 16 December 1985, p. 14.
87  Book list, *Centrepoint Magazine*, 12, March/April 1983, p. 33.
88  *HBA Auckland Newsletter*, 36, June 1987, p. 1.
89  Jennie Nicol, 'A Choice of Birthing: Part 1: Homebirth and Domiciliary Midwifery', Wellington, Department of Health, November 1987, p. 22, https://www.moh.govt.nz/notebook/nbbooks.nsf/0/ 6D092B4E4F967CBC4C2565D7000DD6A4/$file/Choice-of-birthing.pdf (accessed 8 September 2022).
90  *Auckland HBA Newsletter*, 37, November 1987, p. 22.
91  'Homebirth: The International Scene', *Parents and Children*, February/March 1988, cited in *HBA Auckland Newsletter*, 42, February – April 1989, p. 14; see also Penny Simkin, 'Tribute: Sheila Kitzinger (1929–2015), *Birth*, vol. 42, 3, September 2015, pp. 199–201.
92  Burgess, Report, *HBA Auckland Newsletter*, 37, November 1987, p. 22.
93  Marjorie Tew, *A Safer Childbirth? A Critical History of Maternity Care*, Springer, New York, 1990.
94  Marjorie Tew, 'Place of Birth and Perinatal Mortality', *Journal of the Royal College of General Practitioners*, vol. 35, 277, 1985, pp. 390–94.
95  Burgess, Report, *Auckland HBA Newsletter*, 37, November 1987, p. 22.
96  Working Group on Safe Options for Low Risk Pregnancy, sixth draft, October 1989, p. 11, in WWAT, http://wwat.nz/wp-content/uploads/20073-91-005.pdf (accessed 10 March 2023).
97  'Homebirth: The International Scene', *Parents and Children*, February/March 1988.
98  Ann Oakley, 'The Sociology of Childbirth: An Autobiographical Journey Through Four Decades of Research', *Sociology of Health & Illness*, vol. 38, 5, 2016, p. 692, doi: 10.1111/1467-9566.12400; Ann Oakley, 'Home Birth: A Class Privilege', *New Society*, 6 November 1987, p. 27; J. Davies, 'Home birth: A class privilege (letter)', ibid., 13 November 1987.
99  *Save the Midwives Newsletter*, 20, August 1989, p. 25; *HBA Auckland Newsletter*, 42, February–April 1989, pp. 11, 12.
100  'Homebirth: The International Scene', *Parents and Children*, February/March 1988.
101  *HBA Auckland Newsletter*, 42, February–April 1989, pp. 11–15.
102  Ibid., 37, November 1987, p. 23.
103  Kate Isherwood, 'Independent Midwifery in the United Kingdom', in Murphy-Black (ed.), *Issues in Midwifery*, p. 26.
104  *HBA Auckland Newsletter*, 39, March 1988, p. 9.
105  Strid, 'Midwifery in Revolt', p. 15.
106  *HBA Auckland Newsletter*, 32, June 1986, p. 3; ibid., 33, September 1986, advertisement, p. 1.

107 Jane Wilson, 'Immaculate deception', *New York Times*, 22 June 1975, https://www.nytimes.com/1975/06/22/archives/immaculate-deception-doing-what-doesnt-always-come-naturally-birth.html (accessed 10 March 2023); *HBA Auckland Newsletter*, 32, June 1986, p. 3; Surtees, 'Midwifery as Feminist Praxis', p. 171 fn 32; Birth and Being Conference, Victoria, Australia, 1979, in WWAT, http://wwat.nz/wp-content/uploads/20072-2-022.pdf (accessed 10 March 2023).

108 New Zealand College of Midwives (Otago Branch), Submission on the Revision of the Nurses Act (1977), R21935511, 1990, 80, W67/NUR/2, 68678, ANZW.

109 *HBA Auckland Newsletter*, 39, March 1988, p. 16.

110 Linda Bryder, *A History of the 'Unfortunate Experiment' at National Women's Hospital*, Auckland, Auckland University Press, 2008, pp. 182–84.

111 Wendy Savage, *A Savage Enquiry: Who Controls Childbirth?*, Virago, London, 1986; Wendy Savage, *Birth and Power: The Savage Enquiry Revisited*, Middlesex University Press, London, 2007.

112 *HBA Auckland Newsletter*, 40, June–September 1988, p. 5.

113 Ibid., 42, February–April 1989, p. 5.

114 Judi Strid, 'Sheila Kitzinger on Motherhood', *Parents Centre Bulletin*, 120, November 1989, pp. 22–23.

115 Karen Guilliland and Julie Hassen, 'Report from the 1990 Midwives Conference', *NZCOMJ*, vol. 3, November 1990, p. 9.

116 Marsden Wagner, 'Appropriate Technology for Birth', ibid., pp. 10–11, 14–15.

117 Bryder, *The Rise and Fall*, pp. 59–60; Jacqueline Wolf, *Deliver Me from Pain: Anaesthesia and Birth in America*, Johns Hopkins University Press, Baltimore, 2009, pp. 176–78.

118 *New Zealand Herald*, 7 August 1990; Wagner, 'Appropriate Technology for Birth', pp. 10–11, 15.

119 New Zealand Planning Council, *First Report of the Social Monitoring Group: From Birth to Death* (convener Peggy Koopman-Boyden), Wellington, July 1985, pp. 21–22.

CHAPTER 3: *Homebirth and maternity services 1970–1990*

1 Maternity Services Committee (MSC), *Mother and Baby at Home: The Early Days*, Board of Health Report Series 30, Government Printer, Wellington, 1982, p. 8.

2 MSC, *Maternity Services in New Zealand: A Report by the Maternity Services Committee Board of Health*, Board of Health Report Series 26, Government Printer, Wellington, 1976, p. 56.

3 Information paper for MSC meeting, 27, 28 March 1979, R20459385, 1978–1981, Box 5, Record no. 29-21, 53139, Archives New Zealand Wellington (ANZW); on the 1977 United Women's Convention see also Maggie Banks, 'Out on a Limb: The Personal Mandate to Practise Midwifery

by Midwives of the Domiciliary Midwives Society of New Zealand (Incorporated), 1974–1986', PhD thesis, Victoria University of Wellington, 2007, p. 175.
4   Information paper for MSC meeting, 1979, R20459385, ANZW.
5   MSC, 'Obstetrics and the Winds of Change', Board of Health, Wellington, 1979; copy in 'Maternity Services', R20459385, ANZW.
6   Carole Wall, 'Midweek for women', *Auckland Star*, 5 September 1979, p. 24.
7   Linda Bryder, *The Rise and Fall of National Women's Hospital*, Auckland University Press, Auckland, 2014, pp. 172–89.
8   Auckland Branch Home Birth Association (HBA), Submission to MSC, 23 September 1979, R20459385, ANZW.
9   'Women "lured" to hospital, says home birth group', *Auckland Star*, 21 September 1979.
10  'Midwife is one of the family', *North Shore Times*, 10 April 1979, p. 15.
11  Margaret Gibson Smith and Yvonne T. Shadbolt (eds), *Objects and Outcomes: New Zealand Nurses' Association 1909–1983*, New Zealand Nurses' Association, Wellington, 1984, p. 82.
12  Gibson Smith and Shadbolt, *Objects and Outcomes*, p. 93; Sally Pairman and Karen Guilliland, 'The Resurgence of Midwifery', in Karen Guilliland and Sally Pairman, *Women's Business: The Story of the New Zealand College of Midwives, 1986–2010*, New Zealand College of Midwives, Christchurch, 2010, p. 66.
13  'Midwifery Teacher Training Workshop', *New Zealand Nursing Journal: Kai Tiaki*, vol. 71, 6, 1978, p. 17.
14  Panel discussion, 'Where to be born', Green Lane Hospital, 10 November 1976, Joan Donley Papers 1933–2003, MSS & Archives, 2007/15, 5/6/A/1, Manuscripts and Archives, University of Auckland Library (JDP).
15  Rachel Veale, 'Hospital is still safest place to have baby', *Auckland Star*, 19 September 1979.
16  Cited in Banks, 'Out on a Limb', p. 155; 'Letter: New Zealand Home Birth Association', *New Zealand Nursing Journal: Kai Tiaki*, vol. 72, 9, September 1979, p. 12.
17  HBA Auckland, submission to MSC, 1979, R20459385, ANZW.
18  Ibid.; 'Home birth proposal seen as attempt to shut down option', *New Zealand Herald (NZH)*, 13 November 1979; Mrs K.M. Rix-Trott, Letter to the editor, 'Home births', ibid., 14 November 1979.
19  Banks, 'Out on a Limb', p. 131.
20  Hospital Boards' Association, submission to MSC, 15 April 1980, R20459385, ANZW.
21  St George's Private Hospital, Christchurch, submission to MSC, 1980, R20459385, ANZW.
22  Canterbury Hospital Board, submission to MSC, 4 March 1980, R20459385, ANZW.
23  Palmerston North Hospital, submission to MSC, 28 February 1980, R20459385, ANZW.

24 C. S. Harison, submission to MSC, 28 February 1980, 11 June 1980, R20459385, ANZW.
25 M.A.H. Baird, Auckland Branch O&G Society, submission to MSC, 21 May 1980; G.H. Henderson GD, Southland Division O&G Society, submission to MSC, 15 May 1980, R20459385, ANZW.
26 Royal College of Obstetricians and Gynaecologists, submission to MSC, 18 March 1980, R20459385, ANZW.
27 NZMA, submission to MSC, 1980, R20459385, ANZW.
28 National Council of Women, submission to MSC, 15 February 1980, R20459385, ANZW; NCW also summarised this submission in its 1990 Submission to the Social Services Committee, Jocelyn Fish and Janet Hesketh, 9 February 1990, R21935512, 1989-1990, 81 W67/NUR/2 68681, ANZW.
29 Pauline Ray, 'Whose body is it? Whose baby is it?', *New Zealand Listener*, 15 March 1980, p. 15.
30 Julia M. Witchalls (Auckland), Letter to the editor, ibid., 5 April 1980.
31 R. Herrick (Hamilton), ibid.
32 Jess Parker (Auckland), ibid., 12 April 1980.
33 'Bert's Talk 30/10/82', *Centrepoint Magazine*, 12, March/April 1983, pp. 4, 8.
34 'Midwife's comment', ibid., p. 21.
35 *HBA Auckland Newsletter*, 1, July 1980, p. 6.
36 Midwives' and Obstetric Nurses' Special Interest Section NZNA (Inc.), 'Policy Statement on Home Confinement, 1980', R20459385, ANZW; Joan Donley to Maggie Lecky-Thompson, 16 January 1996 (capitals in the original). MSS & Archives, 2007/15 7/2/C/1, JDP.
37 Midwives' and Obstetric Nurses' Special Interest Section NZNA (Inc.), 'Policy Statement on Home Confinement, 1980', R20459385, ANZW.
38 Bryder, *The Rise and Fall*, p. 76.
39 House of Commons (UK), *Second Report from the Social Services Committee, Session 1979–80: Perinatal and Neonatal Mortality, Together with the Proceedings of the Committee and the Minutes of Evidence (including evidence taken by the Social Services and Employment Sub-Committee of the Expenditure Committee in Session 1978–79) and Appendices*, Vol. 1, HMSO, London, 1980, pp. 23, 27–28.
40 Mary-Ellen Barker, 'Midweek for women: Giving birth – home or hospital', *Auckland Star*, 28 May 1980.
41 *Mother and Baby at Home*, p. 9.
42 Ibid., pp. 10, 20.
43 Ibid., p. 34.
44 *HBA National Newsletter*, 4, August 1981, p. 6.
45 *Mother and Baby at Home*, p. 9.
46 Ibid., pp. 11–12 (italics in the original).
47 Ibid., p. 6.
48 Ibid., p. 23; on the New Zealand Diploma in Obstetrics, see Bryder, *The Rise and Fall*, p. 50.
49 *Mother and Baby at Home*, p. 25.

50  Ibid., p. 30.
51  'Policy Statement on Maternal and Infant Nursing', *New Zealand Nursing Journal: Kai Tiaki*, vol. 74, 9, September 1981; Banks, 'Out on a Limb', p. 167.
52  Nurses Amendment Act 1983, 147, Clause 54 (1), p. 1477; Clause 54 (3), (4) and (5), p. 1478, Clause 58 (2), p. 1479.
53  NZ Parliamentary Debates (NZPD), 455, Nurses Amendment Bill, 13 December 1983, p. 4828.
54  Pauline Ray, 'Midwives tales', *New Zealand Listener*, 5 November 1983, pp. 16–17.
55  *HBA National Newsletter*, 2, 3, September 1984, p. 15.
56  NZPD, 13 December 1983, p. 4828.
57  Ibid., p. 4826.
58  Ibid., p. 4827.
59  National Council of Women Inc., submission to Department of Health on the Review of the Nurses Act 1977, Jocelyn Fish, Janet Hesketh, 29 August 1989, R4501215, 24, 3, ANZW.
60  Joan Donley, '"What does the New Zealand College of Midwives do for me?" A Response to the New Zealand Nurses Association', *New Zealand College of Midwives Journal*, vol. 19, November 1998, p. 18; Joan Donley, 'Independent Midwifery in New Zealand', in Tricia Murphy-Black (ed.), *Issues in Midwifery*, Churchill Livingstone, Edinburgh, 1995, p. 65.
61  Sally Blundell, 'NZ – the best place to give birth?', *Newsroom*, 3 June 2021, https://www.newsroom.co.nz/page/nz-the-best-place-to-give-birth
62  Samantha Skiff, 'Machine-minders and Handmaidens? Hospital Midwives and Childbirth in New Zealand, 1950–1990', MA thesis, University of Auckland, 2014, p. 60.
63  Ibid., pp. 60–61.
64  Gabrielle Bourke, 'Illuminating the Dark Hour: Auckland's St Helens Hospital, 1906–1990', MA thesis, University of Auckland, 2006, p. 167.
65  NZPD, 377, Nurses Bill, 26 November 1971, p. 4955.
66  Information paper for MSC meeting, 1979, R20459385, ANZW.
67  Legal Section to Gayle O'Brien, Request for Legal Opinion, Presence of Doctors at Childbirth, 5 June 1989, R16664911, 1935, 366-6-10, 69656, ANZW.
68  Information paper for MSC meeting, 1979, R20459385, ANZW.
69  'No smoking – and watch your diet!', *New Zealand Woman's Weekly*, 30 October 1978, p. 30.
70  Bourke, 'Illuminating the Dark Hour', pp. 116, 167 fn 5.
71  Carolyn Young, in Halina Ogonowska-Coates, *Born: Midwives and Women Celebrate 100 Years*, New Zealand College of Midwives, Christchurch, 2004, pp. 12–13.
72  Helen Rodenburg, 'Right Place, Right Time', in Rosy Fenwicke (ed.), *In Practice: The Lives of New Zealand Women Doctors in the 21st Century*, Penguin Random House, Auckland, 2004, p. 117.
73  Barbara Macfarlane, Secretary HBA Auckland, submission to MSC, 23 September 1979, p. 2, R20459385, ANZW; Ray, 'Whose body is it? Whose baby is it?'.

74   *HBA National Newsletter*, 6, July 1982, p. 14; ibid., March 1984, p. 31.
75   Donley, in Murphy-Black (ed.), *Issues in Midwifery*, p. 66.
76   'Writers defend home births', *Auckland Star*, 19 September 1979.
77   Ina May Gaskin, *Spiritual Midwifery*, The Book Publishing Co., The Farm, Summertown, Tennessee, rev. edn, 1978, pp. 23, 25, 36, 235, 395.
78   *HBA National Newsletter*, 2, October 1980, p. 7.
79   Ibid., 4, August 1981, p. 6.
80   Tina Gilbertson, in Ogonowska-Coates, *Born*, p. 23.
81   Bryan Hardie Boys to Helen Clark, 18 July 1990, Hardie Boys to Simon Upton, Minister of Health, re. Nurses Amendment Act, 1 March 1991, R21935510, 1990-1991, 80, W67/NUR/2, 68956, ANZW.
82   Lynley McFarland, in Ogonowska-Coates, *Born*, p. 18.
83   Joan Donley, *Herstory of N.Z. Home Birth Association*, New Zealand Home Birth Association, Auckland, 1992, p. 35; Helen Brown, 'When birth becomes an "occasion" at home', *New Zealand Woman's Weekly*, 7 August 1978, p. 5; Lyn McLean, 'Home Birth in New Zealand', *New Zealand Nursing Journal: Kai Tiaki*, vol. 73, 7, July 1980, p. 7.
84   'Publicity', *HBA National Newsletter*, special national conference edition, May 1983, p. 6.
85   Pamela Stirling, 'Hard labour', *New Zealand Listener*, 12 March 1990, p. 12.
86   'Dr Wallace Metcalfe Pitcairn mutineer descendant obstetrician pilot collapses, dies, in Melbourne', July 2018, https://www.mscnewswire.co.nz/news-sectors/reporters-desk/item/15453-dr-wallace-metcalfe-pitcairn-mutineer-descendent-obstetrician-pilot-collapses-dies-in-melbourne.html (accessed 11 March 2023).
87   Barbara Hasslacher, 'Birth at Home', *New Zealand Nursing Journal: Kai Tiaki*, vol. 81, 4, April 1988, p. 25.
88   Jennie Nicol, *A Choice of Birthing: Part 1: Homebirth and Domiciliary Midwifery*, Department of Health, Wellington, November 1987, pp. 1, 14, 15, 17, 18, https://www.moh.govt.nz/notebook/nbbooks.nsf/0/6D092B4E4F967CBC4C2565D7000DD6A4/$file/Choice-of-birthing.pdf (accessed 11 March 2023).
89   *HBA National Newsletter*, 4, August 1981, p. 3.
90   Ibid., December 1987, p. I, included in *HBA Auckland Newsletter*, 37, November 1987.
91   *Domiciliary Midwives Society (DMS) Newsletter*, 3, July 1986, pp. 8, 9, 11; Donley, Auckland Domiciliary Midwifery Report, May 1988, in Wise Woman Archives Trust Inc. (WWAT), http://wwat.nz/wp-content/uploads/20001-9-015.pdf (accessed 11 March 2023); Minutes of meeting, DMS, 12 May 1989, p. 2, *DMS Newsletter*, October 1989.
92   Carolyn Young, in Ogonowska-Coates, *Born*, pp. 5, 12.
93   *HBA National Newsletter*, 1, July 1980, p. 7.
94   Baird, submission to MSC, 21 May 1980, R20459385, ANZW.
95   Ray, 'Whose body is it? Whose baby is it?', p. 21.

96 T. E. Kjellstrom, 'Home Birth – A Viable Alternative?' A fifth year Community Health project carried out by 10 students under supervision of Dr T. E. Kjellstrom, Department of Community Health, School of Medicine, University of Auckland, 1982, p. 3, MSS & Archives 2007/15, 1638, JDP.
97 Information paper for MSC meeting, 1979, R20459385, ANZW.
98 Banks, 'Out on a Limb', p. 130.
99 *Mother and Baby at Home*, pp. 24–25.
100 Christchurch Medical Officer of Health (W.A. Malpress) and Principal Public Health Nurse (Mrs R. Selby) to Clinical Services Division, Nursing (Community Health) Division, 16 June 1981, R20459385, ANZW.
101 Nursing Division and Clinical Services Division, Reply to Malpress and Selby, 3 July 1981, R20459385, ANZW.
102 *DMS Newsletter*, 2, March 1985, p. 3.
103 Ibid., 3, July 1986, p. 13.
104 Julie Smith, 'Homebirth midwife breaks the law', *Nelson Evening Mail*, 5 November 1988, cited in *HBA Auckland Newsletter*, 41, October 1988–January 1989, pp. 10–11.
105 *DMS Newsletter*, 6, September 1988, pp. 9–10.
106 Ibid., pp. 10–11.
107 Julie Smith, 'Homebirth midwife breaks the law', *Nelson Evening Mail*, 5 November 1988, cited in *HBA Auckland Newsletter*, 41, October 1988–January 1989, pp. 10–11.
108 *HBA Auckland Newsletter*, 45, December 1989, p. 9; see also Stirling, 'Hard labour', p. 11.
109 Legal Section to Gayle O'Brien, Request for Legal Opinion, Presence of Doctors at Childbirth, 5 June 1989, R16664911, 1935, 366-6-10, 69656, ANZW.
110 Minutes of meeting 12 May 1989, p. 3, *DMS Newsletter*, October 1989.
111 Stirling, 'Hard labour', p. 11.
112 Ibid., p. 12.
113 Secretary's letter, *DMS Newsletter*, October 1989, p. 1.

## CHAPTER 4: *The meaning of autonomy for homebirth midwives in the 1980s*

1 Helen Clark, handwritten note, 30 April 1989, on memorandum from Sheryl Smail, Proposed Review of the Nurses Act 1977, 18 April 1989, R21935507, 80, W67/NUR/2, 68677, Archives New Zealand Wellington (ANZW).
2 Joan Donley, *Herstory of N.Z. Home Birth Association*, New Zealand Home Birth Association (HBA), Auckland, 1992, p. 9.
3 *Home Birth Association (HBA) National Newsletter*, 28, July 1985, p. 1.
4 *Domiciliary Midwives Society (DMS) Newsletter*, 3, July 1986, p. 2.
5 Joan Donley, Author's Preface, *Save the Midwife*, New Women's Press, Auckland, 1986, p. 11.

*Notes*

6   Maggie Banks, 'Out on a Limb: The Personal Mandate to Practise Midwifery by Midwives of the Domiciliary Midwives Society of New Zealand (Incorporated), 1974–1986', PhD thesis, Victoria University of Wellington, 2007, pp. i, 3.
7   HBA Auckland, Submission to Maternity Services Committee, July 1982, Joan Donley Papers, 1933-2003, MSS & Archives 2007/15, 10/6/b/2, Manuscripts and Archives, University of Auckland Library (JDP).
8   Lyn McLean, 'Home Birth in New Zealand', *New Zealand Nursing Journal: Kai Tiaki*, vol. 73, 7, July 1980, p. 7.
9   Pamela Stirling, 'Hard labour', *New Zealand Listener*, 12 March 1990, p. 14.
10  Samantha Skiff, 'Machine-minders and Handmaidens? Hospital Midwives and Childbirth in New Zealand, 1950–1990', MA thesis, University of Auckland, 2014, p. 72.
11  Ibid., p. 46.
12  Gabrielle Bourke, 'Illuminating the Dark Hour: Auckland's St Helen's Hospital, 1906–1990', MA thesis, University of Auckland, 2006, pp. 123, 126, 127, 128, 163, 167, 228.
13  Ibid., p. 128.
14  Ibid., p. 127.
15  *New Zealand Herald*, 13 October 1971.
16  Lynley McFarland, in Halina Ogonowska-Coates, *Born: Midwives and Women Celebrate 100 Years*, New Zealand College of Midwives, Christchurch, 2004, p. 17.
17  Margaret F. Myles, *Textbook for Midwives*, New York, Churchill Livingstone, 9th edn, 1981, pp. xx, 2; 10th edn, 1985, pp. v, vi; on Myles, see E. J. C. Scott, 'Myles, Margaret Fraser (1892–1988)', *Oxford Dictionary of National Biography*, http://www.oxforddnb.com/view/article/74549 (accessed 11 March 2023); 'Obituary: Mrs Margaret Fraser Myles 1892–1988', *Midwifery*, vol. 4, 1988, pp. 95–96; on her 1969 visit to New Zealand, see Donley, *Save the Midwife*, p. 103.
18  Madonna May Grehan, 'Professional Aspirations and Consumer Expectations: Nurses, Midwives, and Women's health', PhD thesis, University of Melbourne, 2009, pp. 3, 254, 312, 319.
19  Karen Guilliland and Sally Pairman, *Women's Business: The Story of the New Zealand College of Midwives, 1986–2010*, New Zealand College of Midwives, Christchurch, 2010, p. 70; Donley, *Herstory*, p. 16.
20  'Policy Statement on Maternal and Infant Nursing', *New Zealand Nursing Journal: Kai Tiaki*, vol. 74, 9, September 1981, p. 19; Valerie E. M. Fleming, 'Midwifery in New Zealand: Responding to Changing Times', *Health Care for Women International*, vol. 17, 1996, pp. 343–59, 351. The definition of a midwife as a 'person' had been adopted by the WHO in 1966, and in 1972 by the International Council of Midwives, but it was not until the 1980s that it was commonly referred to within the homebirth movement in New Zealand, in response to the Nursing Association description of the midwife as a 'nurse' who practised midwifery. See *Save the Midwives Newsletter*, 2, 1984, p. 25.
21  Banks, 'Out on a Limb', p. 165.
22  Donley, *Herstory*, pp. 16, 20–22.

23  'The Nurses Amendment Bill', *New Zealand Listener*, 5 November 1983.
24  Joan Donley, 'Midwives or Moas?', p. 3, presented to the National Midwives Conference, Auckland, August 1988, 6 pages, reproduced in *DMS Newsletter*, 6, September 1988, between pages 6 and 8.
25  *HBA National Newsletter*, March 1984, p. 10; Donley, *Herstory*, p. 26.
26  'Nursing Education in New Zealand', Department of Education, Wellington, 1982, pp. 15, 16.
27  Autonomy of Midwives – Notes for Minister's report, 22 June 1989, R16664911, 1935, 366-6-10, 69656, ANZW; on Plunket nurses, see Linda Bryder, *A Voice for Mothers: The Plunket Society and Infant Welfare 1907–2000*, Auckland University Press, Auckland, 2003; Lynda Exton, *The Baby Business: What's Happened to Maternity Care in New Zealand?*, Craig Potton Publishing, Nelson, 2008, p. 130.
28  Michael Bassett, New Zealand Parliamentary Debates (NZPD), 455, Nurses Amendment Bill, 13 December 1983, p. 4825; one out of the 12 domiciliary midwives in Auckland would be affected according to *HBA National Newsletter*, March 1984, p. 8.
29  *HBA Auckland Newsletter*, 37, September 1987, p. 20.
30  Ibid., 29, September 1985, pp. 3, 4; Auckland HBA, submission to Board of Health Committee on Women's Health, 1985, p. 6, in Wise Woman Archives Trust Inc. (WWAT), http://wwat.nz/wp-content/uploads/20073-91-0401.pdf (accessed 11 March 2023); *HBA Auckland Newsletter*, 29, September 1985, p. 4.
31  Fleming, 'Midwifery in New Zealand', pp. 349–50.
32  Joy Bickley, 'Attempting to Involve Consumers in Midwifery Policy Development: A paper presented at the National Midwifery Conference, Auckland, August 1988', *New Zealand College of Midwives Journal (NZCOMJ)*, vol. 1, September 1989, p. 11.
33  Report on Direct Entry Task Force Collective Round Table Discussion & Planning Meeting, 29 November 1987, with Marilyn Waring, in WWAT, http://wwat.nz/wp-content/uploads/20001-113-009.pdf (accessed 11 March 2023).
34  Helen Carpenter, 'An Improved System of Nursing Education in New Zealand', Department of Health, Wellington, 1971.
35  Margaret Gibson Smith and Yvonne T. Shadbolt (eds), *Objects and Outcomes: New Zealand Nurses' Association 1909–1983*, New Zealand Nurses' Association, Wellington, 1984, p. 92.
36  Ibid.
37  Judy Hedwig and Valerie Fleming, 'Midwifery Practice in New Zealand: A Dynamic Discipline', in Tricia Murphy-Black (ed.), *Issues in Midwifery*, Churchill Livingstone, Edinburgh, 1995, p. 215.
38  Exton, *Baby Business*, p. 43; Donley *Save the Midwife*, p. 102.
39  Skiff, 'Machine-minders and Handmaidens', p. 62.
40  Ibid.
41  Bourke, 'Illuminating the Dark Hour', p. 116.

42  Sheryl Smail, Chief Nursing Officer, Workforce Development, to Eugenie Sage, 22 May 1989; Save the Midwives Direct Entry Midwifery Task Force (Judi Strid) to Helen Clark, 27 August 1989, R4501215, 24, 3, ANZW.
43  Donley, *Save the Midwife*, p. 91.
44  *Otago Daily Times*, 23 May 1989, in R16664911, ANZW.
45  DMS, Minutes of meeting 12 May 1989, p. 2, *DMS Newsletter*, October 1989.
46  Save the Midwives Submission on Nurses Act, Judi Strid, 14 August 1989, R16664911, ANZW.
47  Caroline Flint, 'Should Midwives Train as Florists?', *Nursing Times*, 1986, cited in Strid, Submission, 14 August 1989, p. 3, R16664911, ANZW.
48  *HBA Auckland Newsletter*, 36, June 1987, p. 4; ibid., 37, September 1987, p. 21.
49  NZNA Midwifery Policy Statement May 1988, R16664911, ANZW; on the title of the section, see *DMS Newsletter*, 6, September 1988, p. 1.
50  Guilliland, in Ogonowska-Coates, *Born*, p. 60.
51  Sally Pairman, 'Workforce to Profession: An Exploration of New Zealand Midwifery's Professionalising Strategies from 1986 to 2005', Doctor of Midwifery thesis, University of Technology Sydney, 2005, pp. 6–8.
52  Sally Pairman, 'Educating Midwives for Autonomous Practice', in Guilliland and Pairman, *Women's Business*, p. 499.
53  Guilliland and Pairman, *Women's Business*, p. 68.
54  Wendy Kline, 'Communicating a New Consciousness: Countercultural Print and the Home Birth Movement in the 1970s', *Bulletin of the History of Medicine*, vol. 89, 3, 2015, p. 554.
55  Maggie Lecky-Thompson, 'Independent Midwifery in Australia', in Murphy-Black (ed.), *Issues in Midwifery*, p. 46. Lecky-Thompson was later charged and found guilty of professional misconduct in a disciplinary hearing in 1997–98 which became a cause célèbre within the homebirth movement. See MSS & Archives 2007/15, 1, 1 /2, 7/2/C/1, JDP; Karen Stott, 'Standards of practice regarding home births in Australia', *Plaintiff*, December 1998, pp. 27–30, http://classic.austlii.edu.au/au/journals/PlaintiffJlAUPLA/1998/152.pdf (accessed 21 November 2022); Alan Hewson, 'The History of Obstetrics and Gynaecology in Australia from 1950 to 2010', PhD thesis, University of Newcastle, Australia, 2016, p. 131.
56  'Branch round-up', *HBA Auckland Newsletter*, 44, September 1989, p. 3.
57  Ibid., 37, September 1987, p. 23.
58  'Home birth helpers may be prosecuted', *Northern News*, 20 April 1989, in WWAT, http://wwat.nz/wp-content/uploads/1989-4.pdf (accessed 11 March 2023).
59  DMS, Minutes of meeting 12 May 1989, p. 1, in *DMS Newsletter*, October 1989.
60  Stirling, 'Hard labour', p. 11.
61  'Getting by: Marilyn Garson Looks at Life for Women in the Hokianga', *Broadsheet*, 182, October 1990, pp. 18–19.
62  *Northern News*, 20 April 1989, WWAT.
63  Kali [sic] Judd, Annie Gordan, Mandy Waata, Letter to the editor, *NZCOMJ*, vol. 2, March 1990, p. 4.
64  *Northern News*, 20 April 1989, WWAT.

65  HBA National Newsletter, 33, September 1986, Branch reports: Hokianga, p. 6N.
66  DMS Newsletter, 6, September 1988, p. 3.
67  DMS, Minutes of meeting 12 May 1989, p. 3, DMS Newsletter, October 1989.
68  Joan Donley, Report on College Working Party held 9 October 1988, 20 October 1988, p. 4, MSS & A 2007/2 NZCOM Auckland Region 1985-2002, R300388602, Item 6, Special Collections, University of Auckland Library (NZCOM ARP).
69  Cheryl Smail, Memo for Minister of Health, 23 May 1989, 'Autonomy of Midwives – Notes for Minister's Report', 23 May 1989, p. 5, R21935507, ANZW.
70  Working Group on Safe Options for Low Risk Pregnancy, Policy recommendations for care for pregnancy and childbirth, Sixth Draft, October 1989, in WWAT, http://wwat.nz/wp-content/uploads/20073-91-005.pdf (accessed 11 March 2023); Save the Midwives Newsletter, 4, Spring 1984, p. 8.
71  DMS, Minutes of meeting 12 May 1989, p. 1, DMS Newsletter, October 1989.
72  Stirling, 'Hard labour', p. 11.
73  Minutes of meeting of the national committee of the College of Midwives, 5 May 1990, p. 13, R300388602, Item 5, NZCOM ARP.
74  HBA Auckland Newsletter, 39, March 1988, pp. 5–6.
75  Save the Midwives (Strid) to Helen Clark, 27 August 1989, R4501215, ANZW.
76  Joan Donley, 'Opposition to Home Birth – Fact or Fiction? Conference Address', HBA National Newsletter, 6, July 1982, p. 5.
77  Joan Donley, 'Women in Partnership', Broadsheet, 182, October 1990, p. 8.
78  'Direct Entry Midwives provide positive benefit for patients', NHS Management Bulletin, July 1987, pp. 4–5, in WWAT, http://wwat.nz/wp-content/uploads/20001-113-033b.pdf (accessed 11 March 2023); Kate Isherwood, 'Independent Midwifery in the United Kingdom', in Murphy-Black (ed.), Issues in Midwifery, p. 24.
79  Rea Daellenbach, 'The Paradox of Success and the Challenge of Change: Home Birth Associations of Aotearoa/New Zealand', PhD thesis, University of Canterbury, 1999, p. 99; Donley, Save the Midwife, pp. 50–51, 115.
80  Maternity Services Committee, Mother and Baby at Home: The Early Days: A Report of the Board of Health Maternity Services Committee, Board of Health Report Series 30, Government Printer, Wellington, 1982, p. 22.
81  Norma Campbell and Karen Guilliland, 'Accountability: Midwifery Standards Review and Resolution Committees', in Guilliland and Pairman, Women's Business, p. 377.
82  Report, Domiciliary Midwives' Standards Review Committee Pilot Committee, April 1989, R300388602, Item 6, NZCOM ARP; HBA Auckland Newsletter, 43, June 1989, p. N11.
83  Domiciliary Midwives Standards, Submission to the 1990 Nurses Amendment Bill, 76A, R21935512, 1989-1990, 81, W67/NUR/2, 68681, ANZW.
84  Nurses Review, Yvonne Dorbecker, Minutes of Meeting of Health Department with the NZCOM, 18 October 1989, p. 13, R21935509, 1989, 80,

W67/NUR/2, 68349, ANZW; Joan Donley, meeting of the Auckland Region of the New Zealand College of Midwives, 11 December 1989, p. 3, R300388602, Item 4, NZCOM ARP.

85  G. D. D. Cable to Domiciliary Midwives Standards Review Committee, 23 February 1989, Item 6, NZCOM ARP; *HBA Auckland Newsletter*, 43, June 1989, pp. N11–12.

86  Tony Baird to Joan Donley and Carol Peterson, 8 May 1989, *HBA Auckland Newsletter*, 44, September 1989, p. N14.

87  Donley to Baird, 30 June 1989, ibid., p. N15.

88  Ibid., 35, March 1987, p. 8.

89  Ibid., 45, December 1989, p. 5.

90  NZCOM AGM, 14 July 1990, p. 6; NZCOM Annual Report 1989–90 appendix 1, p. 11, Item 5, NZCOM ARP.

91  *Mother and Baby at Home*, p. 22.

92  Bronwen Pelvin to David Caygill, 5 October 1988, *DMS Newsletter*, October 1988, np.

93  *HBA Auckland Newsletter*, 35, March 1987, p. 10N.

94  Ibid., 36, June 1987, pp. 12, 13 (capitals in the original).

95  On 'Birthcare', see Kim Paterson, 'Birth . . . the way you want it', *New Zealand Woman's Weekly*, 13 July 1987, pp. 56–57.

96  Roger A. Rosenblatt, Judith Reinken and Phil Shoemack, 'Is Obstetrics Safe in Small Hospitals? Evidence from New Zealand's Regionalised Perinatal System', *The Lancet*, vol. 326, 8452, 1985, pp. 429–32.

97  *Northern Advocate*, 22 September 1989, p. 5, in WWAT, http://wwat.nz/wp-content/uploads/20072-3-027.pdf (accessed 13 February 2023).

98  *HBA Auckland Newsletter*, 45, December 1989, p. 3; Marion McLauchlan and Carey Virtue, 'Domino Midwives Wellington', in Guilliland and Pairman, *Women's Business*, p. 353.

99  Donley, *Herstory*, pp. 5, 57, 65; Joan Donley, 'Independent Midwifery in New Zealand', in Murphy-Black (ed.), *Issues in Midwifery*, p. 75; Joan Donley, 'Midwifery Independence?', *NZCOMJ*, vol. 5, October 1991, p. 10.

100  Robert Mannion, 'Focus: The great home birth debate hots up again', *Dominion Sunday Times*, 23 December 1990, p. 9. The article was sparked by: Maria Crotty, Andrew T. Ramsay, Rosemary Smart and Annabelle Chan, 'Planned Homebirths in South Australia 1976–1987', *Medical Journal of Australia*, vol. 153, 1990, pp. 664–71, which found the perinatal death rate five times higher among homebirths than hospital births, even though women choosing homebirth generally came from a higher socio-economic bracket.

101  H. Bastian and P. A. L. Lancaster, *Home Births in Australia 1985–1987*, National Perinatal Statistics Unit and Homebirth Australia, Sydney, 1990, ISSN 1034-7178 (covering 3,400 planned homebirths between 1985–87); see also H. Bastian and P. A. L. Lancaster, *Home Births in Australia, 1988–1990*, AIHW National Perinatal Statistics Unit, Sydney, 1992; Hilda Bastian, Marc J. N. C. Keirse and Paul A. L. Lancaster, 'Perinatal Death Associated with Planned Home Birth in

Australia: Population Based Study', *British Medical Journal*, vol. 317, 8 August 1998, pp. 384–88.
102  Mannion, 'Focus: The great home birth debate hots up again'.
103  Stirling, 'Hard labour', p. 11.
104  *DMS Newsletter*, 6, September 1988, p. 3.
105  Joy Bickley, 'Watchdogs or Wimps? Nurses' Response to the Cartwright Report', in Sandra Coney (ed.), *Unfinished Business: What Happened to the Cartwright Report*, Women's Health Action, Auckland, 1993, pp. 132–33; Joy Bickley, Professional Officer, New Zealand Nurses' Association, Submission to Social Services Select Committee on Nurses Amendment Act, 1 December 1989, R21935507, 1989, 80, W67/NUR/2, 68677, ANZW.
106  *DMS Newsletter*, October 1989, p. 3.
107  Joan Donley to Maggie Lecky-Thompson, 14 December 1986, 1, 1/2, 7/2/C/1, JDP.
108  Donley, 'Midwives or Moas?', p. 1.
109  Tina Gilbertson, in Ogonowska-Coates, *Born*, p. 23.
110  Donley, *Herstory*, p. 30.
111  Joan Donley to Maggie Lecky-Thompson, 16 January 1996, 1, 1/2, 7/2/C/1, JDP.
112  Caroline Flint, 'To My Dear Sisters in New Zealand', *NZCOMJ*, vol. 1, September 1989, p. 9.
113  *DMS Newsletter*, 6, September 1988, p. 1 (underlining in the original).
114  *New Zealand Herald*, 18 August 1988, reproduced in *DMS Newsletter*, 6, 1988, p. 5.
115  *New Zealand Nurses' Association Midwives Section Auckland Region Newsletter*, January 1989, p. 1, R300388602, Item 4, NZCOM ARP.
116  Karen Guilliland, 'Guest Editorial', *NZCOMJ*, vol. 1, September 1989, p. 4.
117  Maggie Lecky-Thompson, 'Independent Midwifery in Australia', in Murphy-Black (ed.), *Issues in Midwifery*, pp. 48–49.
118  Kereen Reiger, 'The Politics of Midwifery in Australia: Tensions, Debates and Opportunities', *Annual Review of Health Social Sciences*, vol. 10, 1, 2000, p. 58.
119  Donley, 'Midwives or Moas?', p. 4.


## CHAPTER 5: 'A highly focused and effective campaign': Homebirth as a political movement in the 1980s

1  Transcript of interview of Joan Donley by Sally Abel, 6 July 1994, p. 1, Joan Donley Papers, MSS & Archives 2007/15, 1638, Manuscripts and Archives, University of Auckland Library (JDP).
2  Joan Donley, *Save the Midwife*, New Women's Press, Auckland, 1986, preface, p. 12; Joan Donley, *Herstory of N.Z. Home Birth Association*, Auckland, New Zealand Home Birth Association (HBA), 1992, p. 20.
3  Joan Donley, *Birthrites: Natural vs Unnatural Childbirth in New Zealand*, Full Court

Press in association with the New Zealand College of Midwives, Auckland, 1998 (reprint of *Save the Midwife* with a new introduction), p. 10.
4   *HBA National Newsletter*, March 1984, p. 8.
5   Ibid., July 1980, p. 1.
6   Ibid., March 1984, p. 31.
7   Listed on back cover, *HBA Auckland Newsletter*, 37, September 1987.
8   Branch contacts, ibid., 43, June 1989, p. 10.
9   Lynda's story, in Karen Guilliland and Sally Pairman, *Women's Business: The Story of the New Zealand College of Midwives, 1986–2010*, New Zealand College of Midwives, Christchurch, 2010, p. 179. On the value attached to the newsletters, see also Donley, *Herstory*, p. 20; Rea Daellenbach, 'The Paradox of Success and the Challenge of Change: Home Birth Associations of Aotearoa/New Zealand', PhD thesis, University of Canterbury, 1999, pp. 110, 126; *HBA National Newsletter*, 2, October 1980, p. 15; ibid., 2, 2, June 1984, p. 1; ibid., 32, June 1986, p. 2.
10  Carolyn Young, 'The Honouring of Joan Donley, O.B.E', *New Zealand College of Midwives Journal (NZCOMJ)*, vol. 2, March 1990, p. 11; Daellenbach, 'The Paradox of Success', pp. 111, 138.
11  Young, 'The Honouring of Joan Donley', pp. 10–11.
12  Carolyn Young, 'Joan – the Midwife Friend', in Halina Ogonowska-Coates, *Born: Midwives and Women Celebrate 100 Years*, New Zealand College of Midwives, Christchurch, 2004, p. 6.
13  *HBA National Newsletter*, 32, June 1986, p. 4.
14  *HBA Auckland Newsletter*, 37, September 1987, pp. 21–22; ibid., 36, June 1987, p. 6.
15  Donley to Maggie Lecky-Thompson, 14 December 1986, MSS & Archives 2007/15, 1, 1/2, 7/2/C/1, JDP.
16  See, for instance, Mary-Ellen Barker, 'Midweek for women: Giving birth – home or hospital', *Auckland Star*, 28 May 1980.
17  Pauline Ray, 'Whose body is it? Whose baby is it?', *New Zealand Listener*, 15 March 1980, pp. 20–24.
18  Joan Donley, 'Healthy Women', *Broadsheet*, 93, October 1981, p. 40.
19  'Home Birth Week, 1982', MSS & Archives 2007/15, 1, 1/3, 17/12/2007, JDP.
20  *HBA National Newsletter*, May 1983, p. 9.
21  'Bert's Talk 30/10/82', *Centrepoint Magazine*, 12, March/April 1983, p. 2.
22  *HBA Auckland Newsletter*, December 1987, p. III, included in ibid., 37, November 1987.
23  *HBA National Newsletter*, May 1983, p. 10.
24  Joan Donley, 'Having the baby at home', *Broadsheet*, 132, September 1985, p. 17.
25  Report on Direct Entry Task Force Collective Round Table Discussion & Planning Meeting, 29 November 1987, with Marilyn Waring, in Wise Woman Archives Trust Inc. (WWAT), http://wwat.nz/wp-content/uploads/20001-113-009.pdf (accessed 11 March 2023).
26  *HBA Auckland Newsletter*, 32, June 1986, p. 2; Mary Dobbie, *The Trouble with*

*Women: The Story of Parents Centre New Zealand*, Cape Catley, Whatamongo Bay, 1990, p. 127; Ray, 'Whose body is it?', p. 24; 'Lynda's Story', in Guilliland and Pairman, *Women's Business*, p. 182.
27  *HBA National Newsletter*, 6, July 1982, p. 1.
28  Ibid., p. 3.
29  Ibid., 1, July 1980, p. 2.
30  Ibid., 4, August 1981, p. 4.
31  Ibid., 6, July 1982, p. 15.
32  Ibid., May 1983, pp. 6, 9.
33  Mary Nacey, address to 1983 conference, *HBA National Newsletter*, in ibid., p. 2.
34  'Home birth devotees fight to keep option open', *Dominion*, 18 November 1982, in WWAT, http://wwat.nz/wp-content/uploads/1982-5.pdf (accessed 20 March 2023).
35  *HBA National Newsletter*, May 1983, p. 6.
36  Ibid., p. 5.
37  Donley's speech at 1983 national conference, in ibid., pp. 12–13.
38  Ibid., March 1984, pp. 1–2.
39  Joan Donley, 'The New Women's Board of Health', *New Zealand Women's Health Network Newsletter*, April 1985 and August 1985; *HBA Auckland Newsletter*, 29, September 1985, p. 17; Women's Health Committee, Report to the Board of Health 1985–1988, Wellington, March 1988, p. 31, https://www.moh.govt.nz/notebook/nbbooks.nsf/0/BB312B216ECC779A4C2565D7000DD7D9/$file/women's-health-nz-85-88.pdf (accessed 20 February 2023).
40  *HBA Auckland Newsletter*, 35, March 1987, p. 1.
41  Ibid., 37, September 1987, p. 23.
42  Donley, Report on Direct Entry Task Force Collective Round Table Discussion & Planning Meeting, WWAT.
43  Doris Gordon, *Back-Blocks Baby-Doctor: An Autobiography*, Faber & Faber, London, 1955, p. 170.
44  Donley, Report on Direct Entry Task Force Collective Round Table Discussion & Planning Meeting, WWAT.
45  Sally Pairman, 'Developing & Crafting a Vision: A Strategic Plan for Midwifery', *NZCOMJ*, vol. 18, April 1998, p. 5. Waring's lobbying advice was also acknowledged in Guilliland and Pairman, *Women's Business*, p. 30.
46  Jacqui Anderson, in Ogonowska-Coates, *Born*, p. 50.
47  College of Midwives National Committee, Minutes, 1 April 1989, MSS & Archives 2007/2 NZCOM Auckland Region 1985-2002, R300388602, Item 4, Special Collections, University of Auckland Library (NZCOM ARP).
48  Guilliland and Pairman, *Women's Business*, pp. 28–29.
49  Save the Midwives, Submission on Nurses Act, Judi Strid, 14 August 1989, R4501215, 24, 3 (Associate Health Katherine O'Regan files, Series 7838), Archives New Zealand Wellington (ANZW).
50  Rob Munro to Katherine O'Regan, 13 September 1989, R4501215, ANZW.
51  Maurice McTigue to O'Regan, 29 August 1989, R4501215, ANZW.

52 Report on Direct Entry Task Force Collective Round Table Discussion and Planning Meeting, WWAT.
53 Daellenbach, 'The Paradox of Success', p. 108.
54 Maggie Banks, 'Out on a Limb: The Personal Mandate to Practise Midwifery by Midwives of the Domiciliary Midwives Society of New Zealand (Incorporated), 1974–1986', PhD thesis, Victoria University of Wellington, 2007, p. 250.
55 *HBA Auckland Newsletter*, 43, June 1989, p. 2.
56 Donley, *Herstory*, pp. 48–51.
57 *HBA Auckland Newsletter*, 47, Winter 1990, p. 3.
58 Ibid., pp. 1–2.
59 Ibid., p. 7.
60 Rachel Schmidt, 'A Voyage to Motherhood: Pacific Mothers' Lived Experiences of Pregnancy, Childbirth, Postnatal Care and Early Motherhood, 1950–1995', MA thesis, University of Auckland, 2020.
61 National Health Committee, *Review of Maternity Services in New Zealand*, National Health Committee, Wellington, September 1999, pp. 45, 55, 59, 99, https://www.moh.govt.nz/notebook/nbbooks.nsf/0/9B3D7BB224CAEC6C4C25681B006EE921/$file/mands2.pdf (accessed 20 February 2023).
62 *HBA National Newsletter*, 7, November 1982, p. 2.
63 *Parents Centre Bulletin*, 9, February 1984, p. 9, cited in Daellenbach, 'The Paradox of Success', p. 141.
64 *HBA National Newsletter*, 6, July 1982, p. 10.
65 Ibid., 7, November 1982, p. 12.
66 Ibid., May 1983, pp. 3, 5.
67 Ibid., 32, June 1986, p. 2; Donley, *Herstory*, p. 29.
68 Donley, Report of conference, in *HBA National Newsletter*, 6, July 1982, pp. 2–3; ibid, May 1983, pp. 8, 10; Donley, *Herstory*, p. 15.
69 'Lynda's Story', in Guilliland and Pairman, *Women's Business*, p. 179.
70 *HBA National Newsletter*, March 1984, p. 8.
71 Ibid., 2, 2, June 1984, p. 13.
72 Ibid., March 1984, p. 7.
73 New Zealand Parliamentary Debates (NZPD), 455, 1983 Nurses Amendment Act, 13 December 1983, p. 4838.
74 *HBA National Newsletter*, May 1983, p. 5.
75 Health Benefits Review, *Choices for Health Care: Report of the Health Benefits Review*, Health Benefits Review, Wellington, 1986, p. 118.
76 Ibid., pp. 55–56.
77 *HBA Auckland Newsletter*, 35, March 1987, p. 12; Health Benefits Review, *Choices for Health Care*, pp. 153–57.
78 Health Benefits Review, pp. 120–21.
79 Jennie Nicol, *A Choice of Birthing: Part 1: Homebirth and Domiciliary Midwifery*, Department of Health, Wellington, November 1987, p. 4, https://www.moh.govt.nz/notebook/nbbooks.nsf/0/6D092B4E4F967CBC4C2565D7000DD6A4/$file/

Choice-of-birthing.pdf (accessed 20 February 2023); see also Daellenbach, 'The Paradox of Success', p. 160.
80 Sally Pairman and Karen Guilliland, 'The Resurgence of Midwifery', in Guilliland and Pairman, *Women's Business*, p. 67.
81 Peggy Anne Field, 'Impressions of Women's Health in New Zealand', *Midwifery*, vol. 6, 4, 1990, pp. 185–92, 185.
82 Field, 'Impressions', p. 192.
83 Ibid., May 1983, p. 5.
84 Wellington HBA report, Letter from Michael Bassett, 31 March 1987, *HBA Auckland Newsletter*, 37, 1987, pp. 10–11.
85 Joan Donley and Brenda Hinton, 'Home Birth Associations, 1978–', first published in 1993, updated in 2019 by Elizabeth Cox, https://nzhistory.govt.nz/women-together/home-birth-associations (accessed 20 February 2023).
86 *HBA Auckland Newsletter*, 36, June 1987, p. 5.
87 Nicol, *A Choice of Birthing*, p. 1.
88 Ibid., p. 6.
89 Donley to Nicol, 4 February 1988, MSS & Archives 2007/15, 1, 1/3, 11/4/A/4, JDP.
90 Guilliland, Meeting with David Caygill, 28 November 1987, 20001-113-031, in WWAT, http://wwat.nz/wp-content/uploads/20001-113-031.pdf (accessed 20 February 2023).
91 Caygill to Guilliland, 15 January 1988, 2001-113-029a, in WWAT, http://wwat.nz/wp-content/uploads/20001-113-029a.pdf (accessed 20 February 2023).
92 David Caygill, Memorandum for the Social Equity Committee: Report on Easing Current Legislative Restrictions on Midwives, 12 April 1988: R21935507, 1989, 80, W67/NUR/2, 68677, ANZW.
93 Caygill to Lynda Williams, 12 August 1988, cited in Joan Donley, 'Professionalism: The Importance of Consumer Control Over Childbirth', *NZCOMJ*, vol. 1, September 1989, p. 6.
94 Reported in *HBA Auckland Newsletter*, 41, October 1988–January 1989, p. 12.
95 Guilliland, meeting with Caygill, 28 November 1987, WWAT.
96 Sally Abel, 'Midwifery and Maternity Services in Transition: An Examination of Change following the Nurses Amendment Act 1990', PhD thesis, University of Auckland, 1997, pp. 97–99. Clark's husband, Dr Peter Davis, was Abel's second supervisor for her PhD thesis.
97 Sally Pairman, 'Educating Midwives for Autonomous Practice', in Guilliland and Pairman, *Women's Business*, p. 500.
98 Claudia Pond Eyley and Dan Salmon, *Helen Clark: Inside Stories*, Auckland University Press, Auckland, 2015, p. 84.
99 Helen Clark, panellist, webinar: 'Emancipating Midwifery – Reflecting on 30 years of midwifery autonomy', 3 September 2020 (time: 18.11.29–18.13.00), hosted by Alison Eddy, Chief Executive, New Zealand College of Midwives, https://www.midwife.org.nz/news/webinar-emancipating-midwifery-reflecting-on-30-years-of-midwifery-autonomy/ (accessed 20 February 2023).

100 Helen Clark to Donley, 26 March 1985, MSS & Archives 2007/15, 5/6/A/1, JDP. See also Linda Bryder, *The Rise and Fall of National Women's Hospital*, Auckland University Press, Auckland, 2014, p. 200.
101 Donley, Editorial, *HBA Auckland Newsletter*, 42, February–April 1989, pp. 1–2.
102 DMS to Minister of Health, letter reproduced in *Domiciliary Midwives Society (DMS) Newsletter*, April 1989, np.
103 Helen Clark, handwritten note, 30 April 1989, on memo from Sheryl Smail, Chief Nursing Officer, Proposed Review of the Nurses Act 1977, 18 April 1989, R21935507, ANZW.
104 Smail, Notes for Minister's report, 22 May 1989, R21935507, ANZW.
105 Smail, 'Autonomy of Midwives – Notes for Minister's Report', 22 May 1989, p. 7, R21935507, ANZW.
106 Bronwen Pelvin, Secretary's letter to members, p. 2, *DMS Newsletter*, April 1989.
107 Maternity Services Committee, *Special Care Services for the Newborn in New Zealand: A Report of the Maternity Services Committee*, Board of Health Report Series 29, Wellington, 1982, pp. 8, 9, 11; see also Bryder, *The Rise and Fall*, pp. 133–41.
108 Helen Clark, Speech notes to open the NZCOM National Conference, 18 August 1990, pp. 1, 6, 8, R21935508, 1990, 80 W67/NUR/2 68680, ANZW; reproduced in full in *NZCOM Newsletter*, 3, 3, February 1991; also in MSS & Archives 2007/15, 5/6/A/1, JDP.
109 Helen Clark, Speech notes to New Zealand Nurses' Union 16th AGM and Conference, 9 June 1989, p. 2, R16664911, 1989, 1935, 366-6-10, 69656, ANZW.
110 Pamela Stirling, 'Hard labour', *New Zealand Listener*, 12 March 1990, p. 13.
111 *HBA National Newsletter*, March 1984, p. 12.
112 Health Benefits Review, *Choices for Health Care*, p. 2.
113 Daellenbach, 'The Paradox of Success', pp. 161–63; see also Christine Cheyne, Michael O'Brien and Michael Belgrave, *Social Policy in Aotearoa New Zealand: A Critical Introduction*, Oxford University Press, Auckland, 1997, pp. 223–26.
114 *HBA Auckland Newsletter*, 29, September 1985, p. 18.
115 Donley, Editorial, ibid., 42, February–April 1989, p. 1.
116 Ibid.
117 'Mother and baby bond best in home birth', *Northern News*, 20 April 1989, in WWAT, http://wwat.nz/wp-content/uploads/1989-4.pdf (accessed 20 February 2023).
118 *HBA Auckland Newsletter*, 30, November 1985, p. 4; Nicol, *A Choice of Birthing*, p. 8.
119 Auckland Women's Health Council, 5 August 1989, R300388602, Item 4, NZCOM ARP.
120 *HBA Auckland Newsletter*, 45, December 1989, p. 20.
121 Working Group to Prepare Policy Recommendations on Choices for Safe Options for Low Risk Pregnancy, Draft terms of reference (20 April 1989), R16664911, ANZW; also Donley, 'Working Party on Low Risk Pregnancies', *HBA Auckland Newsletter*, 42, February–April 1989, p. 10.

122 Sheryl Smail, Chief Nursing Officer, Workforce Development, to Eugenie Sage, 22 May 1989, R16664911, ANZW; Bronwen Pelvin, Secretary's letter to members, p. 2, *DMS Newsletter*, April 1989, np.
123 Media Release, Minister of Health, 8 November 1989, R21935507, ANZW.
124 'Midwives form professional organisation', *New Zealand Doctor*, 17 April 1989.
125 *DMS Newsletter*, 6, September 1988, p. 1.
126 Karen Guilliland, 'Maintaining the Links: A History of the Formation of the NZCOM', *NZCOMJ*, vol. 1, September 1989, p. 14; Maternity Action Alliance was a coalition of Auckland and Wellington Maternity Action.
127 *Education Effects: Magazine of Childbirth Educators NZ*, Summer 2003, p. 5; see also 'Sharron's Story', in Guilliland and Pairman, *Women's Business*, pp. 186–95.
128 Midwifery Council of New Zealand, *Annual Report for year to 31 March*, 2008, p. 6, https://www.midwiferycouncil.health.nz/common/Uploaded%20files/Annual%20reports/Midwifery%20Council%20Annual%20Report%202008.pdf (accessed 20 February 2023).
129 Guilliland, 'Maintaining the Links', p. 14.
130 See Linda Bryder, *A History of the 'Unfortunate Experiment' at National Women's Hospital*, Auckland University Press, Auckland, 2009; Angela E. Raffle, Anne Mackie and J. A. Muir Gray, *Screening: Evidence and Practice*, Oxford, Oxford University Press, 2nd edn, 2019, pp. 190–204; Angela E. Raffle and J. A. Muir Gray, 'Review: The 1960s Cervical Screening Incident at National Women's Hospital, Auckland, New Zealand: Insights for Screening Research, Policy Making and Practice', *Journal of Clinical Epidemiology*, vol. 122, June 2020, pp. A8–A13; Iain Chalmers, 'Commentary: The "Unfortunate Experiment" That Was Not, and the Indebtedness of Women and Children to Herbert ("Herb") Green (1916–2001)', *Journal of Clinical Epidemiology*, vol. 122, June 2020, pp. A13–A19.
131 *Northern Advocate*, 26 September 1988, cited in Bryder, *A History of the 'Unfortunate Experiment'*, p. 200.
132 *Ministry of Women's Affairs Newsletter*, 7, December 1987–January 1988, cited in Bryder, *A History of the 'Unfortunate Experiment'* p. 137.
133 'Midwives go it alone', *NZ News UK*, 17 April 1989, in WWAT, http://wwat.nz/wp-content/uploads/20001-113-033b.pdf (accessed 20 February 2023).
134 *New Zealand Herald*, 21 November 1987; *Report of the Committee of Inquiry into Allegations Concerning the Treatment of Cervical Cancer at National Women's Hospital and into Other Related Matters* (chair Silvia Cartwright), Government Printing Office, Auckland, 1988, p. 172; Bryder, *A History of the 'Unfortunate Experiment'*, p. 141.
135 Bryder, *A History of the 'Unfortunate Experiment'*, p. 141.
136 Ibid.
137 *Report of the Committee of Inquiry*, p. 96; Bryder, *A History of the 'Unfortunate Experiment'*, p. 195.
138 Jacqui Anderson, Del Lewis, Julie Hasson and Karen Guilliland, 'Doctors Need No Defending', *New Zealand Nursing Journal: Kai Tiaki*, vol. 81, 12, December/January 1989, p. 3.

139  Jan Corbett, 'Second thoughts on the unfortunate experiment at National Women's', *Metro*, July 1990, p. 61; Bryder, *A History of the 'Unfortunate Experiment'*, p. 158.
140  *Time* magazine, Summer 1990, p. 22.
141  David McLoughlin, 'The politics of childbirth', *North & South*, August 1993, p. 59.
142  Philippa Mein Smith, 'Midwifery Re-innovation in New Zealand', in J. Stanton (ed.), *Innovations in Health and Medicine: Diffusion and Resistance in the Twentieth Century*, Routledge, New York, 2002, p. 179.
143  Young, 'The Honouring of Joan Donley', pp. 10–11; see also BH, 'Joan Donley OBE', *HBA Auckland Newsletter*, 46, Autumn 1990, p. 16.
144  Joan Donley, 'Women in Partnership, Report on 1990 Conference', *Broadsheet*, 182, October 1990, p. 7; Joan Donley, 'Political Comment: Autonomy for Midwives', *NZCOMJ*, vol. 3, November 1990, p. 7.
145  Donley, 'Political Comment: Autonomy for Midwives', p. 9; Clark, Speech notes to open the NZCOM National Conference, Dunedin, 18 August 1990, p. 1; Sally Pairman, 'Educating Midwives for Autonomous Practice', in Guilliland and Pairman, *Women's Business*, p. 557 fn 71; Daellenbach, 'The Paradox of Success', p. 168.
146  Marsden Wagner, 'Appropriate Technology for Birth', *NZCOMJ*, vol. 3, November 1990, pp. 10–15.
147  Karen Guilliland, 'NZCOM (Inc.) Annual Report', ibid., 5, October 1991, pp. 17–19.
148  NZPD, 510, 21 August 1990, pp. 304–33.
149  Sally Pairman and Danielle Cameron, 'Editorial: Women in Partnership', *NZCOMJ*, vol. 3, November 1990, p. 4.
150  Karen Guilliland, 'Women & Midwives – Maintaining the Links', speech at 1990 NZCOM conference, p. 4, MSS & Archives, 2007/15, 1638, JDP.
151  C. P. Grigg and S. K. Tracy, 'New Zealand's Unique Maternity System', *Women and Birth*, vol. 26, 1, March 2013, pp. e59–e64, doi: http://dx.doi.org/10.1016/j.wombi.2012.09.006
152  Claire Sweetman, 'Safe Deliveries? A Review of New Zealand's Midwifery Regulation Through the Lens of the Health and Disability Commissioner', Laws 513 – Law and Medicine Research Paper, Victoria University of Wellington, 2013, p. 26.
153  Eyley and Salmon, *Helen Clark: Inside Stories*, p. 84.
154  Donley and Hinton, 'Home Birth Associations'.

## CHAPTER 6: *The 1990 Nurses Amendment Act and midwife autonomy*

1  Jonathan Hunt, New Zealand Parliamentary Debates (NZPD), 502, 9 November 1989, p. 13465.
2  Helen Clark, ibid., 502, 9 November 1989, pp. 13479–80 (Clause 1 was the short title).

3   Jenny Kirk (Birkenhead), ibid., 502, 9 November 1989, p. 13484.
4   *NZCOM Newsletter*, 3, 3, February 1991, p. 3 of speech, in Wise Woman Archives Trust Inc. (WWAT), http://wwat.nz/wp-content/uploads/20061-1991Vol3No3Feb.pdf (accessed 11 March 2023).
5   Katherine O'Regan (Waipa), NZPD, 502, 9 November 1989, p. 13483.
6   Submission 27W, Ruth Martis, Palmerston North, R21935512, 1989-1990, 81, W67/NUR/2 68681, Archives New Zealand Wellington (ANZW).
7   Joan Donley, 'Women in Partnership, *Broadsheet*, 182, October 1990, p. 8; Joan Donley, 'Independent Midwifery in New Zealand', in Tricia Murphy-Black (ed.), *Issues in Midwifery*, Churchill Livingstone, Edinburgh, 1995, p. 75.
8   David McLoughlin, 'The politics of childbirth: Midwives versus doctors', *North & South*, August 1993, p. 65.
9   Submission 80W, Celeste McCoy, 7 February 1990, R21935511, 80, W67/NUR/2, 68678, ANZW. Others making this point included: Submission 59W, Elizabeth Scott, Motueka District Women's Electoral Lobby Inc.; Submission 77, Nelson Home Birth Association; Submission 57W, NZ College of Midwives Canterbury/West Coast Region; Submission 22W, NZ College of Midwives Southland Region; Submission 17W, Linda Gilmore, Waihi; Submission 89W, Auckland Home Birth Association Inc., R21935511, ANZW.
10  Submission 76, Domiciliary Midwives Society of New Zealand, Bronwen Pelvin, R21935511, ANZW.
11  Submission 83, National Council of Women (NCW) of NZ Inc., Jocelyn Fish and Janet Hesketh, 9 February 1990, p. 6, R21935512, ANZW; Clark, NZPD, 502, 9 November 1989, p. 13480.
12  Ibid., p. 13480; NZ Planning Council, *First Report of the Social Monitoring Group: From Birth to Death* (chair Peggy Koopman-Boyden), Wellington, July 1985, pp. 21–22.
13  Kirk, NZPD, 502, 9 November 1989, p. 13484.
14  Clark, NZPD, 502, 9 November 1989, p. 13485.
15  Bryan Hardie Boys to Helen Clark, 18 July 1990; Clark to Hardie Boys, 20 August 1990, R21935510, 1990-1991, 80, W67/NUR/2, 68956, ANZW.
16  Clark, NZPD, 502, 9 November 1989, p. 13485.
17  McKinnon and Anne Collins (Labour MP, East Cape), NZPD, 502, 9 November 1989, p. 13481.
18  Margaret Shields, ibid., 455, 13 December 1983, p. 4828.
19  Peter Tapsell, ibid., 455, 13 December 1983, p. 4827.
20  McKinnon, ibid., 507, 29 May 1990, p. 1806.
21  Clark, ibid., 507, 29 May 1990, p. 1808.
22  *Home Birth Association (HBA) Auckland Newsletter*, 45, December 1989, p. 1.
23  Ms J. Myers, Submission 1W, 14 November 1989, R21935507, 1989, 80, W67/NUR/2, 68677, ANZW.
24  Submissions 96W, 97W, 98W, R21935512, ANZW.
25  Motueka District Women's Electoral Lobby Inc., Elizabeth Scott, Submission 59W, 6 February 1990, R21935512, ANZW; for other short submissions see also R21935511, ANZW.

26  Figures given in Nelson HBA Submission 57W, R21935511, ANZW.
27  Sarah Boyle to Gail Longmore, Nurses Amendment Bill, 6 March 1990, R21935511, ANZW.
28  Submission 76, Domiciliary Midwives Society of New Zealand, Riverside Community, Upper Moutere, Submission 54W, Auckland Domiciliary Midwives Society, R21935511, ANZW.
29  Submission 8, New Zealand Nurses' Association, Professional Officer Joy Bickley, 1 December 1989, R21935507, ANZW.
30  Joy Bickley, 'Watchdogs or Wimps? Nurses' Response to the Cartwright Report', in Sandra Coney (ed.), *Unfinished Business, What Happened to the Cartwright Report*, Women's Health Action, Auckland, 1993, pp. 132–33.
31  Sharron Cole, National Executive member, Parents Centre NZ, 30 July 1990, R21935508, 80 W67/NUR/2 68680, ANZW.
32  Submission 82W, Women's Division Federated Farmers of New Zealand Inc., J. McIntyre, Health Convener, February 1990, R21935512, ANZW.
33  Submission 83, NCW, pp. 2–4, R21935512, ANZW.
34  Submission 58W, Nurses and Midwives of the Waikato AHB region (Maureen Lawton), R21935511, ANZW.
35  Submission 9, RNZCOG, R.J. Seddon, H.K. Sill, 1 December 1989, R21935507, ANZW (NZCOG founded 1982, with 'Royal' prefix from 1984).
36  On Diana Edwards (1923–2014), see *New Zealand Medical Journal*, vol. 127, 1403, 26 September 2014, p. 76. This obituary describes her as a pioneer of women's health.
37  Rea Daellenbach, 'The Paradox of Success and the Challenge of Change: Home Birth Associations of Aotearoa/New Zealand', PhD thesis, University of Canterbury, 1999, p. 170.
38  Submission 91, NZMA (Lewis King, Chair of Council), 12 February 1990, R21935512, ANZW.
39  Clark, NZPD, 510, 21 August 1990, p. 305.
40  Clark, Speech notes to open the NZCOM National Conference, 18 August 1990, p. 3, R21935508, ANZW; also in *NZCOM Newsletter*, 3, 3, February 1991 (p. 3 of speech), p. 10, in WWAT, http://wwat.nz/wp-content/uploads/20061-1991Vol3No3Feb.pdf (accessed 11 March 2023).
41  Judy Keall (Glenfield), NZPD, 507, 29 May 1990, p. 1804. Report of the Social Services Committee on the Nurses Amendment Bill May 1990, NZ House of Representatives, p. 10, R21935512, ANZW.
42  Daellenbach, 'The Paradox of Success', p. 170.
43  Ibid., p. 171.
44  O'Regan, NZPD, 507, 29 May 1990, p. 1809; Geoffrey Palmer, *Unbridled Power? An Interpretation of New Zealand's Constitution and Government*, Oxford University Press, Wellington, 1979.
45  Murray McCully (East Coast Bays), NZPD, 507, 29 May 1990, p. 1811; McCully, ibid., 510, 21 August 1990, pp. 318, 330.
46  Kirk, ibid., 507, 29 May 1990, p. 1809.
47  McKinnon, ibid., 507, 29 May 1990, p. 1806.

48  Ibid., 510, 21 August 1990, pp. 306, 309.
49  McCully, ibid., 510, 21 August 1990, pp. 319, 321.
50  Keall, ibid., 510, 21 August 1990, p. 316; *Evening Post*, 27 June 1990, R21935508, ANZW.
51  McKinnon, NZPD, 502, 9 November 1989, p. 13481; Clark, ibid., 502, 9 November 1989, p. 13485.
52  'Bill to give midwives more scope: Parliament', *Evening Post*, 9 November 1989; 'Midwives win sole role', *New Zealand Herald*, 10 November 1989, section 1, p. 2.
53  NZCOM Annual Report 1989–90, Appendix 1, p. 3, Item 5, MSS & Archives-2007/2, New Zealand College of Midwives Auckland Region records, Special Collections, University of Auckland Library.
54  NZGPA to J. Kirk, Social Services Select Committee, 20 July 1990, R21935508, ANZW.
55  Jude Henry, CEO, NZMA, to Katherine O'Reagan [sic], Social Services Select Committee, 24 July 1990, R21935508, ANZW; also in R4501215, 1989-1990, 24, 3, ANZW.
56  M. A. H. Baird to O'Reagan [sic], 24 July 1990, R4501215, ANZW.
57  Maureen Lawton, Director of Nursing Practice, Waikato AHB, on behalf of senior nurses and midwives, Waikato AHB to Helen Clark, copies sent to Teenah Handiside, Acting Chief Nursing Officer, Workforce Development Department of the Department of Health, 16 July 1990, WWAT, http://wwat.nz/wp-content/uploads/20073-91-003.pdf (accessed 23 February 2023).
58  Karen Guilliland response to Lawton, 30 July 1990, WWAT, http://wwat.nz/wp-content/uploads/20073-91-003.pdf (accessed 23 February 2023).
59  Lois Robertson, National Secretary NCW, to Jonathan Hunt, 4 September 1990, R21935510, ANZW.
60  Keall, NZPD, 510, 21 August 1990, pp. 315–16.
61  Helen Clark to Lois Robertson, 12 October 1990, R21935510, ANZW.
62  Helen Clark, format of letter on NA Act, 29 August 1990, R21935508, ANZW; Clark, Speech notes to open NZCOM Conference, 18 August 1990, p. 5, R21935508, ANZW.
63  Jacqui Anderson (pp Karen Guilliland) NZCOM to Sue Scobie, Nurse Advisor Department of Health, 1 November 1989, R21935509, 1989, 80, W67/NUR/2, 68349, ANZW.
64  Sheryl Smail, Chief Nursing Officer, 20 June 1989, 'Issues arising from Amendment to the Nurses Act 1977, autonomy of Midwives', R21935507, ANZW.
65  Sue Scobie and Yvonne Dorbecker to Sally Shaw, General Manager, Population Health Policy – re autonomy of midwives, 12 September 1989, R21935514, 1986-1989, 81, W67/NUR/2, 68348, ANZW.
66  Smail memo, 22 June 1989, p. 3, R21935507, ANZW.
67  See Caroline Flint, Polly Poulengeris and Adrian Grant, 'The "Know Your Midwife" Scheme: A Randomised Trial of Continuity of Care by a Team

of Midwives', *Midwifery*, vol. 5, 1, March 1989, pp. 11–16, doi: https://doi.org/10.1016/S0266-6138(89)80059-2
68   Bob Boyd, Primary Health Care, Appendix 2 Autonomy of Midwives, R21935507, ANZW.
69   Chris Harrington, Assistant Manager, Medicines and Benefits Unit, 13 October 1989, R21935509, 1989, 80, W67/NUR/2, 68349, ANZW.
70   Ibid.
71   Teenah Handiside, Acting Chief Nursing Officer, Workforce Management, Department of Health, to Clark, 19 December 1989, and margin notes by Clark, R21935507, ANZW.
72   Pamela Stirling, 'Hard labour', *New Zealand Listener*, 12 March 1990, p. 11.
73   Helen Clark, Memo to Social Equity Committee, 17 July 1989, R21935507, ANZW; R21935514, ANZW.
74   Helen Clark to MPs Elizabeth Tennet, 21 July 1989, Margaret Shields, 25 July 1989, R21935514, ANZW.
75   Clark, NZPD, 502, 9 November 1989, p. 13486.
76   Sally Pairman and Karen Guilliland, 'Reinstating Midwifery Autonomy', in Karen Guilliland and Sally Pairman, *Women's Business: The Story of the New Zealand College of Midwives, 1986–2010*, New Zealand College of Midwives, Christchurch, 2010, p. 36.
77   O'Regan, NZPD, 510, 21 August 1990, pp. 313, 314.
78   Kirk, ibid., 502, 9 November 1989, p. 13485.
79   O'Regan, ibid., 510, 21 August 1990, p. 311.
80   Ibid., p. 314.
81   Jeff Grant (Awarua), ibid., 510, 21 August 1990, p. 321.
82   Grant, ibid., 510, 21 August 1990, p. 333.
83   Clark, ibid., 510, 21 August 1990, p. 306.
84   McCully, ibid., 510, 21 August 1990, p. 321.
85   Submission 83, NCW, p. 5, R21935512, ANZW.
86   Lois Robertson, National Secretary NCW, to Jonathan Hunt, 4 September 1990, R21935510, ANZW.
87   Guilliland and Pairman, *Women's Business*, p. 33.
88   Keall, NZPD, 507, 29 May 1990, p. 1805; see also, Judy Keall (chair), Report of the Social Services Committee on the Nurses Amendment Act May 1990, p. 6, R21935512, ANZW.
89   Submission 5, NZCOM, R21935507, ANZW.
90   Submission 27W, Martis, R21935512, ANZW.
91   O'Regan, NZPD, 502, 9 November 1989, p. 13483.
92   Kirk, ibid., 507, 29 May 1990, p. 1810.
93   Ibid., 510, 21 August 1990, p. 311.
94   Keall, ibid., 510, 21 August 1990, pp. 316, 327.
95   Sally Shaw to Mary O'Regan, Ministry of Women's Affairs, 3 December 1987, WWAT, http://wwat.nz/wp-content/uploads/20001-113-029.pdf (accessed 23 February 2023).

96   David Caygill to Wendy Stevens, 27 November 1987, 2001-113-008 (underlining in original report), WWAT, http://wwat.nz/wp-content/uploads/20001-113-008.pdf (accessed 23 February 2023).
97   Guilliland, Meeting with David Caygill, 28 November 1987, 20001-113-031, WWAT, http://wwat.nz/wp-content/uploads/20001-113-031.pdf (accessed 23 February 2023).
98   Smail, Memo for Minister of Health, 23 May 1989, 'Autonomy of Midwives – Notes for Minister's Report', p. 7, R21935514, ANZW; copy also in R16664911, 1989, 1935, 366-6-10, 69656, ANZW; and R21935507, ANZW.
99   Gayle O'Brien, Memo to Karen Poutasi, re. Midwifery (Direct Entry), 24 May 1989, R16664911, 1935, 366-6-10, 69656, ANZW; Sheryl Smail, 'Autonomy of Midwives – Notes for Minister's Report', 22 May 1989, p. 8, R21935507, ANZW.
100  Smail, 22 June 1989, p. 5, R21935507, ANZW.
101  Handwritten comments by Clark, 20 February 1990, to Smail's Draft Policy Paper for Review of Nurses Act, 16 February 1990, R21935511, ANZW.
102  Maureen Lawton to Helen Clark, 16 July 1990, p. 3, point 2.
103  Lawton to Clark, p. 5.
104  Brian Edwards, *Helen: Portrait of a Prime Minister*, Exisle Publishers, Auckland, 2001, pp. 203, 209.
105  Claudia Pond Eyley and Dan Salmon, *Helen Clark: Inside Stories*, Auckland University Press, Auckland, 2015, p. 80.
106  Helen Clark, webinar: 'Emancipating Midwifery – reflecting on 30 years of midwifery autonomy', 3 September 2020 (time: 18.13.42), hosted by Alison Eddy, Chief Executive, New Zealand College of Midwives, https://www.midwife.org.nz/news/webinar-emancipating-midwifery-reflecting-on-30-years-of-midwifery-autonomy/ (accessed 23 February 2023); see also Sally Abel, 'Midwifery and Maternity Services in Transition: An Examination of Change Following the Nurses Amendment Act 1990', PhD thesis, University of Auckland, 1997, p. 99.
107  Press Statement, Rt Hon Helen Clark, Minister of Health, embargoed until 18 August 1990, R21935508, ANZW.
108  Clark, Speech notes to open the NZCOM National Conference, 18 August 1990, p. 10, R21935508, ANZW; see also Guilliland and Pairman, *Women's Business*, p. 33.
109  Clark, NZPD, 502, 9 November 1989, p. 13480.
110  Ibid., p. 13485.
111  Keall, ibid., 510, 21 August 1990, p. 328.
112  Daellenbach, 'The Paradox of Success', p. 2.
113  Abel, 'Midwifery and Maternity Services in Transition', pp. 84, 106.
114  Department of Health, 'Part 1: What Everyone Should Know', *Nurses Amendment Act 1990: Information for Health Providers*, Department of Health, Wellington, October 1990, p. 5, https://www.moh.govt.nz/notebook/nbbooks.nsf/0/7e9811383ed959b34c2565d7000de831/$FILE/Nurses%20Amendment%20Act%201990%20-%20information%20for%20health%20providers.pdf (accessed 23 February 2023); copy in R21935510, ANZW.

115 E.M. Shepherd, Manager O&G Services, to Sheilah O'Sullivan and John Holmes, 21 November 1991, R21935506, 1991-1992, 80, W67/NUR/2, ANZW.
116 Guilliland and Pairman, *Women's Business*, p. 41.
117 Abel, 'Midwifery and Maternity Services in Transition', p. 124.
118 See Diane M. Fraser and Margaret A. Cooper (eds), *Myles' Textbook for Midwives*, https://www.fishpond.com.au/Books/Myles-Textbook-for-Midwives-Diane-M-Fraser-Margaret-A-Cooper/9780443072345 (accessed 23 February 2023).
119 Preface, in Sally Pairman, Jan Pincombe, Carol Thorogood and Sally Tracy (eds), *Midwifery: Preparation for Practice*, Churchill Livingston Elsevier, Marrickville NSW, 2006, p. viii.
120 Bronwen Pelvin, 'Life Skills for Midwifery Practice', in Pairman et al., *Midwifery: Preparation for Practice*, p. 229; Sally Pairman and Judith McAra-Couper, 'Theoretical Frameworks for Midwifery Practice', in ibid., p. 249.
121 O'Regan, NZPD, 510, 21 August 1990, p. 328.
122 'Lynda's Story', in Guilliland and Pairman, *Women's Business*, p. 183.

## CHAPTER 7: *Midwifery autonomy and partnership in the 1990s*

1 Helen Clark, 'Address to the New Zealand College of Midwives National Conference, Thursday 29 August 1996,' *New Zealand College of Midwives Journal* (*NZCOMJ*), vol. 15, October 1996, p. 8.
2 Stacy Gregg, 'The hand that stocks the cradle', *Sunday Star-Times*, 4 May 1997.
3 Alice Coyle, 'Six Years of Independent Midwifery in London', *NZCOMJ*, vol. 7, December 1992, p. 19.
4 Lesley Page, 'Editorial', ibid., vol. 13, October 1995, p. 4.
5 Diony Young, 'The Midwifery Revolution in New Zealand: What We Can Learn', *Birth*, vol. 23, 3, 1996, pp. 125–27.
6 Beverley A. Lawrence Beech, 'User Views of Maternity Care', *NZCOMJ*, vol. 19, November 1998, p. 16.
7 Sarah Stewart, 'Midwifery in New Zealand: A Cause for Celebration', *MIDIRS Midwifery Digest*, vol. 11, 3, September 2001, p. 319.
8 Beverley Crombie, '"A Midwife's Gift – Love, Skill and Knowledge": The Theme for the International Confederation of Midwives 22nd International Conference', *NZCOMJ*, vol. 4, May 1991, p. 19.
9 Helen Manoharan, 'Book review: Tricia Murphy-Black, *Issues in Midwifery*, Churchill Livingstone, Edinburgh 1995', *NZCOMJ*, vol. 13, October 1995, p. 4 (the two others had higher degrees – Judy Hedwig MA (1990) and Valerie Fleming (PhD 1994).
10 *Home Birth Association (HBA) Auckland Newsletter*, 56, Summer 1992–93, inside front cover.
11 Karen Guilliland and Sally Pairman, 'International Confederation of Midwives 23rd Triennial Congress Vancouver, Canada, 4–14 May 1993', *NZCOMJ*, vol. 9, October 1993, pp. 6, 8.
12 *HBA Auckland Newsletter*, 56, Summer 1992–93, front cover.

13   Sally Pairman, 'Workforce to Profession: An Exploration of New Zealand Midwifery's Professionalising Strategies from 1986 to 2005', Doctor of Midwifery thesis, University of Technology Sydney, 2005, pp. 194–95.
14   Ibid., p. 175.
15   Sally Pairman, 'Opening Address at Conference', *NZCOMJ*, vol. 15, October 1996, p. 5.
16   Karen Guilliland, 'National Directors Forum', *New Zealand College of Midwives National Newsletter*, November/December 1997, p. 9.
17   Index of NZCOM Journals, *NZCOMJ*, vol. 39, October 2008, pp. 16–25.
18   Joan Donley, *Birthrites: Natural vs Unnatural Childbirth in New Zealand*, Full Court Press in association with New Zealand College of Midwives, Auckland, 1998.
19   Pairman, 'Workforce to Profession', pp. 188, 205; Karen Guilliland and Sally Pairman, *Women's Business: The Story of the New Zealand College of Midwives, 1986–2010*, New Zealand College of Midwives, Christchurch, 2010, p. 153.
20   Joan Donley, 'Women in Partnership', *Broadsheet*, 182, October 1990, p. 8; Joan Donley, 'Political Comment: Midwifery Independence?, *NZCOMJ*, vol. 5, October 1991, p. 10.
21   Joan Donley, 'Political Comment: Protocols?', ibid., vol. 7, December 1992, pp. 10–11.
22   Inquest, included in High Court hearing of *Matthews v Hunter*, 10 September 1991, pp. 7–8, http://coroniallaw.org.nz/wp-content/uploads/2019/01/Matthews-v-Hunter-unreported-version.pdf (accessed 20 January 2019); 'Branch Roundup: Nelson', *HBA Auckland Newsletter*, 50, Autumn 1991, p. 35.
23   'Coroner calls for homebirth review', *New Zealand Doctor (NZD)*, 15 July 1991.
24   Inquest, High Court hearing, pp. 7–8.
25   Donley, 'Political Comment: Protocols?', p. 10; Inquest, High Court hearing, pp. 7–8; Joan Donley, 'Independent Midwifery in New Zealand', in Tricia Murphy-Black (ed.), *Issues in Midwifery*, Churchill Livingstone, Edinburgh, 1995, p. 72.
26   Submission 1990, R21935511, 80, W67/NUR/2, 68678, Archives New Zealand Wellington (ANZW); Diana Edwards to O'Regan, 27 June 1991, R21935506, 1991-1992, Box 80, W67/NUR/2, ANZW.
27   Donley, 'Political Comment: Protocols?', p. 10.
28   Joan Donley, *Herstory of N.Z. Home Birth Association*, New Zealand Home Birth Association, Auckland, 1992, p. 65.
29   Helen Murdoch, 'Coroner urges backup midwives', *Press*, 3 November 2010, http://www.stuff.co.nz/national/4301071/Coroner-urges-backup-midwives
30   David McLoughlin, 'The politics of childbirth', *North & South*, August 1993, pp. 68–69; Cate Brett, 'Midwife crisis', *HQ Magazine*, March/April 1996, p. 86.
31   Pairman, 'Workforce to Profession', pp. 178, 194–95, 197.
32   Bronwen Pelvin, 'Midwifery Issues: Highlighted by the Recent "Frontline" Programme', *NZCOMJ*, vol. 7, December 1992, p. 13.
33   McLoughlin, 'The politics of childbirth', p. 66.
34   Report of the South Australian Maternal, Perinatal and Infant Mortality Committee, 2011; Melissa Sweet, 'Concerns continue about unsafe home birth

practices: Dr Andrew Pesce', *Croakey Health Media*, 11 November 2011, https://www.croakey.org/concerns-continue-about-unsafe-home-birth-practices-dr-andrew-pesce/ (accessed 6 September 2022).
35   McLoughlin, 'The politics of childbirth', p. 69.
36   Guilliland and Pairman, *Women's Business*, p. 150.
37   McLoughlin, 'The politics of childbirth', p. 56; 'Mother Care: Maternity Care funding provisions', *Consumer*, 356, January/February 1997, p. 5.
38   These figures are taken from the *HBA Auckland Newsletter*, 1989–1997.
39   Brett, 'Midwife crisis', p. 90.
40   McLoughlin, 'The politics of childbirth', p. 65.
41   Ibid., p. 59.
42   Carolyn Young, in Halina Ogonowska-Coates, *Born: Midwives and Women Celebrate 100 Years*, New Zealand College of Midwives, Christchurch, 2004, p. 15.
43   *HBA Auckland Newsletter*, 64, Winter/Spring 1995, pp. 1, 6.
44   Donley, 'Political Comment: Midwifery Independence?', p. 10; Joan Donley, 'Speech at 1992 NZCOM Conference', *HBA Auckland Newsletter*, 56, Summer 1992–93, p. 6; Donley, *Birthrites*, p. 11.
45   Joan Donley, 'Political Comment: Informed Consent', *NZCOMJ*, vol. 10, April 1994, p. 20.
46   Valerie Fleming, 'New Zealand's First Doctorate in Midwifery! Partnership, Power and Politics: Feminist Perceptions of Midwifery Practice: Interview by Andrea Gilkison', *NZCOMJ*, vol. 12, April 1995, p. 11; Valerie Fleming, 'Midwives No Joke', *Broadsheet*, 175, February 1990, p. 6.
47   Maggie Banks, 'Out on a Limb: The Personal Mandate to Practise Midwifery by Midwives of the Domiciliary Midwives Society of New Zealand (Incorporated), 1974–1986', PhD thesis, Victoria University of Wellington, 2007, p. 11.
48   Sally Abel, 'Midwifery and Maternity Services in Transition: An Examination of Change Following the Nurses Amendment Act 1990', PhD thesis, University of Auckland, 1997, p. 127.
49   Banks, 'Out on a Limb', p. 11.
50   Penny St John, 'News: Harsh words from women', *NZD*, 11 October 2000; the paper was also cited in Ruth Joy Surtees, 'Midwifery as Feminist Praxis in Aotearoa/New Zealand', PhD thesis, University of Canterbury, 2003, p. 45.
51   Surtees, 'Midwifery as Feminist Praxis', p. 170.
52   Denise Black, 'Letter to the editor', *NZCOMJ*, vol. 26, April 2002, p. 26; on Black as a homebirth midwife, see Banks, 'Out on a Limb', p. 117.
53   See also Abel, 'Midwifery and Maternity Services in Transition', p. 121.
54   'Your Choices in Childbirth', *Consumer*, 324, March 1994, p. 7; 'New Zealand Mothers and Babies: An Analysis of National Maternity Data', Health Funding Authority, Wellington, June 1999, p. 32, https://www.moh.govt.nz/notebook/nbbooks.nsf/0/191031B6A410B99ACC256B520070A4BA/$file/New%20Zealand%20mothers%20and%20babies.pdf (accessed 24 February 2023). See also Lynda Exton, *Baby Business: What's Happened to Maternity Care in New Zealand?*, Craig Potton Publishing, Nelson, 2008, p. 167.

55  Judy Hedwig and Valerie Fleming, 'Midwifery Practice in New Zealand: A Dynamic Discipline', in Murphy-Black (ed.), *Issues in Midwifery*, p. 219.
56  Brett, 'Midwife crisis', p. 88.
57  Karen Guilliland and Sally Pairman, 'The Midwifery Partnership – A Model for Practice: A paper for presentation at the NZCOM Conference, Rotorua, 12–14 August 1994', *NZCOMJ*, vol. 11, October 1994, p. 5.
58  Karen Guilliland, 'Midwifery in New Zealand', paper presented at the 'Future Birth: The Place to be Born Conference', Australia, for Birth International, an Organisation of Childbirth Educators, February 1999,w https://birthinternational.com/midwifery-in-new-zealand/ (accessed 24 February 2023).
59  Banks, 'Out on a Limb', p. 22.
60  Guilliland and Pairman, 'The Midwifery Partnership', pp. 5–9.
61  Sally Pairman, 'Developing & Crafting a Vision: A Strategic Plan for Midwifery', *NZCOMJ*, vol. 18, April 1998, p. 7.
62  Pairman, 'Workforce to Profession', pp. 1, 6; Sally Pairman, 'Partnership Revisited: Towards Midwifery Theory', *NZCOMJ*, vol. 21, October 1999, p. 6.
63  Joan Skinner was included in the 1991 HBA list of 'Domiciliary Midwives Currently Accepting Homebirth Bookings', *HBA Auckland Newsletter*, 50, Autumn 1991, p. 14.
64  Joan Skinner, 'Partnership: Individualism, Contractualism or Feminist Praxis', *NZCOMJ*, vol. 21, October 1999, pp. 14–17.
65  Karen Guilliland and Sally Pairman, Letter to the editor, 'Response, Midwifery Partnership', ibid., 12, April 1995, p. 6.
66  Pairman, 'Workforce to Profession', p. 68.
67  Ibid., p. 108 (draft of a chapter 'Midwifery Partnership: Working "With" Women', for 2nd edition of Lesley Page and Rona McCandlish (eds), *The New Midwifery: Science and Sensitivity in Practice*, Churchill Livingstone, Edinburgh, 2006).
68  Nicky Leap and Sally Pairman, 'Working in Partnership', in Sally Pairman, Jan Pincombe, Carol Thorogood and Sally Tracy (eds), *Midwifery: Preparation for Practice*, Churchill Livingstone Elsevier, Marrickville NSW, 2006, p. 259.
69  Ibid., p. 265.
70  Helen Manoharan, *NZCOMJ*, vol. 15, October 1996, p. 4; Sally Pairman, 'Opening Address at Conference', ibid., p. 5.
71  Speech reported in 'News: Medical model takes a hammering at conference', *NZD*, 18 September 1996; see also B. K. Rothman, *Recreating Motherhood: Ideology and Technology in a Patriarchal Society*, W. W. Norton, New York, 1989.
72  Nurses Review, Yvonne Dorbecker, Minutes of Meeting of Health Department with NZCOM, 18 October 1989, p. 8, R21935509, 1989, 80, W67/NUR/2, 68349, ANZW.
73  Leap and Pairman, 'Working in Partnership', in Pairman et al. (eds), *Midwifery: Preparation for Practice*, p. 265.
74  Pelvin, 'Midwifery Issues: Highlighted by the Recent "Frontline" Programme', pp. 12–13.
75  Exton, *Baby Business*, p. 141.

76  Bronwen Pelvin, 'Midwifery Issues', *NZCOMJ*, vol. 7, December 1992, p. 13 (italics in the original).
77  'New rules on birth referrals welcome', Christchurch *Press*, 5 June 1995.
78  Lisa Mannion, Letter to the editor, *New Zealand Herald*, 11 July 1995.
79  'Midwife inquiry over baby death', *Sunday Star-Times*, 20 September 1998.
80  Amanda Cropp, 'Who will deliver your baby?', *Next*, September 2000, p. 102.
81  Helen Newnham and Jackie Pearse, 'Legal Frameworks for Practice in Australia and New Zealand', in Pairman et al. (eds), *Midwifery: Preparation for Practice*, p. 199.
82  Kate Isherwood, 'Independent Midwifery in the United Kingdom', in Murphy-Black (ed.), *Issues in Midwifery*, pp. 34–35.
83  Anne-Marie Boxall and Kathy Flitcroft, 'Debate: Open Access: From Little Things, Big Things Grow: A Local Approach to System-wide Maternity Services Reform in the Absence of Definitive Evidence', *Australia and New Zealand Health Policy*, vol. 4, 18, 2007, doi: https://doi.org/10.1186/1743-8462-4-18
84  Andrew F. Pesce, 'Editorial: Planned Home Birth in Australia: Politics or Science?', *Medical Journal of Australia*, vol. 192, 2, 18 January 2010, pp. 60–61.
85  Peter D. G. Skegg, 'English Medical Law and "Informed Consent": An Antipodean Assessment and Alternative', *Medical Law Review*, vol. 7, 2, Summer 1999, p. 161.
86  Joan Donley, '"What does the New Zealand College of Midwives do for me?" A Response to the New Zealand Nurses Organisation', *NZCOMJ*, vol. 19, November 1998, p. 21.
87  Lynda Williams to Ron Paterson, Health and Disability Commissioner, 9 August 2001, *Maternity Services Consumer Council Newsletter*, 44, September 2001, and response from Paterson, 12 December 2001, ibid., 45, December 2001.
88  Bronwen Pelvin, 'On the Edge: Midwifery and the Art of Knowing', *NZCOMJ*, vol. 15, October 1996, p. 14.
89  Bernadette Rae, 'Room for choice', *New Zealand Herald*, 20 July 1993, section 2, p. 1.
90  Barbara Clotworthy, Letter to the editor, *NZCOMJ*, vol. 12, April 1995, p. 4.
91  Edna Rose, Letter to the editor, *NZCOMJ*, vol. 12, April 1995, pp. 4–5.
92  Kim Wheeler, Letter to the editor, ibid., vol. 11, October 1994, p. 10.
93  Barbara Churcher, ibid., vol. 12, April 1995, p. 5.
94  Deborah Earl, Eileen Gibson, Trish Isa, Judith McAra-Couper, Betty McGregor and Helen Thwaites, 'Core Midwifery: The Challenge Continues', *NZCOMJ*, vol. 27, October 2002, p. 30.
95  Donley to Maggie Lecky-Thompson, 24 November 1996, MSS & Archives 2007/15, 1, 1/2, 7/2/C/1, Joan Donley Papers, Special Collections, University of Auckland Library (JDP).
96  Karen Guilliland, 'Learning from Midwives', *Kai Tiaki: Nursing New Zealand*, October 1996, p. 23; Karen Guilliland, 'Section 51: Contract for Autonomy', *NZCOMJ*, vol. 16, April 1997, p. 8.
97  Guilliland, 'Learning from Midwives', p. 23; Guilliland, 'Section 51', p. 8.
98  Sally Pairman, Editorial, *NZCOMJ*, vol. 11, October 1994, p. 4.

99 Stewart, 'Midwifery in New Zealand: A Cause for Celebration', p. 321.
100 Guilliland and Pairman, 'The Midwifery Partnership', p. 5.
101 Skinner, 'Partnership: Individualism, Contractualism or Feminist Praxis', pp. 15–16.
102 Karen Guilliland, Women & Midwifes – Maintaining the Links', speech at 1990 NZCOM conference, p. 8, MSS & Archives, 2007/15, 1638, JDP.
103 Ibid., p. 10.
104 Karen Guilliland and Sally Pairman, 'Midwifery Education – a National Perspective – the New Zealand College of Midwives', *NZCOMJ*, vol. 4, May 1991, p. 6.
105 Guilliland and Pairman, *Women's Business*, p. 204; representatives from La Leche League and Plunket were added in 2002.
106 Ibid., p. 86.
107 Deena Coster, 'Taranaki woman's lifetime of work in Maori health and midwifery celebrated', *Stuff*, 8 January 2016, https://www.stuff.co.nz/taranaki-daily-news/news/75677251/taranaki-womans-lifetime-of-work-in-maori-health-and-midwifery-celebrated
108 Karen Guilliland, 'Wise woman graciously bridged worlds of Maori and midwifery profession', *NZD*, 1 February 2017.
109 Simon Upton, 'Conference Opening Speech', *NZCOMJ*, vol. 7, December 1992, p. 14; Abel, 'Midwifery and Maternity Services in Transition', p. 259.
110 Ibid., p. 260.
111 Jean Te Huia, 'Nga Maia Maori Midwives Aotearoa 1993–', *Women Together: A History of Women's Organisations in New Zealand*, 2019, https://nzhistory.govt.nz/women-together/nga-maia-maori-midwives-aotearoa (accessed 24 February 2023).
112 Hope Tupara, 'Meeting the Needs of Maori Women: The Challenge for Midwifery Education', *NZCOMJ*, vol. 25, October 2001, p. 8.
113 Abel, 'Midwifery and Maternity Services in Transition', pp. 260–61; 'Nga Maia O Aotearoa's India Experience', *NZCOMJ*, vol. 18, April 1998, p. 28.
114 Ibid., pp. 28–29; Guilliland and Pairman, *Women's Business*, pp. 208–9.
115 'Nga Maia O Aotearoa's India Experience', p. 28.
116 Home Birth Aotearoa Conference, 14 July 2015, Speakers, https://homebirth.org.nz/conference2015-2/ (accessed 24 February 2023).
117 'Calls to address shortage of Māori midwives', RNZ, 1 October 2015, https://www.rnz.co.nz/news/te-manu-korihi/285826/calls-to-address-shortage-of-maori-midwives; Te Huia, 'Nga Maia'.

## CHAPTER 8: *The politics of maternity services and 'shared care' after 1990*

1 Lesley Page, Editorial, *New Zealand College of Midwives Journal (NZCOMJ)*, vol. 13, October 1995, p. 4.
2 Not all GPs chose to provide childbirth services; those who regularly did so were generally known as GP obstetricians and many held the Diploma of Obstetrics (Dip Obs) from National Women's Hospital.

3   David McLoughlin, 'The politics of childbirth: Midwives versus doctors', *North & South*, August 1993, p. 56.
4   Ibid., p. 58.
5   Donna Chisholm, 'Maternity bills skyrocketing', *Sunday Star*, 24 February 1991; see also Lynda Exton, *The Baby Business: What's Happened to Maternity Care in New Zealand?*, Craig Potton Publishing, Nelson, 2008, p. 70.
6   Maggie Banks, 'Out on a Limb: The Personal Mandate to Practise Midwifery by Midwives of the Domiciliary Midwives Society of New Zealand (Incorporated), 1974–1986', PhD thesis, Victoria University of Wellington, 2007, p. 1.
7   Joan Donley, *Herstory of N.Z. Home Birth Association*, New Zealand Home Birth Association, Auckland, 1992, pp. 33, 35.
8   Joan Donley and Brenda Hinton (updated by Elizabeth Cox, 2019), 'Home Birth Associations, 1978–', https://nzhistory.govt.nz/women-together/home-birth-associations (accessed 24 February 2023).
9   Donley, *Herstory*, pp. 35–36.
10  McLoughlin, 'The politics of childbirth', p. 60.
11  Joan Donley, 'Independent Midwifery in New Zealand', in Tricia Murphy-Black (ed.), *Issues in Midwifery*, Churchill Livingstone, Edinburgh, 1995, p. 74; Barbara Katz Rothman, *In Labor: Women and Power in the Birthplace*, W. W. Norton, New York, 1982.
12  Sally Abel, 'Midwifery and Maternity Services in Transition: An Examination of Change following the Nurses Amendment Act 1990', PhD thesis, University of Auckland, 1997, pp. 140–43.
13  Glenn Blanchette, 'The Changing Landscape of Maternity Services', in Robin Gauld (ed.), *Continuity and Chaos: Health Care Management and Delivery in New Zealand*, University of Otago Press, Dunedin, 2003, p. 138; 'Your Choices in Childbirth', *Consumer*, 324, March 1994, p. 7; 'Mother Care: Maternity Care Funding Provisions', *Consumer*, 365, January/February 1997, p. 5.
14  Bruce Ansley, 'Babes at risk', *New Zealand Listener*, 5 April 1997, p. 22.
15  'Your Choices in Childbirth', p. 8.
16  William Ferguson, Letter to the editor, *Sunday Star-Times*, 11 July 2004.
17  Homebirth doctors in Auckland included John Hilton, William Ferguson, Phil Railton, Sean McGarry, Adrian Gane, Alistair Leggat, Diana Nash and Graham Gulbransen, *Home Birth Association (HBA) Auckland Newsletter*, 50, Autumn 1991, p. 22.
18  Ibid., 62, Spring 1994, p. 1.
19  Veronica Muller, Sian Burgess, Maggie Cropper and Heather Waugh, ibid., 57, Autumn 1993, p. 12.
20  McLoughlin, 'The politics of childbirth', p. 58.
21  *HBA Auckland Newsletter*, 57, Autumn 1993, p. 12.
22  Ibid., p. 11.
23  Jan Thompson and Rose Vos, ibid., 62, Spring 1994, p. 15; ibid., 64, Winter/Spring 1995, pp. 15, 16, 18, 19.

24  Abel, 'Midwifery and Maternity Services in Transition', p. 127.
25  Jo Coco, 'Midwives increase childbirth options', *New Zealand Herald* (*NZH*), 26 July 1993.
26  Philip Rushmer, 'Midwives raise the cost of childbirth', ibid., 19 July 1993.
27  Fiona Barber, 'Doctors argue for teamwork with midwives', ibid., 7 August 1995; also reported in *HBA Auckland Newsletter*, 64, Winter/Spring 1995, pp. 33–34; Amanda Cropp, 'Who will deliver your baby?', *Next*, September 2000, p. 103.
28  Barber, 'Doctors argue for teamwork with midwives'.
29  *HBA Auckland Newsletter*, 64, Winter/Spring 1995, p. 34; Barber, *NZH*, 8 August 1995.
30  Coopers & Lybrand, 'First Steps Towards an Integrated Maternity Services Framework: Working Papers of the Report', Regional Health Authorities Maternity Services Project, Ministry of Health, Wellington, November 1993, p. 17, https://www.moh.govt.nz/notebook/nbbooks.nsf/0/9F9AE7A8B59317794C2565D700186156/$file/first%20steps%20towards%20an%20integrated%20maternity%20services%20framework.pdf (accessed 25 February 2023).
31  Abel, 'Midwifery and Maternity Services in Transition', pp. 191–92.
32  Ansley, 'Babes at risk', p. 21.
33  Helen Rodenburg, in Rosy Fenwicke (ed.), *In Practice: The Lives of New Zealand Women Doctors in the 21st Century*, Random House, Auckland, 2004, p. 117.
34  Kathryn McNeil, 'Midwives get political support from the top', *New Zealand Doctor* (*NZD*), 18 September 1996.
35  Sally Pairman, 'Opening Address at Conference', *NZCOMJ*, vol. 15, October 1996, pp. 5–7.
36  Karen Guilliland, 'Section 51: Contract for Autonomy', ibid., 16, April 1997, p. 8.
37  Karen Bartholomew, 'The Realities of Choice and Access in the Lead Maternity Carer System: Operationalising Choice Policy in the New Zealand Maternity Reforms', Master of Public Health thesis, University of Auckland, 2010, pp. 44, 45, 47.
38  National Health Committee, *Review of Maternity Services in New Zealand*, National Health Committee, Wellington, September 1999, p. 83, https://www.moh.govt.nz/notebook/nbbooks.nsf/0/9B3D7BB224CAEC6C4C25681B006EE921/$file/mands2.pdf (accessed 25 February 2023).
39  Susannah Hill, 'Rural groups keep up fight for shared care', *NZD*, 12 April 2000.
40  Tony Fitchett, 'Viewpoint: Return to S88 recipe for obstetric disaster', ibid., 6 June 2001.
41  'Birth Notices', *HBA Auckland Newsletter*, 68, Winter/Spring 1997, pp. 19–24.
42  Male doctors were: Gulbransen, Railton, Ferguson and Leon (Lee) Nixon; Female: Alison Copland, Alison Denyer, Erica Lauder, Jackie Mills, Diana (Di) Nash and Janice (Jan) Raymond, *HBA Newsletter*, 69, Summer/Autumn 1998, p. 25. Other female GPs mentioned in *HBA Newsletters* were Lynne Coleman, Jan Singer, Margaret Karetai and Monica Yusak.

*Notes*

43   Martin Johnston, 'Dejected GP quits babies', *NZH*, 1 October 1999; Diana Nash, Foreword, in Joan Donley, *Save the Midwife*, New Women's Press, Auckland, 1986, pp. 7–9.
44   *HBA Auckland Newsletter*, 36, June 1987, p. 5.
45   Susannah Hill, 'Conference: Where to from here?', *NZD*, 21 November 2001.
46   On this closure see Linda Bryder, *The Rise and Fall of National Women's Hospital*, Auckland University Press, Auckland, 2014, pp. 231–33.
47   Margaret Shanks, 'Mothers in for shock giving birth', *NZH*, 18 September 2003, p. A15.
48   Liane Topham-Kindley, 'Two southern GPOs throw in the towel', *NZD*, 20 October 2004, p. 2.
49   Carroll Du Chateau, 'Sweet William's bitter choice: One of few remaining GPs handling deliveries quits', *NZH*, 19 November 2005, online 18 November 2005, https://www.nzherald.co.nz/nz/one-of-few-remaining-gps-handling-deliveries-quits/SK247S24W7FZHT5D4UCIKZLRBU/
50   Bruce Ansley, 'Another unfortunate experiment?', *New Zealand Listener*, 14 August 1999, p. 21; Ansley, 'Babes at risk', p. 22.
51   Martin Johnston, 'Doctors drop out of baby business', *NZH*, 30 September 1999.
52   Guilliland, 'Section 51: Contract for Autonomy', p. 6.
53   Penny St John, 'Patients dissatisfied with new maternity system', *NZD*, 12 November 1997.
54   Karen Guilliland, 'National Directors Forum', *New Zealand College of Midwives National Newsletter*, 7, December 1997, p. 8.
55   Catherine Masters, 'Squalling loudest before the birth', *NZH*, 18 November 1998.
56   Exton, *Baby Business*, p. 143.
57   Bartholomew, 'The Realities of Choice and Access', pp. 51–52.
58   Bryder, *The Rise and Fall*, p. 216.
59   Lynda Williams, 'Charging women not answer to maternity', *NZD*, 26 May 1999.
60   Lynda Williams, 'Mothers missing out in maternity negotiations', ibid., 30 April 1997.
61   'News, Petition for postnatal care', ibid., 20 August 1997; see also Kathy Glasgow, 'Maternity "Shambles"', *New Zealand Health Review*, vol. 1, 1, Autumn 1998, pp. 9–12.
62   Kareen Floyd, 'Postnatal ability goes unrewarded', *NZD*, 29 April 1998.
63   Catherine Masters, 'How did the government's maternity services scheme get so out of control?', *NZH*, 18 November 1998.
64   Andrew Laxon, 'News review: Women hurt in maternity care crossfire', *NZH Sunday*, 12 August 1997, A11.
65   Susannah Hill, 'GPOs drop out at increasing rates', *NZD*, 12 May 1999.
66   New Zealand General Practitioners' Association, 'Maternity Survey Proof of Lost Services', *GP Focus: The Newsletter of the New Zealand General Practitioners' Association*, 1997; Susannah Hill, 'News: Fleeing in droves from maternity', *NZD*, 10 December 1997.
67   Williams, 'Charging women not answer to maternity'.

68   Peter Dukes, 'Letter to the editor: NZMA on the case with maternity', *NZD*, 23 June 1999.
69   Martin Johnston, 'News review: Maternity system has many admirers', *NZH*, 30 April 1999, A11.
70   Susannah Hill, 'Maternity recalled', *NZD*, 8 December 1999.
71   National Health Committee, *Review of Maternity Services*, pp. 6, 18.
72   Ibid., pp. 87–89.
73   Hill, 'Maternity recalled'.
74   Sandra Coney, 'Focus: Creech milking risky scheme', *Sunday Star-Times*, 10 October 1999, C4; Maggie Barry, 'Letter to the editor: Coney's columns', ibid., 24 October 1999.
75   National Health Committee, *Review of Maternity Services*, p. 87.
76   Ibid., pp. 6, 33.
77   Ibid., pp. 7, 54.
78   Ibid., p. 33.
79   Ibid., p. ii.
80   Ibid., p. 102.
81   Ibid., pp. 9, 69; Susannah Hill, 'Professions united in report condemnation', *NZD*, 13 October 1999.
82   National Health Committee, *Review of Maternity Services*, pp. 82, 83.
83   Martin Johnston, 'Doctors drop out of baby business', *NZH*, 30 September 1999.
84   Cited in Exton, *Baby Business*, p. 98.
85   Susannah Hill, 'Obstetrics delivers for committed GPOs: Profile', *NZD*, 29 August 2001; Staff Reporters (SR), 'Rationale for closing non S88 deals flawed', ibid., 23 May 2001.
86   Barbara Fountain, 'Well, you asked HFA, November 2000, 2000; Maternity Services: A Reference Document, November 2000 HFA, pp. 8, 16, 17, 36, 42, 50, 57; SR, 'Rationale for closing non S88 deals flawed', *NZD*, 23 May 2000.
87   'MATPRO encouraged by Health Minister's endorsement', *Scoop*, 9 March 2001, https://www.scoop.co.nz/stories/PO0103/S00040.htm; Susannah Hill, 'NZCOM seeks "equity"', *NZD*, 23 May 2001; Barbara Fountain, 'Editorial: Victims of their success' and Susannah Hill, 'MP attacks MOH', ibid.,, 23 May 2001.
88   Kerry Prendergast, 'New Section 88 move keeps group guessing', *NZD*, 15 August 2001.
89   Rodenburg, in Fenwicke, *In Practice*, p. 118.
90   SR, 'LMC shortage grows', *NZD*, 13 February 2002; St John, 'News brief', ibid., 28 July 2004; Review of the Quality, Safety and Management of Maternity Services in the Wellington Area, Commissioned by the Ministry of Health, October 2008, p. 44, https://www.health.govt.nz/system/files/documents/publications/maternity-services-review-oct08-v2.pdf (accessed 25 February 2023).
91   Rodenburg, in Fenwicke, *In Practice*, p. 118.
92   Exton, *Baby Business*, p. 104.
93   IPAs were GP collectives, set up around the country from 1993 following health reforms relating to budget-holding, with about 30 in existence by

1999: Laurence Malcolm and Nicholas Mays, 'New Zealand's Independent Practitioner Associations: A Working Model of Clinical Governance in Primary Care?', *British Medical Journal*, vol. 319, 7221, 20 November 1999, pp. 1340–42, doi: 10.1136/bmj.319.7221.1340

94   Susannah Hill, 'Larger schemes under threat from S51 move', *NZD*, 29 March 2000.
95   Susannah Hill, 'News: GPOs launch daring plan', ibid., 20 December 2000.
96   Liane Topham-Kindley, 'Southern maternity scheme a lifesaver', ibid., 28 February 2001.
97   Fountain, 'Editorial: Victims of their success'.
98   Hill, 'NZCOM seeks "equity"'.
99   SR, 'Rationale for closing non S88 deals flawed', ibid.
100  Karine Baker, Letter to the editor, 'Stats challenge prevailing birth care ideology', ibid., 19 December 2001.
101  William Ferguson, Letter to the editor, 'Ministry should reveal agenda against GPs', ibid., 6 June 2001.
102  Hill, 'GPOs launch daring plan'; A .E. J. Fitchett, Letter to the editor, 'Ideology deals blow to GPOs', ibid., 31 January 2001.
103  Fitchett, 'Viewpoint'.
104  Blanchette, 'The Changing Landscape', pp. 144, 145.
105  Susannah Hill, 'Where to from here?: Conference', *NZD*, 21 November 2001.
106  Susannah Hill, 'Women should be told choice isn't cheap', ibid., 26 September 2001.
107  Exton, *Baby Business*, p. 93.
108  Blanchette, 'The Changing Landscape', p. 139.
109  Penny St John, 'Major maternity risks still going unheeded', *NZD*, 19 July 2000.
110  Amanda Sheddan, 'Maternal mental health stretched', ibid., 30 August 2000.
111  Annette King, 'Guest Editorial', *NZCOMJ*, vol. 25, October 2001, p. 5.
112  Exton, *Baby Business*, pp. 105, 107.
113  'Feature: King for 1804 days', *NZD*, 17 November 2004, p. 10.
114  Greg Meylan, 'PHO casts cloud over the Hokianga', ibid., 25 February 2004.
115  National Health Committee, *Review of Maternity Services*, p. 68.
116  Christine Elizabeth O'Rourke Hendry, 'Midwifery in New Zealand 1990–2003: The Complexities of Service Provision', Doctor of Midwifery thesis, University of Technology Sydney, 2003, pp. 190, 200, 206; Sally Pairman, 'Developing & Crafting a Vision: A Strategic Plan for Midwifery', *NZCOMJ*, vol. 18, April 1998, p. 9; Chris Hendry and Karen Guilliland, 'The Midwifery and Maternity Providers Organisation: A Strategy for Future-proofing Midwifery in New Zealand', in Karen Guilliland and Sally Pairman, *Women's Business: The Story of the New Zealand College of Midwives, 1986–2010*, New Zealand College of Midwives, Christchurch, 2010, pp. 427–34.
117  Karen Guilliland, Sally K. Tracy and Carol Thorogood, 'Australian and New Zealand Health and Maternity Services', in Sally Pairman, Jan Pincombe,

Carol Thorogood and Sally Tracy (eds), *Midwifery: Preparation for Practice*, Churchill Livingstone Elsevier, Marrickville NSW, 2006, p. 15.
118 Liane Topham-Kindley, 'Maternity pilots call for GP midwife teams', *NZD*, 28 March 2001.
119 Liane Topham-Kindley, 'Oamaru GPOs throw in towel', ibid., 10 October 2001.
120 Susannah Hill, 'New mothers' group supports co-payment', ibid., 23 October 2002.
121 Rodenburg, in Fenwicke, *In Practice*, p. 119.
122 Jon Gadsby, 'Broken Dolls', *Avenues*, September 2004, pp. 17–31; cited in Exton, *Baby Business*, p. 129.
123 Susannah Hill, 'Big wail at Gadsby over maternity', *NZD*, 3 November 2004, p. 4.
124 SR, 'Wairarapa women keen to keep GPOs', ibid., 9 March 2005, p. 9.
125 Rodenburg, in Fenwicke, *In Practice*, pp. 117–18.
126 Du Chateau, 'One of few remaining GPs handling deliveries quits'; Liane Topham-Kindley, 'Never say die: GPOs meet for CME talks', *NZD*, 6 October 2004, p. 9.
127 William Ferguson, 'Letter to the editor: Minister misunderstands demise of GPOs', ibid., 11 August 2004, p. 19.
128 Claire Sweetman, 'Safe Deliveries? A Review of New Zealand's Midwifery Regulation Through the Lens of the Health and Disability Commissioner', Laws 513 – Law and Medicine Research Paper, Faculty of Law, Victoria University of Wellington, 2013, p. 27.
129 Chrystal Jaye, Zara Mason and Dawn Miller, '"Tossing Out the Baby with the Bath Water": New Zealand General Practitioners on Maternity Care', *Medical Anthropology*, vol. 32, 5, 2013, pp. 448–66; Lucy Ratcliffe, 'Still catching babies: Last of the GPOs', *NZD*, 14 August 2013, pp. 8–9; see also Hanna Preston and Dawn Miller, 'Final-year Medical Students' Perceptions of Maternity Care in General Practice', *New Zealand Medical Journal*, vol. 125, 1352, March 2012, pp. 39–47.
130 Jacqueline Wolf, *Deliver Me from Pain: Anaesthesia and Birth in America*, Johns Hopkins University Press, Baltimore, 2009, p. 193.
131 Malatest International Consulting and Advisory Services, 'Report: Comparative Study of Maternity Systems, Prepared for the Ministry of Health', November 2012, pp. 62, 97, 98, https://www.health.govt.nz/system/files/documents/publications/comparative-study-of-maternity-systems-nov13.pdf (accessed 25 February 2023).
132 Hendry, 'Midwifery in New Zealand', pp. 102, 135.
133 Susannah Hill, 'NZMA to help Kaipara win maternity services', *NZD*, 29 September 1999.
134 Malatest International, 'Report', pp. 62, 97, 98.
135 Susannah Hill, 'NZ loses skilled O&G to Middle East perks', *NZD*, 3 July 2002.
136 Blanchette, 'The Changing Landscape', pp. 147, 148.
137 Ibid., pp. 145, 148.
138 Anne-Marie Boxall and Kathy Flitcroft, 'Debate: Open Access: From Little Things, Big Things Grow: A Local Approach to System-wide Maternity Services

Reform in the Absence of Definitive Evidence', *Australia and New Zealand Health Policy*, vol. 4, 18, 2007, doi:10.1186/1743-8462-4-18
139 Susannah Hill, 'Consensus reached on rural maternity rights', *NZD*, 20 December 2000; Susannah Hill, 'Rural message to doctor', ibid., 31 January 2001.
140 Liane Topham-Kindley, 'Midwife shortage hard on rural women', ibid., 10 March 2004.
141 Liane Topham-Kindley, 'Rural maternity plight investigated', ibid., 11 August 2004, p. 8.
142 Don Simmers, 'The Few: New Zealand's Diminishing Number of Rural GPs Providing Maternity Services', *New Zealand Medical Journal*, vol. 119, 1241, September 2006, pp. 1–3, U2151.
143 Ibid.
144 Chris Hendry, 'Report on Mapping the Rural Midwifery Workforce in New Zealand for 2008', *NZCOMJ*, vol. 41, October 2009, pp. 12–19.
145 Ibid., p. 13.
146 Ibid., pp. 14–15, 18.
147 *Improving Maternity Services in Australia: The Report of the Maternity Services Review*, Department of Health, Commonwealth of Australia, February 2009, p. 43.
148 Leonie Howie and Adele Robertson, *Island Nurses: Stories of Birth, Life and Death on Remote Great Barrier Island*, Allen & Unwin, Auckland, 2017.
149 Adele M. Robertson, 'Rural Women and Maternity Services', in Jean Ross (ed.), *Rural Nursing: Aspects of Practice*, Rural Health Opportunities, Ministry of Health, Dunedin, 2008, pp. 179–200, https://www.health.govt.nz/system/files/documents/publications/rural-nursing-aspects-of-practice-mar08.pdf (accessed 25 February 2023).
150 Liane Topham-Kindley, 'Midwife shortage hard on rural women', *NZD*, 10 March 2004.
151 Malatest International, 'Report', pp. 79, 80.
152 'Delivery "botch-up" claim examined', *NZH*, 15 March 2001, https://www.nzherald.co.nz/nz/delivery-botch-up-claim-examined/X4MYSZ5PQIPK4GYNDQOCX6N76Q/
153 Penny St John, 'Major maternity risks still going unheeded', *NZD*, 19 July 2000.
154 'Maternity Services: A Reference Document', November 2000, p. 64.
155 Liane Topham-Kindley, 'Conference: Midwifery referrals in line with norm', *NZD*, 28 July 2004, p. 12.
156 Lucy Ratcliffe, 'Still catching babies: Last of the GPOs', ibid., 14 August 2013, p. 9.

## CHAPTER 9: *The practice of midwifery and the 'midwifery model' in the 1990s*

1 Irene Calvert, *Birth in Focus: Midwifery in Aotearoa*, Dunmore Press, Palmerston North, 1998, p. 12.
2 Joan Donley, 'Political Comment: Protocols?', *New Zealand College of Midwives Journal (NZCOMJ)*, vol. 7, December 1992, p. 10.
3 Cate Brett, 'Midwife crisis', *HQ Magazine*, March/April 1996, p. 86.

4   David McLoughlin, 'The politics of childbirth: Midwives versus doctors', *North & South*, August 1993, p. 66.
5   Karen Guilliland, 'Midwifery in New Zealand', paper presented at the Future Birth: The Place to be Born Conference, Australia, February 1999, *Birth International*, https://birthinternational.com/midwifery-in-new-zealand/ (accessed 2 March 2023).
6   Ibid.
7   'NZCOM Position Statement: Ultrasound', *NZCOMJ*, vol. 5, October 1991, p. 12; Karen Guilliland, 'National Directors Forum', *New Zealand College of Midwives National Newsletter*, November/December 1997, p. 9.
8   Reported in Wan Tinn and Stephen Tong, 'Intrapartum Fetal Monitoring: Yesterday, Today and Tomorrow', *O&G Magazine*, vol. 11, 4, Summer 2009, p. 36.
9   McLoughlin, 'The politics of childbirth', p. 66.
10  Sally Abel, 'Midwifery and Maternity Services in Transition: An Examination of Change Following the Nurses Amendment Act 1990', PhD thesis, University of Auckland, 1997, pp. 133–34.
11  Ibid.
12  Mark Henaghan, *Health Professionals and Trust: The Cure for Healthcare Law and Policy*, Routledge-Cavendish, London, 2011, p. 89.
13  Ibid.; see also Abel, 'Midwifery and Maternity Services in Transition', p. 135.
14  McLoughlin, 'The politics of childbirth', p. 66; Adelia Ferguson, 'Babies dying for need of proper care says doctor', *New Zealand Herald (NZH)*, 3 January 1995.
15  Karen Guilliland, 'Birthing: Danger in "mindless activity"', *NZH*, 26 January 1995.
16  Hilda Bastian, Marc J. N. C. Keirse and Paul A. Lancaster, 'Perinatal Death Associated with Planned Home Birth in Australia: Population Based Study', *British Medical Journal*, vol. 317, 7155, 8 August 1998, pp. 384–88, doi: 10.1136/bmj.317.7155.384
17  'Pressure on midwives', *Sunday News*, 9 February 1997.
18  'Concern over birth rules', *NZH*, 17 June 1995, section 1, p. 16; *Home Birth Association (HBA) Auckland Newsletter*, 64, Winter/Spring 1995, p. 32.
19  Ibid., p. 33.
20  Brett, 'Midwife crisis', p. 89.
21  Karen Guilliland, Sally K. Tracy and Carol Thorogood, 'Australian and New Zealand Health and Maternity Services', in Sally Pairman, Jan Pincombe, Carol Thorogood and Sally Tracy (eds), *Midwifery: Preparation for Practice*, Churchill Livingstone Elsevier, Marrickville NSW, 2006, p. 17.
22  Stephen Robson, 'Attempting Vaginal Birth After a Previous Caesarean Section: How Should We Counsel Women and Their Families?', *O&G Magazine* vol. 12, 2, Winter 2010, pp. 23, 25.
23  Nick Smith, 'Specialists push mother's choice', *NZH*, 8 December 1998, A16; see also Nicky Leap and Sally Pairman, 'Working in Partnership', in Pairman et al. (eds), *Midwifery: Preparation for Practice*, p. 264.
24  Maggie Banks, 'Breech Birth Women-wise', *NZCOMJ*, vol. 15, October 1996, pp. 17–19.

25 Ina May Gaskin, *Spiritual Midwifery*, The Book Publishing Co., The Farm, Summertown, Tennessee, rev. edn, 1978, pp. 325, 395.
26 Banks, 'Breech Birth Women-wise', p. 19; Maggie Banks, *Breech Birth Woman-Wise*, Birthspirit Books, Hamilton, 1998, p. 49.
27 Maggie Banks, 'Out on a Limb: The Personal Mandate to Practise Midwifery by Midwives of the Domiciliary Midwives Society of New Zealand (Incorporated), 1974–1986', PhD thesis, Victoria University of Wellington, 2007, p. 18.
28 Inquest into the death of Isabell Grace Riddell 970506 Hamilton District Coroner 24 April 1997; Rhonda Powell, Shawn Walker and Alison Barrett, 'Informed Consent to Breech Birth in New Zealand', *New Zealand Medical Journal*, vol. 128, 1418, 24 July 2015, pp. 85–92; Henaghan, *Health Professionals and Trust*, p. 92.
29 Banks, *Breech Birth Woman-Wise*, p. 50.
30 Sian Burgess, 'Commentary on: Practice Wisdom', *NZCOMJ*, vol. 30, April 2004, p. 5. (Burgess did, however, critique Banks's guidelines on fetal heart monitoring: see above, p. 223).
31 Karen Guilliland, 'Midwifery Autonomy in New Zealand: How Has It Influenced Birth Outcomes of New Zealand Women?', ibid., 23, January 2001, p. 7.
32 Guilliland, Tracy and Thorogood, 'Australian and New Zealand Health and Maternity Services', p. 15.
33 Celia P. Grigg, Sally K. Tracy, Mark Tracy, Virginia Schmied and Amy Monk, 'Transfer from Primary Maternity Unit to Tertiary Hospital in New Zealand – Timing, Frequency, Reasons, Urgency and Outcomes: Part of the Evaluating Maternity Units Study', *Midwifery*, vol. 31, September 2015, pp. 879–87.
34 'Birth system dangerous says expert', *NZH*, 20 December 1997; 'Broken dad's anguish: Coroner calls for shake-up', *Sunday Star-Times*, 5 April 1998.
35 Sarah Catherall, 'Maternity death worries', *Sunday Star-Times*, 12 April 1998.
36 Ibid.
37 'Birth allegation', *NZH*, 2 April 1988; 'Midwife to pay', ibid., 27 April 1998; 'Striking off midwife "exceptionally harsh"', ibid., 28 May 1998.
38 Guilliland, 'National Directors Forum', p. 9.
39 Penny St John, 'O&Gs say bye bye baby', *New Zealand Doctor (NZD)*, 27 September 2000.
40 Deborah Earl, Eileen Gibson, Trish Isa, Judith McAra-Couper, Betty McGregor and Helen Thwaites, 'Core Midwifery: The Challenge Continues', *NZCOMJ*, vol. 27, October 2002, p. 30.
41 Ibid.
42 Evan J. Begg, Senior Lecturer in Clinical Pharmacology, Christchurch School of Medicine, and President ASCEP NZ, to Simon Upton, Minister of Health, 30 November 1990; also J.A. Millar, Senior Lecturer in Clinical Pharmacology, University of Otago, to Katherine O'Regan, 28 November 1990, and response, 22 January 1991, and Helen McKinnon, President, NZ Hospital Pharmacists' Association, to Simon Upton, 16 November 1990, R21935510, 1990-1991, 80, W67/NUR/2, 68956, Archives New Zealand Wellington (ANZW).

43  Judi Strid to Simon Upton, 26 December 1990, R21935510, ANZW.
44  Department of Health, Nurses Amendment Act: Information for health providers, Wellington, October 1990, R21935510, ANZW.
45  Marion Hunter and Jackie Gunn, 'Pharmacology and Prescribing', in Pairman et al. (eds), *Midwifery: Preparation for Practice*, p. 525.
46  Ibid.
47  Ibid., pp. 525, 530, 540.
48  Marie E. Burgess, *A Guide to the Law for Nurses and Midwives*, Pearson Education New Zealand, Auckland, 4th edn, 2008, p. 158.
49  Karen Guilliland and Sally Pairman, 'Midwifery Education – A National Perspective, the New Zealand College of Midwives (continued from page 6)', *NZCOMJ*, vol. 4, May 1991, p. 15.
50  Ibid., p. 5.
51  Sally Pairman, Editorial, ibid., vol. 11, October 1994, p. 4.
52  Lynda Exton, *The Baby Business: What's Happened to Maternity Care in New Zealand?*, Craig Potton Publishing, Nelson, 2008, p. 130.
53  Sally Pairman, 'Education Framework, November 1999', *NZCOMJ*, vol. 22, June 2000, p. 9; Sally Pairman, 'From Autonomy and Back Again: Educating Midwives Across a Century, Part 2', ibid., vol. 34, April 2006, p. 14.
54  Jackie Gunn, 'Diploma in Midwifery (3 year Direct Entry) Auckland', ibid., *vol.* 6, June 1992, p. 6; Joan Donley, 'Political Comment: Direct Entry Midwifery (DEM)', ibid., vol. 6, June 1992, p. 10.
55  Sally Pairman, 'Diploma in Midwifery (3 year Direct Entry) Otago', ibid., *vol.* 6, June 1992, p. 7.
56  New Zealand Nurses and Midwives 2000, Table 21, p. 33, New Zealand Health Information Service, May 2002, Ministry of Health, https://www.moh.govt.nz/notebook/nbbooks.nsf/0/7f63f6c0628f96994c25686d0007423b/$FILE/nurses2000.pdf (accessed 2 March 2023).
57  Sally Pairman, 'Direct Entry Midwifery', *NZCOMJ*, vol. 11, October 1994, p. 26.
58  Ibid.
59  Karen Lane, 'Understanding World Views for Midwifery', in Pairman et al. (eds), *Midwifery: Preparation for Practice*, pp. 48–60.
60  Sally Pairman, 'Developing & Crafting a Vision: A Strategic Plan for Midwifery', *NZCOMJ*, vol. 18, April 1998, p. 9.
61  Pairman et al. (eds), *Midwifery: Preparation for Practice*: Part A: Partners, pp. 3–223, and Part B: Practice, Section one: Partnership, pp. 237–80.
62  Sally Pairman, 'Partnership Revisited: Towards Midwifery Theory', *NZCOMJ*, vol. 21, October 1999, p. 6.
63  Exton, *Baby Business*, pp. 46–47.
64  Pairman, 'Diploma in Midwifery', 1992, p. 7.
65  Pairman, 'Direct Entry Midwifery', 1994, p. 26.
66  Bronwen Pelvin, 'Life Skills for Midwifery Practice', in Pairman et al. (eds), *Midwifery: Preparation for Practice*, p. 234; Sally Pairman and Judith McAra-Couper, 'Theoretical Frameworks for Midwifery Practice', in Pairman et al., *Midwifery: Preparation for Practice*, p. 255.

67  Rosemary Methven, review of Caroline Flint, *Sensitive Midwifery*, in *Midwifery*, vol. 3, 1987, p. 101.
68  Bronwyn Hegarty and Zab Frankin, 'How Useful Is Bioscience Knowledge in Midwifery and Is It Necessary for Safe Practice?', *NZCOMJ*, vol. 14, April 1996, pp. 7–9.
69  Abel, 'Midwifery and Maternity Services in Transition', p. 258.
70  See comments by Wellington Area Review in Chapter 11, above, p. 234.
71  Dawn Holland, 'Practice Wisdom: Mentoring – A Personal Analysis', *NZCOMJ*, vol. 23, January 2001, p. 17.
72  Ibid., p. 15.
73  Pairman, 'Direct Entry Midwifery', 1994, p. 26.
74  New Zealand Nurses and Midwives 2000, Table 23, pp. 34, 35.
75  'Student faces suspension over baby', *Sunday Star-Times*, 27 June 1999.
76  Diana Nash, 'Foreword', in Joan Donley, *Save the Midwife*, New Women's Press, Auckland, 1986, p. 8.
77  Abel, 'Midwifery and Maternity Services in Transition', p. 259. In contrast, Guilliland and Pairman claimed in 2010 there were 72 Māori midwives in 1994: Karen Guilliland and Sally Pairman, *Women's Business: The Story of the New Zealand College of Midwives, 1986–2010*, New Zealand College of Midwives, Christchurch, 2010, p. 206.
78  New Zealand Nurses and Midwives 2000, Tables 22 and 23, p. 34.
79  Abel, 'Midwifery and Maternity Services in Transition', p. 260.
80  Hope Tupara, 'Meeting the Needs of Māori Women: The Challenge for Midwifery Education', *NZCOMJ*, vol. 25, October 2001, p. 7.
81  Elaine Papps and Irihapeti Ramsden, 'Cultural Safety in Nursing: The New Zealand Experience', *International Journal for Quality in Health Care*, vol. 8, 5, October 1996, pp. 491–97; Tupara, 'Meeting the Needs of Māori Women', p. 7.
82  Irihapeti Merenia Ramsden, 'Cultural Safety and Nursing Education in Aotearoa and Te Waipounamu', PhD thesis, Victoria University of Wellington, 2002.
83  Anne Barlow, 'Evaluation of Educational Aspects of NZCOM: Standards Review Process', *NZCOMJ*, vol. 24, April 2001, p. 15. The Tohunga Suppression Act was passed in 1907.
84  Lis Ellison-Loschmann, Letter to the editor, *NZCOMJ*, vol. 25, October 2001, p. 38; Irihapeti Ramsden, 'Improving Practice Through Research', *Kai Tiaki: Nursing New Zealand*, vol. 7, 2001, pp. 23–26.
85  Report of Committee of Inquiry into Maternity Services, *Appendices to the Journals of the House of Representatives (AJHR)*, H31A, 1938, p. 96. See also Linda Bryder, 'They do what you wish; they like you; you the good nurse!': Colonialism and Native Health Nursing in New Zealand, 1900–1940', in Helen Sweet and Sue Hawkins (eds), *Colonial Caring: A History of Colonial and Post-colonial Nursing*, Manchester University Press, Manchester, 2015, pp. 96–97.
86  Anne Barlow, Letter to the editor, *NZCOMJ*, vol. 25, October 2001, p. 38.
87  Pamela Wood, 'Guest Editorial', ibid., vol. 31, October 2004, p. 4.
88  Pairman, 'From Autonomy and Back Again, p. 4.

89   Christina A. Jeffery, 'Whanautanga: The Experiences of Māori Women Who Gave Birth at National Women's Hospital 1958–2004', MA thesis, University of Auckland, 2005, p. 87.
90   Donley, *Save the Midwife*, p. 124.
91   Tupara, 'Meeting the Needs of Māori Women', pp. 6–9.
92   Reena Kainamu, 'Students' Corner: E Mahara Ana Te Whanau The Family Remembers', *NZCOMJ*, vol. 23, January 2001, pp. 24–26.
93   Sally K. Tracy and Suzanne Miller, 'Working in Collaboration', in Pairman et al. (eds), *Midwifery: Preparation for Practice*, p. 273.
94   She referenced this to a 1981 letter she had received from a UK homebirth society. Joan Donley, 'Ultrasound Use in New Zealand', *NZCOMJ*, vol. 3, November 1990, pp. 19–21.
95   *HBA Newsletter*, 47, Winter 1990, p. 3; Joan Donley, 'Women in Partnership', *Broadsheet*, 182, October 1990, p. 7; NZCOM, 'Position Statement: Ultrasound', *NZCOMJ*, vol. 5, October 1991, p. 12.
96   Suzanne Hope Suarez, 'Midwifery Is Not the Practice of Medicine', *Yale Journal of Law and Feminism*, vol. 5, 1993, p. 339.
97   *HBA Auckland Newsletter*, 62, Spring 1994, pp. 28, 30; 'From the Newspapers: NZH, 11 December 2001', *Maternity Services Consumer Council Newsletter*, 45, December 2001.
98   Malcolm Nicolson and John E. E. Fleming, *Imaging and Imagining the Fetus: The Development of Obstetric Ultrasound*, Johns Hopkins University Press, Baltimore, 2013, p. 260.
99   Joan Donley, 'Political Comment: Routine Pregnancy Testing', *NZCOMJ*, vol. 14, April 1996, p. 13.
100  Caroline de Costa, *The Women's Doc: True Stories from My Five Decades Delivering Babies and Making History*, Allen & Unwin, Sydney, 2021, pp. 186, 189–90.
101  Adelia Ferguson, 'Babies dying for need of proper care says doctor', *NZH*, 3 January 1995.
102  Transcript of interview of Joan Donley by Sally Abel, 6 July 1994, p. 7, Joan Donley Papers, MSS & Archives, 2007/15, 1638, Manuscripts and Archives, University of Auckland Library (JDP).
103  Abel, 'Midwifery and Maternity Services in Transition', p. 127.
104  *HBA Auckland Newsletter*, 54, Winter 1992, p. 12; ibid., 64, Winter/Spring 1995, p. 6.
105  Transcript of interview of Donley by Abel, p. 7, JDP.
106  'A Consensus Statement Vitamin K Prophylaxis in the Newborn', *NZCOMJ*, vol. 23, January 2001, pp. 33–34 (underlining in the original).
107  Amanda Cropp, 'Who will deliver your baby?', *Next*, September 2000, p. 100; Administration of Vitamin K to newborn baby, HDC Decision 11HDC00957, 10 June 2013, pp. 1, 7, https://www.hdc.org.nz/decisions/search-decisions/2013/11hdc00957/
108  Yvonne Zurynski, Cameron J. Grover, Bin Jalaludin and Elizabeth J. Elliott, 'Vitamin K Deficiency Bleeding in Australian Infants 1993–2017: An Australian

Paediatric Surveillance Unit Study', *Archives of Disease in Childhood*, vol. 105, 5, 2006, https://adc.bmj.com/content/105/5/433

109   See, for example, *HBA Auckland Newsletter*, 64, Winter/Spring 1995, p. 29; ibid., 69, Summer/Autumn 1998, p. 36.

110   Robert Strecker video, ibid., 56, Summer 1992–93, inside front cover.

111   'Vaccinations: A Guide to Healthy Pregnancy, Auckland HBA 1993', reprint, ibid., 61, Winter 1994, pp. 5–9.

112   'Mandatory Choice for Vaccination becomes a reality for N.Z.', ibid., 63, Summer/Autumn 1995, p. 23.

113   Joan Donley 'Immunisation', *NZCOMJ*, vol. 11, October 1994, p. 15.

114   Ibid., pp. 14–15.

115   Advertisement: 'International Symposium', ibid., p. 15.

116   Gillian Durham, 'Immunisation', ibid., vol. 12, April 1995, p. 13.

117   Donley, 'Response', ibid., pp. 14–15.

118   Karen Guilliland, 'College Response' and 'Editor's Note', ibid., pp. 15, 27.

119   *NZCOM National Newsletter*, June/July 1995, pp. 42–46 (her disclaimer was on the back inside cover, Wise Woman Archives Trust Inc. (WWAT), http://wwat.nz/wp-content/uploads/20061-1995JunJul.pdf (accessed 2 March 2023). On the conference details and report, see also MSS & Archives 2007/15, 7/1/A/1 Part 2, JDP.

120   Erwin Alber, Letter to the editor, 'Vaccination Information', *NZCOMJ*, vol. 13, October 1995, p. 5.

121   See Bruce Hamilton, 'Williams, Ulric Gaster', *Dictionary of New Zealand Biography, Te Ara – the Encyclopedia of New Zealand*, https://teara.govt.nz/en/biographies/4w19/williams-ulric-gaster (accessed 2 March 2023). On Erwin Alber, see also http://encyclopediaantivaccinemovement.blogspot.com/2014/01/erwin-alber.html (accessed 2 March 2023).

122   'Audio Tape Review', *NZCOMJ*, vol. 13, October 1995, p. 26.

123   Erwin Alber, Letter to the editor, 'Vaccination Awareness', ibid., vol. 14, April 1996, pp. 4, 28.

124   Erwin Alber, 'A Travel Report and a Look at Vaccination', ibid., p. 22.

125   Erwin Alber, Letter to the editor, 'Vaccination Awareness', ibid., vol. 15, October 1996, p. 4; Department of Nursing and Midwifery, Otago Polytechnic, Letter to the editor, 'Receipt of Book', ibid., p. 19.

126   Orma Bradfield, 'Book Review, Neil Z. Miller', ibid., p. 24.

127   Alber to Guilliland, 10 November 1999, MSS & Archives 2007/15, 4, 2/6/B/1 Part 1, JDP.

128   Guilliland to Alber, 25 November 1999, MSS & Archives 2007/15, 4, 2/6/B/1 Part 1, JDP (underlining in the original).

129   Erwin Alber, Letter to the editor, 'The Female Principle', *NZCOMJ*, vol. 22, June 2000, p. 4.

130   Teresa Cameron, Letter to the editor, ibid., vol. 23, January 2001, p. 30.

131   Elaine Boyd and Coralie Zimmer, Letters to the editor, ibid., p. 31.

132   Susannah Hill, 'NZMA to help Kaipara win maternity services', *NZD*, 29 September 1999.

133  National Health Committee, *Review of Maternity Services in New Zealand*, National Health Committee, Wellington, September 1999, pp. 6, 14, 27, 35, https://www.moh.govt.nz/notebook/nbbooks.nsf/0/9B3D7BB224CAEC6C4C25681B006EE921/$file/mands2.pdf (accessed 2 March 2023).
134  Sally Pairman, in Halina Ogonowska-Coates, *Born: Midwives and Women Celebrate 100 Years*, New Zealand College of Midwives, Christchurch, 2004, p. 66.

## CHAPTER 10: *The new century: 'When things go wrong'*

1  Helen Newnham and Jackie Pearse, 'Legal Frameworks for Practice in Australia and New Zealand', in Sally Pairman, Jan Pincombe, Carol Thorogood, Sally Tracy (eds), *Midwifery: Preparation for Practice*, Churchill Livingstone Elsevier, Marrickville NSW, 2006, pp. 195–96.
2  Te Tatau o te Whare Kahu Midwifery Council, 'Competencies for Entry to the Register of Midwives', 2007, https://www.midwiferycouncil.health.nz/common/Uploaded%20files/Midwifery%20Leaders/Competencies%20for%20Entry%20to%20the%20register%20of%20Midwives%202007.pdf (accessed 3 March 2023).
3  Marie E. Burgess, *A Guide to the Law for Nurses and Midwives*, Pearson Education New Zealand, Auckland, 4th edn, 2008, p. 99.
4  Martin Johnston and Natalie Akoorie, 'Babies' deaths reignite maternity row', *Weekend Herald*, 23 June 2012, p. A22, https://www.nzherald.co.nz/nz/babies-deaths-reignite-maternity-row/GDROFD7RHGC4ZGXUIHS6AULMCY/
5  'Sharron's Story', in Karen Guilliland and Sally Pairman, *Women's Business: The Story of the New Zealand College of Midwives, 1986–2010*, New Zealand College of Midwives, Christchurch, 2010, p. 195.
6  'Wellington coroner Garry Evans reflects on 18 years of sad deaths', *Dominion Post*, 12 November 2015, https://www.stuff.co.nz/dominion-post/news/73738804/wellington-coroner-garry-evans-reflects-on-18-years-of-sad-deaths
7  Donna Chisholm, 'Stand and deliver', *New Zealand Listener*, 14 February 2015, p. 20.
8  'Home birth deaths prompt call for midwifery review', *New Zealand Herald (NZH)*, 6 November 2005, https://www.nzherald.co.nz/nz/home-birth-deaths-prompt-call-for-midwifery-review/5G32M7ZQRKMY3EORMS3CRWV2JU/
9  Karen Guilliland, 'Midwifery Autonomy in New Zealand: How Has it Affected Birth Outcomes of New Zealand Women', *New Zealand College of Midwives Journal (NZCOMJ)*, vol. 23, January 2001, p. 7.
10  Perinatal and Maternal Mortality Review Committee (PMMRC), Report on Recommendation One by the Wellington Coroner resulting from two cases of perinatal death, 21 December 2005, to Pete Hodgson, AD20-82-2-1, p. 2, https://www.hqsc.govt.nz/assets/PMMRC/Publications/pmmrchealthreport.pdf

(accessed 1 February 2022); reported widely in the press: 'Home birth deaths prompt call for midwifery review', *NZH*, 6 November 2005; Martin Johnston, 'Midwives discovered babies' breech positions too late', ibid., 8 November 2005, https://www.nzherald.co.nz/nz/midwives-discovered-babies-breech-positions-too-late/WRQ66QOZXK2VFV5YK74P6Q265E/; Deborah Coddington, 'Minister acts on baby deaths report', *Herald on Sunday*, 13 November 2005, https://www.nzherald.co.nz/nz/minister-acts-on-baby-deaths-report/WAX5XAV3Z3TZO3M64VTL5CKWTQ/

11  'Home birth deaths prompt call for midwifery review', *NZH*, 6 November 2005.
12  PMMRC, Report on Recommendation One, 2005, p. 3.
13  Lynda Exton, *The Baby Business: What's Happened to Maternity Care in New Zealand?*, Craig Potton Publishing, Nelson, 2008, pp. 117–18. White's experience in homebirth is taken from her credentials listed in *NZCOMJ*, vol. 5, October 1991, p. 13.
14  Leah Haines, 'Another unfortunate experiment', *New Zealand Listener*, 31 January 2009, p. 18.
15  Ibid.
16  Maggie Banks, 'Practice Wisdom: Active Breech Birth: The Point of Least Resistance', *NZCOMJ*, vol. 36, April 2007, p. 6.
17  PMMRC, *Eighth Annual Report*, June 2014, p. 126, https://www.hqsc.govt.nz/assets/Our-work/Mortality-review-committee/PMMRC/Publications-resources/eighth-PMMRC-report-June-2014.pdf (accessed 3 March 2023).
18  Michael Bassett, 'Time to ditch patch warfare', *Press*, 22 November 2005, p. A11; Exton, *The Baby Business*, pp. 119–20.
19  Teresa O'Connor, 'Midwifery – A Workforce Under Pressure: The past 15 years have been turbulent for the midwifery profession. What's the state of play for the workforce now?', *Kai Tiaki: Nursing New Zealand*, vol. 12, 3, April 2006, p. 18.
20  'Baby death avoidable tragedy says coroner: Health – Women's Health', *Dominion Post*, 7 July 2007, https://www.pressreader.com/new-zealand/the-dominion-post/20070707/281676840501142
21  See above, Chapter 7, pp. 140–41.
22  'Coroner: Home births need two midwives', *Stuff*, 2 November 2010, http://www.stuff.co.nz/editors-picks/4299061/Coroner-Home-births-need-two-midwives; 'Call for backup after home birth death', *NZH*, 2 November 2010, https://www.nzherald.co.nz/nz/news/article.cfm?c_id=1&objectid=10684823; Helen Murdoch, 'Coroner urges backup midwives', *Press*, 3 November 2010, http://www.stuff.co.nz/national/4301071/Coroner-urges-backup-midwives
23  Karen Guilliland, Sally K. Tracy and Carol Thorogood, 'Australian and New Zealand Health and Maternity Services', in Pairman et al. (eds), *Midwifery: Preparation for Practice*, p. 15.
24  James Ihaka, 'Midwife says baby's death rare event', *NZH*, 9 February 2011, https://www.nzherald.co.nz/nz/midwife-says-babys-death-rare-event/HCTLWRAFBQ4SV6GT2BNRZ2TBLU/; 'Midwife blamed for baby's death', ibid., 8 February 2011, https://www.nzherald.co.nz/nz/midwife-blamed-for-

babys-death/2QBERIDKXG2LZPWMZD36576UOA/; 'Grieving parents push for midwifery changes', ibid., 12 February 2011, https://www.nzherald.co.nz/nz/grieving-parents-push-for-midwifery-changes/6CSXHPI7OELYFENZZ2WDEXELTM/

25  Johnston and Akoorie, 'Babies' deaths reignite maternity row'.
26  'Grieving parents push for midwifery changes'.
27  Maryanne Twentyman, 'Midwife provided "reasonable care"', 17 February 2011, *Waikato Times*, http://www.stuff.co.nz/waikato-times/4668058/Midwife-provided-reasonable-care
28  Martin Johnston, 'Tighter rules aim to stop new midwives picking up "bad habits"', *NZH*, 23 June 2012, p. A2, https://www.nzherald.co.nz/nz/tighter-rules-aim-to-stop-new-midwives-picking-up-bad-habits/LMN4VVC45QL4JD4UACAUR4LGWY/
29  Johnston and Akoorie, 'Babies' deaths reignite maternity row'; APNZ, 'Report into horrific labour released', *NZH*, 5 February 2014, https://www.nzherald.co.nz/nz/report-into-horrific-labour-released/EF7EYJHR7JLGYO7OITRF75CAGQ/
30  Johnston and Akoorie, 'Babies' deaths reignite maternity row'.
31  Ibid.
32  Maryanne Twentyman, 'Midwife's failures left off record', *Waikato Times*, 4 September 2012, http://www.stuff.co.nz/national/7604776/Midwifes-failures-left-off-record
33  Guilliland et al., 'Australian and New Zealand Health and Maternity Services', in Pairman et al. (eds), *Midwifery: Preparation for Practice*, p. 15.
34  Maryanne Twentyman, 'Charlotte eases couple's pain', *Waikato Times*, 19 July 2010, http://www.stuff.co.nz/waikato-times/news/3932452/Charlotte-eases-couples-pain
35  Natalie Akoorie, 'Dad's shock after partner and baby die', *NZH*, 24 May 2012, https://www.nzherald.co.nz/nz/dads-shock-after-partner-and-baby-die/JT5H2V2UYUYFRW7BJBABSBSEOU/
36  'Midwives' complaint not upheld', *Waikato Times*, 30 August 2012, http://www.stuff.co.nz/waikato-times/news/7575674/Midwives-complaint-not-upheld
37  'Fatal birth inquest: "I hope there's change"', *NZH*, 26 February 2014, https://www.nzherald.co.nz/nz/fatal-birth-inquest-i-hope-theres-change/S2LSGFQCAH5EHKH4VXJOEFGSYA/
38  Ibid.; 'Inquest begins into Huntly deaths', *Stuff*, 17 February 2014, http://www.stuff.co.nz/waikato-times/news/9730544/Inquest-begins-into-Huntly-deaths; Natalie Akoorie, 'Inquest into deaths of mother and newborn begin', *NZH*, 17 February 2014, https://www.nzherald.co.nz/nz/inquest-into-deaths-of-mother-and-newborn-begin/VWOE5EB6JT57KPLUJHJIYVQABY/; 'Delivery dilemma – the birthing centre debate', *Bay of Plenty Times*, 8 December 2014, https://www.nzherald.co.nz/bay-of-plenty-times/news/delivery-dilemma-the-birthing-centre-debate/YSVT7DXDKNO7BEZSSRPI3Z5NQE/

39  Belinda Feek, 'Expert midwife shocked mother "fainted"', *Waikato Times*, 25 February 2014, http://www.stuff.co.nz/waikato-times/9759003/Expert-midwife-shocked-mother-fainted.
40  Libby Wilson, 'New midwives should not lead care – coroner', *Stuff*, 30 January 2015, https://www.stuff.co.nz/national/health/65621844/new-midwives-should-not-lead-care---coroner; Chisholm, 'Stand and deliver', p. 21.
41  Wilson, 'New midwives should not lead care – coroner'; also cited in AIM Submission the Health Select Committee, Consumer concerns with the recently strengthened Midwifery First Year of Practice for new graduate midwives, 24 November 2015, p. 17, https://www.parliament.nz/resource/en-NZ/51SCHE_EVI_51DBHOH_PET66361_1_A458322/1e6c981d1f978e7e8fac593cae7ba567f092764e (accessed 3 March 2023).
42  AIM Submission to the Health Select Committee, 2015, p. 17.
43  Tony Baird, Letter to the editor, 'Death in childbirth', *New Zealand Listener*, 14 March 2015, p. 6; Rose Collins, Letter to the editor, 'Midwifery's place', ibid., 28 February 2015, p. 6.
44  Libby Wilson, Nancy EL-Gamel and Aaron Leaman, 'Mum and baby deaths: Coroner slams midwife', *Stuff*, 30 January 2015, https://www.stuff.co.nz/national/health/65621504/mum-and-baby-deaths-coroner-slams-midwife
45  Ibid.
46  Chisholm, 'Stand and deliver', p. 20.
47  Wilson, 'New midwives should not lead care – coroner'.
48  Ibid.
49  Home Birth Aotearoa, 'Media release on Coroner Report into deaths of Casey Nathan and son Kymani', 3 February 2015, https://homebirth.org.nz/media-release-on-coroner-report-into-deaths-of-casey-nathan-and-son-kymani/
50  Cited in Chisholm, 'Stand and deliver', pp. 21–22.
51  Ibid.
52  Linda Bryder, *The Rise and Fall of National Women's Hospital*, Auckland University Press, Auckland, 2014, pp. 117–41.
53  Chisholm, 'Stand and deliver', p. 22.
54  Margaret Guthrie, Letter to the editor, *New Zealand Listener*, 21 February 2015, p. 6.
55  Deb Pittam and Sue Bree, Letter to the editor, ibid., 7 March 2015, p. 6.
56  Newnham and Pearse, 'Legal Frameworks for Practice in Australia and New Zealand', in Pairman et al. (eds), *Midwifery: Preparation for Practice*, p. 198.
57  'Baby death avoidable tragedy says coroner: Health – Women's Health', *Dominion Post*, 7 July 2007, https://www.pressreader.com/new-zealand/the-dominion-post/20070707/281676840501142
58  'Report into horrific labour released'; 'Baby death brings apology', *Otago Daily Times*, 6 February 2014, https://www.odt.co.nz/news/national/baby-death-brings-apology
59  Donna Chisholm, 'Failure to deliver', *North & South*, August 2011, pp. 38–50.

60   Ibid.
61   Rosemary Godbold, 'Informed Consent and Midwifery Practice in New Zealand: Lessons from the Health and Disability Commissioner', *NZCOMJ*, vol. 42, May 2010, p. 12.
62   Ibid., p. 15; Health and Disability Commissioner (HDC) Decision 06HDC08238: 'Death of baby several hours after home birth', 2 July 2007, https://www.hdc.org.nz/decisions/search-decisions/2007/06hdc08238-decision/
63   Midwifery Council, 'Competencies for Entry to the Register of Midwives'.
64   Joan Skinner, 'Risk and Safety', in Pairman et al. (eds), *Midwifery: Preparation for Practice*, p. 66.
65   Godbold, 'Informed Consent', pp. 12–16.
66   Claire Sweetman, 'Safe Deliveries? A Review of New Zealand's Midwifery Regulation through the Lens of the Health and Disability Commissioner', Laws 513 – Law and Medicine Research Paper, Faculty of Law, Victoria University of Wellington, 2013, pp. 1, 30, https://researcharchive.vuw.ac.nz/xmlui/bitstream/handle/10063/3327/thesis.pdf?sequence=1 (accessed 3 March 2023).
67   Ibid., p. 59.
68   Ibid., p. 46.
69   Ibid., p. 30.
70   Ibid., p. 31; HDC Decision 07HDC03243, 'Inadequate documentation and standard of care during labour', 28 November 2007, https://www.hdc.org.nz/decisions/search-decisions/2007/07hdc03243-decision/, p. 17. An Apgar score is used to ascertain and record the condition of the baby, looking at colour, respiratory effort, heart rate, muscle tone and reflex response, with a maximum/optimal score of 10.
71   HDC Decision 07HDC03243, p. 23.
72   Ibid., pp. 10–11; hypoxic ischaemic encephalopathy is damage to cells in the central nervous system (the brain and spinal cord) from inadequate oxygen.
73   Sweetman, 'Safe Deliveries?' p. 35; HDC Decision 05HDC01760, 'Provision of antenatal and labour care', November 2006, https://www.hdc.org.nz/decisions/search-decisions/2006/05hdc01760-decision/; HDC Decision 10HDC00267, 'Provision of antenatal care, labour care and postnatal support', May 2012, pp. 2, 5, 8, https://www.hdc.org.nz/decisions/search-decisions/2012/10hdc00267/
74   HCD Decision 09HDC01311, 'Care and documentation relating to a woman with symptoms of pre-eclampsia', https://www.hdc.org.nz/decisions/search-decisions/2010/09hdc01311/
75   HDC Decision 11HDC00957, 'Administration of Vitamin K to newborn baby', 10 June 2013, pp. 1, 7, https://www.hdc.org.nz/decisions/search-decisions/2013/11hdc00957/
76   Ibid., pp. 1, 3; also reported in Nicole Pryor, 'Midwife fails in baby care', *Stuff*, 24 June 2013, http://www.stuff.co.nz/ipad-editors-picks/8835030/Midwife-fails-in-baby-care
77   Sweetman, 'Safe Deliveries?', p. 38; HDC Decision 00HDC08628, 'Death of baby following obstructed home labour and delayed referral to specialist

care', 30 July 2002, p. 36, https://www.hdc.org.nz/media/3798/00hdc08628-midwife.pdf
78 On Muir, see Maggie Banks, 'Out on a Limb: The Personal Mandate to Practise Midwifery by Midwives of the Domiciliary Midwives Society of New Zealand (Incorporated), 1974–1986', PhD thesis, Victoria University of Wellington, 2007, p. 125.
79 HDC Decision 00HDC08628, p. 35.
80 Sweetman, 'Safe Deliveries?', p. 38; HDC Decision 00HDC08628, pp. 34–38.
81 Ibid., p. 67.
82 Ibid., pp. 3, 36.
83 Sweetman, 'Safe Deliveries?', pp. 39, 40; Decision 06HDC18721, 'Death of baby following prolonged pregnancy', 14 May 2008, https://www.hdc.org.nz/media/1880/06hdc18721midwife.pdf
84 Ibid., p. 9.
85 Ibid., p. 29.
86 Ibid., p. 9.
87 Nicky Leap and Sally Pairman, 'Working in Partnership', in Pairman et al. (eds), *Midwifery: Preparation for Practice*, p. 263.
88 HDC Decision 06HDC18721, pp. 6, 7.
89 Ibid., Addendum, pp. 37–38.
90 Sweetman, 'Safe Deliveries?', pp. 40–41; HDC Decision 07HDC15908, 'Abnormalities missed during labour', 5 December 2008, p. 15, https://www.hdc.org.nz/search-site?keywords=07HDC15908
91 Sweetman, 'Safe Deliveries?', p. 41.
92 Maggie Banks, 'Practice Wisdom: Utilising the Unborn Baby's In-labour Movements', *NZCOMJ*, vol. 29, October 2003, p. 6.
93 Rhondda Davis, Sian Burgess and Maggie Banks, 'Practice Wisdom', ibid., vol. 30, April 2004, p. 5.
94 Deborah Davis, Sally Baddock, Sally Pairman et al., 'Planned Place of Birth in New Zealand: Does It Affect Mode of Birth and Intervention Rates Among Low Risk Women?' *Birth*, vol. 38, 2, 2011, pp. 111–19, doi: 10.1111/j.1523-536X.2010.00458.x
95 Robyn Mary Maude, 'Intelligent Structured Intermittent Auscultation (ISIA): A Mixed Methods Evaluation of an Informed Decision-making Framework for Fetal Heart Rate Monitoring', PhD thesis, Victoria University of Wellington, 2012, pp. 3–6, 28, 60, 265.
96 HDC Decision 12HDC00214, 'Midwifery care provided during labour', 25 February 2014, pp. 4, 14, https://www.hdc.org.nz/decisions/search-decisions/2014/12hdc00214/
97 Ibid., p. 12.
98 Ibid., p. 14.
99 Sweetman, 'Safe Deliveries?', p. 42; HDC Decision 07HDC08615, 'Inadequate newborn resuscitation technique and post-partum haemorrhage monitoring', 17 September 2008, https://www.hdc.org.nz/search-

site?keywords=07HDC08615, p. 9; 'Midwives told to apologise after botched birth', *NZH*, 14 October 2008, https://www.nzherald.co.nz/nz/midwives-told-to-apologise-for-botched-birth/JELPZZCJYSD2KIKASY2V26YA2U/

100   HDC Decision 07HDC08615, pp. 14, 34.
101   Ibid., pp. 28, 42.
102   Ibid., pp. 17–18.
103   Sweetman, 'Safe Deliveries?', p. 43; HDC Decision 11HDC00521, 'Delay in requesting assistance when fetal heart rate inadequate', 10 June 2013, https://www.hdc.org.nz/decisions/search-decisions/2013/11hdc00521/; HDC Decision 12HDC00301, 'Care provided to young pregnant woman', 9 July 2013, https://www.hdc.org.nz/search-site?keywords=12HDC00301
104   HDC Decision 11HDC00521, pp. 2, 17.
105   HDC Decision 12HDC00301, p. 2.
106   'Midwife fails teen mother: report', *Stuff*, 3 September 2013, http://www.stuff.co.nz/national/health/9120526/Midwife-fails-teen-mother-report
107   HDC Decision 12HDC00301, pp. 1, 8, 20.
108   'Midwife fails teen mother: report'.
109   Selina Powell, '"Sub-optimal" midwife still working under new name', *Marlborough Express*, 19 March 2015, https://www.stuff.co.nz/marlborough-express/news/67440701/sub-optimal-midwife-still-working-under-new-name
110   Sweetman, 'Safe Deliveries?', p. 44.
111   Ibid., p. 46.
112   On the 'Notice', see Wellington Area Review in above, Chapter 11, pp. 233–34.
113   Sweetman, 'Safe Deliveries?', p. 49; a press request for information from the Ministry of Health on homebirths led to quoted figures of around 2,000 home births for 2005 and 2006, but the LMC claim form from 2007 did not ask the LMC to state if the birth was at home: Janine Rankin, 'Health Ministry doesn't collect home birth data', *Manawatu Standard*, 26 November 2010, http://www.stuff.co.nz/manawatu-standard/4392647/Health-Ministry-doesn-t-collect-home-birth-data
114   Sweetman, 'Safe Deliveries?', p. 50. Exton, *Baby Business*, p. 112, referred to dramatic reduction in homebirths from 5% in 1999 to 1.7% in 2002.
115   Jon Wilcox, 'Battle lines drawn in "The good fight"', *NZD*, 17 November 2010, p. 22.
116   Davis, Baddock, Pairman, et al., 'Planned Place of Birth'.
117   Chisholm, 'Failure to deliver'.
118   Karen Guilliland, Letter to the editor, 'For babies' sake', *New Zealand Listener*, 21 March 2015, p. 9.
119   Mark Henaghan, *Health Professionals and Trust: The Cure for Healthcare Law and Policy*, Routledge-Cavendish, London, 2011, pp. 91–92; HDC Decision 07HDC16053, 'Transfer to secondary services after prolonged second stage of labour', 10 June 2008, https://www.hdc.org.nz/decisions/search-decisions/2008/07hdc16053-decision/; https://www.midwiferycouncil.health.nz/common/Uploaded%20files/Annual%20reports/Midwifery%20Council%20Annual%20Report%202016.pdf bridge

120 'Boy's birth injury "reveals divisions in maternity care"', *Dominion Post*, 31 January 2009, http://www.stuff.co.nz/national/health/524566/Boys-birth-injury-reveals-divisions-in-maternity-care
121 Henaghan, *Health Professionals and Trust*, p. 90; HDC Decision 04HDC05503, 'Management of labour and subsequent death of baby', 28 November 2006, https://www.hdc.org.nz/media/3455/04hdc05503midwives.pdf; 'Midwife "asked to keep quiet"', *NZH*, 8 March 2006, https://www.nzherald.co.nz/nz/news/article.cfm?c_id=1&objectid=10371569
122 'Midwife found not guilty of manslaughter', *NZH*, 21 March 2006, https://www.nzherald.co.nz/nz/news/article.cfm?c_id=1&objectid=10373747
123 HDC Decision 04HDC05503, pp. 22, 29, 30.
124 Martin Johnston, 'Government ready to tighten controls on midwives', *NZH*, 6 February 2006, https://www.nzherald.co.nz/nz/government-ready-to-tighten-controls-on-midwives/HJ42IHG4TCEJMJTDNEH726QKQA/
125 HDC Decision 06HDC08238, 'Death of baby several hours after home birth', 2 July 2007, p. 22, https://www.hdc.org.nz/decisions/search-decisions/2007/06hdc08238-decision/
126 HDC Decision 11HDC00957, 'Administration of Vitamin K to newborn baby', 10 June 2013, Para. 53, p. 7; See also See Irene Calvert, 'Trauma, Relational Trust and the Effects on the Midwife', PhD thesis, Massey University, 2011, pp. 146–80.
127 'Report into horrific labour released'.
128 Ibid.

## CHAPTER 11: *Maternity system under fire: The Midwifery Council's first decade*

1 *Sunday Star-Times*, 5 February 2006.
2 N. Pattison and R. Teele, 'A Plea for a Comprehensive Perinatal Database', *New Zealand Medical Journal (NZMJ)*, vol. 114, 1141, 12 October 2001, pp. 439–40.
3 Rosemary Reid, Editorial, 'Obstetric Perspectives: Quality Within Choice', *NZMJ*, vol. 117, 1206, 26 November 2004, U1169.
4 Linda Bryder, *The Rise and Fall of National Women's Hospital*, Auckland University Press, Auckland, 2014, pp. 167, 206; Alastair Haslam, 'Maternal Mortality in New Zealand', *O&G Magazine*, vol. 11, 1 Autumn 2009, https://www.ogmagazine.org.au/11/1-11/maternal-mortality-new-zealand-2/; A. Haslam and C. Farquhar, 'Maternal Mortality in New Zealand', *O&G Magazine*, vol. 15, 1, Autumn 2013, https://www.ogmagazine.org.au/15/1-15/maternal-mortality-new-zealand/
5 Coopers and Lybrand, 'First Steps Towards an Integrated Maternity Services Framework', Working Papers for the Report, RHA Maternity Services Project, November 1993, pp. 20, 30, https://www.moh.govt.nz/notebook/nbbooks.nsf/0/9F9AE7A8B59317794C2565D700186156/$file/first%20steps%20towards%20an%20integrated%20maternity%20services%20framework.pdf (accessed 6 March 2023).
6 Perinatal and Maternal Mortality Review Committee (PMMRC), *First Report to the Minister of Health: June 2005 to June 2007*, Wellington,

2007, pp. 3, 22, https://www.moh.govt.nz/notebook/nbbooks. nsf/0/0482427869B6BD5ACC257391006D02C7/$file/Perinatal%20and%20 Maternal%20Mortality%20First%20annual%20report%202005-07.pdf (accessed 6 March 2023).

7   Ibid., pp. 13–14.
8   Cynthia Farquhar, 'Chair's introduction', PMMRC, *Fifth Annual Report (First Report to the Health Quality & Safety Commission New Zealand)*, Wellington, 2011, p. 2, https://ourarchive.otago.ac.nz/bitstream/handle/10523/12432/ Fifth%20Annual%20Report%20of%20the%20Perinatal%20and%20Maternal%20 Mortality%20Review%20Committee?sequence=1&isAllowed=y (accessed 6 March 2023).
9   Introducing the Health Quality & Safety Commission New Zealand, https://pac.org.nz/bpj/2011/june/hqsc.aspx (accessed 6 March 2023).
10  PMMRC, Report on Recommendation One by the Wellington Coroner Resulting from Two Cases of Perinatal Death', 21 December 2005, to Pete Hodgson, AD20-82-2-1, pp. 2–6.
11  'Baby death report fuels call for review', *New Zealand Herald (NZH)*, 5 February 2006, https://www.nzherald.co.nz/nz/baby-death-report-fuels-call-for-review/ AXAAQK6Z2ETUYD7BLI7XMWZ4LM/
12  Lawton was made an Officer of the New Zealand Order of Merit for services to women's health in 2005.
13  Amanda Cameron, 'Maternity audit battle under way', *New Zealand Doctor (NZD)*, 8 February 2006, p. 3.
14  Cameron, 'Maternity audit battle under way'; Teresa O'Connor, 'Midwifery – A Workforce Under Pressure', *Kai Tiaki: Nursing New Zealand*, vol. 12, 3, April 2006, p. 18.
15  'Hodgson argues against review of maternity services', *NZH*, 20 March 2006, https://www.nzherald.co.nz/nz/hodgson-argues-against-review-of-maternity-services/AVGE4P3NCAFEEJAPTESHIT4YNE/
16  Emily Watt, 'Delivery by new midwives "dangerous"', *Dominion Post*, 23 December 2009, http://www.stuff.co.nz/national/3168973/Delivery-by-new-midwives-dangerous
17  'Baby's death the result of midwife incompetence - doctor', *Newshub*, 2 July 2008, https://www.newshub.co.nz/entertainment/babys-death-the-result-of-midwife-incompetence--doctor-2008070218
18  Review of the Quality, Safety and Management of Maternity Services in the Wellington Area, commissioned by the Ministry of Health, October 2008, https:// www.nzno.org.nz/Portals/0/Files/Documents/Activities/Submissions/2008-10%20 %20%20maternity-services-review-Wellington.pdf (accessed 6 March 2023).
19  Ibid., pp. 7, 31, 36, 97.
20  Ibid., p. 14.
21  Ibid., p. 34.
22  Ibid., p. 60.
23  Ibid., p. 61.

24  Anne Barlow, 'Evaluation of Educational Aspects of the New Zealand College of Midwives Standard Review Process', *New Zealand College of Midwives Journal (NZCOMJ)*, vol. 24, April 2001, p. 14.
25  Review, Wellington Area, p. 46.
26  Ibid., pp. 45–46.
27  Ibid., pp. 19, 43, 45, 47.
28  Ibid., p. 42.
29  'Maternity: The mother of all failings', *Scoop Health Independent News*, 8 October 2008, https://www.scoop.co.nz/stories/GE0810/S00038/maternity-the-mother-of-all-failings.htm
30  'GP author undeterred by criticism of book', *NZD*, 22 October 2008, p. 2; 'Maternity Service in Crisis: Doctor', ibid., 8 October 2008, https://www.nzherald.co.nz/nz/maternity-service-in-crisis-doctor/QDQZBJ4SX6UT26N2GORY7AGD6E
31  'Maternity service in crisis: Doctor'; 'Maternity system a scandal says GP', *Press*, 31 January 2009, https://www.stuff.co.nz/the-press/663011/Maternity-system-a-scandal-says-GP
32  PMMRC, *First Report*, p. 6.
33  Book Reviews: *The Baby Business: What's happened to maternity care in New Zealand?*, in *Journal of Primary Health Care*, vol. 1, 1, March 2009, https://www.publish.csiro.au/hc/pdf/HC09082
34  *Improving Maternity Services in Australia: The Report of the Maternity Services Review*, Department of Health, Commonwealth of Australia, February 2009.
35  Leah Haines, 'Another unfortunate experiment', *New Zealand Listener*, 31 January 2009, pp. 14–19, p. 16.
36  Beverley A. Lawton, Abby Koch, James Stanley and Stacie E. Geller, 'The Effect of Midwifery Care on Rates of Caesarean Delivery', *International Journal of Gynecology & Obstetrics*, vol. 123, 3, 2013, pp. 213–16.
37  *Improving Maternity Services in Australia*, p. 19.
38  Ibid., p. 43.
39  Haines, 'Another unfortunate experiment', p. 16.
40  Karen Guilliland and Sally Pairman, *Women's Business: The Story of the New Zealand College of Midwives, 1986–2010*, New Zealand College of Midwives, Christchurch, 2010, p. 627.
41  Ibid., p. 224.
42  C. P. Grigg and S. K. Tracy, 'New Zealand's Unique Maternity System', *Women and Birth*, vol. 26, 1, 2013, pp. e59–e64, doi: http://dx.doi.org/10.1016/j.wombi.2012.09.006
43  Haines, 'Another unfortunate experiment', p. 16.
44  Ben Fawkes, 'Babies stillborn as signs missed', *Dominion Post*, 11 March 2009, http://www.stuff.co.nz/national/1756588/Babies-stillborn-as-signs-missed
45  Haines, 'Another unfortunate experiment', pp. 16–17.
46  Lannes Johnson, 'Experimenting with maternity services: Causes and consequences of another unfortunate experiment', *NZD*, 11 March 2009, p. 12.

47  Kim Thomas, 'Mums petition Govt for review', 4 July 2009, https://www.stuff.co.nz/national/2525023/Mums-petition-Govt-for-review; 'Baby's death reveals system inadequacy', *Press*, 31 January 2009, http://www.stuff.co.nz/national/health/663058/Babys-death-reveals-system-inadequacy

48  'Delivery dilemma – the birthing centre debate', *Bay of Plenty Times*, 8 December 2014, https://www.nzherald.co.nz/bay-of-plenty-times/news/delivery-dilemma-the-birthing-centre-debate/YSVT7DXDKNO7BEZSSRPI3Z5NQE/

49  Ibid.

50  Petition 2008/23 Jennifer Maree Hooper, Report of the Health Committee to Parliament, October 2010, p. 7, https://www.parliament.nz/resource/en-NZ/49DBSCH_SCR4887_1/a3528664733efee6dfbadb8a416cf9c63fd77517 (accessed 6 March 2023).

51  Report of Health Committee, p. 8; Thomas, 'Mums petition Govt for review'; Natalie Akoorie, 'Mum fights good fight over birthing bungles', *Waikato Times*, 26 September 2009, http://www.stuff.co.nz/waikato-times/news/2905296/Mum-fights-good-fight-over-birthing-bungles

52  Thomas, 'Mums petition Govt for review'; Akoorie, 'Mum fights good fight over birthing bungles'.

53  Report of Health Committee, pp. 6, 18.

54  Ibid., p. 7.

55  Ibid., pp. 5, 16.

56  'Meanwhile: Petition seeks longer training for LMC midwives', *NZD*, 11 August 2010, p. 2; Amanda Cameron, 'Internship plan posed for midwives' (first signatory, Linda Depledge-Brooker), ibid., 25 August 2010, p. 19.

57  Maryanne Twentyman, 'Minister looks at midwife training', *Waikato Times*, 24 July 2010, http://www.stuff.co.nz/waikato-times/editors-picks/3953639/Minister-looks-at-midwife-training

58  Maryanne Twentyman, 'Newborn given drug in error', ibid., 3 July 2010, http://www.stuff.co.nz/waikato-times/3880846/Newborn-given-drug-in-error

59  Cameron, 'Internship plan posed for midwives', p. 19; Twentyman, 'Minister looks at midwife training'.

60  Farquhar, 'Chair's Introduction', PMMRC, *Fifth Annual Report*, p. 2; *Report*, pp. 63, 77, 82; Vicki Culling, 'Issues for parents, families and whanau', p. 83.

61  Donna Chisholm, 'Failure to deliver', *North & South*, August 2011, pp. 38–50.

62  Ibid.

63  Ibid.

64  Maryanne Twentyman, 'Group aims to make maternity services safer', *Waikato Times*, 30 March 2011, http://www.stuff.co.nz/waikato-times/news/4826654/Group-aims-to-make-maternity-services-safer; Press release: Action to Improve Maternity, 'Births no safer for Kiwi mothers and babies', 13 June 2013, https://www.scoop.co.nz/stories/GE1306/S00048/births-no-safer-for-kiwi-mothers-and-babies.htm

65  Grigg and Tracy, 'New Zealand's Unique Maternity System'.

66  Sally Pairman and Roslyn Donnellan-Fernandez, 'Professional Frameworks for Practice in Australia and New Zealand', in Sally Pairman, Jan Pincombe, Carol Thorogood and Sally Tracy (eds), *Midwifery: Preparation for Practice*, Churchill Livingstone Elsevier, Marrickville NSW, 2006, p. 175.
67  Jacqueline Wolf, *Deliver Me from Pain: Anaesthesia and Birth in America*, Johns Hopkins University Press, Baltimore, 2009, pp. 187, 189, 192, 195.
68  Caroline de Costa and Hans Pols, 'Shifting Paradigms: Homebirth Special Issue', *O&G Magazine*, vol. 14, 4, Summer 2011, https://www.ogmagazine.org.au/13/4-13/shifting-paradigms/
69  A further 16.6% of all births were emergency caesareans: National Women's Annual Clinical Report 2009, Auckland District Health Board, 2009, p. 24.
70  Jenny Forsyth, 'News review: A pregnant woman has the right to elect a caesarean. But how difficult is it to make that decision?', *NZH*, 12 October 1999.
71  Caroline de Costa, *The Women's Doc: True Stories from My Five Decades Delivering Babies and Making History*, Allen & Unwin, Sydney, 2021, pp. 168–69.
72  'Births no safer for Kiwi mothers and babies'.
73  Chisholm, 'Failure to deliver'; Martin Johnston and Natalie Akoorie, 'Babies' deaths reignite maternity row', *Weekend Herald*, 23 June 2012, p. A23; Donna Chisholm, 'Stand and deliver', *New Zealand Listener*, 14 February 2015, pp. 18–23.
74  'Births no safer for Kiwi mothers and babies'.
75  'Our Network', AIM website, http://aim.org.nz/network/
76  Jenn Hooper, Letter to the editor, 'We want the best for every mother and every baby', *Waikato Times*, 1 May 2013, http://www.stuff.co.nz/waikato-times/opinion/letters/8618602/We-want-the-best-for-every-mother-and-every-baby; original quote was in RedPR, 'NZ College of Midwives disturbed by Waikato Times breaching interim name suppression', Infonews.co.nz, 27 April 2013, https://www.infonews.co.nz/news.cfm?id=103741
77  Margaret Guthrie, Letter to the editor, *New Zealand Listener*, 21 February 2015, p. 6.
78  Pippa MacKay, Letter to the editor, *New Zealand Listener*, 28 February 2015, pp. 6–7.
79  Donna Chisholm, 'Birth control', ibid., 8 October 2016, p. 24.
80  Table 4.5, PMMRC, *Fifteenth Annual Report*, 2022, p. 81, https://www.hqsc.govt.nz/resources/resource-library/fifteenth-annual-report-of-the-perinatal-and-maternal-mortality-review-committee-reporting-mortality-and-morbidity-2020/ (accessed 6 March 2023).
81  'Babies' deaths reignite maternity row'; AIM, 'More deaths and injuries predicted', *Scoop: Health*, 22 August 2011, https://www.scoop.co.nz/stories/GE1108/S00084/more-deaths-and-injuries-predicted.htm
82  Helen M. Barnes, Angela M. Barnes, Joanne Baxter, Sue Crengle, Leonie Pihama, Mihi Ratima and Bridget Robson, 'Hapū Ora: Wellbeing in the Early Stages of Life', Massey University, 2013, p. 51, https://www.massey.ac.nz/massey/fms/Colleges/College%20of%20Humanities%20and%20Social%20Sciences/

Shore/reports/Hapu%20Ora%208%20Nov%202013.pdf (accessed 6 March 2023); Grigg and Tracy, 'New Zealand's Unique Maternity System'.

83   'Delivery dilemma – the birthing centre debate', *Bay of Plenty Times*, 8 December 2014, https://www.nzherald.co.nz/bay-of-plenty-times/news/delivery-dilemma-the-birthing-centre-debate/YSVT7DXDKNO7BEZSSRPI3Z5NQE/

84   John Schibeci (collator), 'Non-pharmacological Pain Management in Childbirth', *O&G Magazine*, vol. 11, 4, Summer 2009, p. 27.

85   Celia P. Grigg, Sally K. Tracy, Virginia Schmied, et al., 'Women's Experiences of Transfer from Primary Maternity Unit to Tertiary Hospital in New Zealand: Part of the Prospective Cohort Evaluating Maternity Units Study', *BMC Pregnancy Childbirth*, vol. 15, 339, 2015, doi: https://doi.org/10.1186/s12884-015-0770-2

86   Adele M. Robertson, 'Rural Women and Maternity Services', in Jean Ross (ed.), *Rural Nursing: Aspects of Practice*, Rural Health Opportunities, Ministry of Health, Dunedin, 2008, p. 184, https://www.health.govt.nz/system/files/documents/publications/rural-nursing-aspects-of-practice-mar08.pdf (accessed 6 March 2023).

87   Chris Hendry, 'Report on Mapping the Rural Midwifery Workforce in New Zealand for 2008', *NZCOMJ*, vol. 41, 2009, pp. 12–19.

88   Ruth Keber, 'Birthing centre transfers revealed', *Bay of Plenty Times*, 18 March 2015, https://www.nzherald.co.nz/bay-of-plenty-times/news/birthing-centre-transfers-revealed/EZD3ACA6WKCS6KPZWYGCOAWHAA/

89   Gerard H. A. Visser, 'Obstetric Care in the Netherlands: Relic or Example?', *Journal of Obstetrics and Gynaecology Canada*, vol. 34, 10, October 2012, pp. 971–75, doi: https://doi.org/10.1016/S1701-2163(16)35410-X

90   Costa and Pols, 'Shifting Paradigms'; Frank A. Chervenak, Laurence B. McCullough, Robert L. Brent, Malcolm I. Levene and Birgit Arabin, 'Planned Home Birth: The Professional Responsibility Response', *American Journal of Obstetrics & Gynecology*, January 2013, p. 33.

91   Maggie Lecky-Thompson, 'Independent Midwifery in Australia', in Tricia Murphy-Black (ed.), *Issues in Midwifery*, Churchill Livingstone, London, 1995, pp. 44–45.

92   Alan Merry, Foreword, PMMRC, *Eighth Annual Report*, 2014, p. 1, https://www.hqsc.govt.nz/resources/resource-library/eighth-annual-report-of-the-perinatal-and-maternal-mortality-review-committee/ (accessed 6 March 2023).

93   PMMRC, *Eighth Annual Report*, p. 10.

94   PMMRC, *Twelfth Annual Report*, 2018, p. 82, https://www.hqsc.govt.nz/resources/resource-library/twelfth-annual-report-of-the-perinatal-and-maternal-mortality-review-committee/ (accessed 6 March 2023).

95   PMMRC, *Eighth Annual Report*, Table 3.7, p. 159.

96   Ruth Zielinski, Kelly Ackerson and Lisa K. Low, 'Planned Home Birth: Benefits, Risks and Opportunities', *International Journal of Women's Health*, vol. 7, 2015, pp. 361–77.

97   Auckland District Health Board and Waitemata District Health Board, *Collaboration Maternity Plan: Working Together to Plan Future Maternity Services to 2025*, Auckland, 2015, p. 12.

98  Robyn M. Kennare, Marc J. N. C. Keirse, Graeme R. Tucker and Annabelle C. Chan, 'Planned Home and Hospital Births in South Australia, 1991–2006: Differences in Outcomes', *Medical Journal of Australia*, vol. 192, 2, 18 January 2010, pp. 76–80.
99  Auckland District Health Board and Waitemata District Health Board, *Collaboration Maternity Plan*, p. 7.
100 Maternity Services, Notice Pursuant to Section 88 of the New Zealand Public Health and Disability Act 2000, *Supplement to New Zealand Gazette*, Wellington, 24 April 2002, 40, p. 1114, https://www.moh.govt.nz/notebook/nbbooks.nsf/0/883C781AEBC58DD0CC257F5300784276/$file/07.%202002%20Section%2088%20Notice.pdf (accessed 6 March 2023).
101 Liane Topham-Kindley, 'LMCs need to toe line', *NZD*, 5 June 2002,
102 Angela Gregory, 'Midwives accused of threat to babies', *NZH*, 19 June 2002, https://www.nzherald.co.nz/nz/midwives-accused-of-threat-to-babies/PJUNT3IBTX63W3MKWHJWVE6XRI/
103 Reported in Liane Topham-Kindley,'Tukuitonga staunch on anti immunisation', *NZD*, 3 July 2002.
104 Erin Hudson and Susan Claridge (IAS), to Collin Tukuitonga, 18 June 2002, MSS-Archives-2007/15, Sub-Series 5/1/9, File 7/1/A/4, Joan Donley Papers, Special Collections, University of Auckland Library (JDP).
105 Lynda Williams to Tukuitonga, 19 June 2002, File 7/1/A/4, JDP.
106 Sian Burgess to Collin Tukuitonga, 18 June 2002, File 7/1/A/4, JDP.
107 Susan K. Claridge, *Investigate Before You Vaccinate: Making an Informed Decision about Vaccination in NZ*, Immunisation Awareness Society, Auckland, 2006.
108 Susan K. Claridge, 'Making INFORMED Decisions about Vaccinating your Child', *Education Effects*, Spring 2002, pp. 15–23.
109 Ibid., pp. 19–20, 21.
110 S. Clendon, Letter to the editor, *Education Effects*, Autumn 2003, p. 41; Helen Petousis-Harris, Letter to the editor, ibid., pp. 43–46.
111 'Become a childbirth educator', *NZCOMJ*, vol. 24, April 2001, p. 6.
112 'Antenatal Classes: A New Zealand Patient's Perspective', *O&G Magazine*, vol. 11, 11, 4, Summer 2009, p. 24.
113 Amanda Cameron, 'What's with my health professional advising against getting jabs?', *NZD*, 21 April 2010, p. 10.
114 Ibid.
115 Ibid.
116 Inquiry into Improving Rates of Childhood Immunisation, 1.6E, Report of the Health Committee, Paul Hutchison Chair, March 2011, p. 32, https://www.parliament.nz/resource/0000157667 (accessed 6 March 2023).
117 'Many midwives shun flu shots', *Herald on Sunday*, 24 March 2013, https://www.nzherald.co.nz/nz/many-midwives-shun-flu-shots/SYAGYTX5X23KOSIC6ANDNBULDE/
118 PMMRC, *Eleventh Annual Report*, 2017, p. 12. https://www.hqsc.govt.nz/resources/resource-library/eleventh-annual-report-of-the-perinatal-and-maternal-mortality-review-committee/ (accessed 6 March 2023).

119  *State of the World's Mothers Report* 2015, p. 60, https://www.savethechildren. org/content/dam/usa/reports/advocacy/sowm/sowm-2015.pdf (accessed 6 March 2023); Submissions to the Health Select Committee, Consumer concerns with the recently strengthened Midwifery First Year of Practice for new graduate midwives, 24 November 2015, AIM, https://www.parliament.nz/resource/en-NZ/51SCHE_EVI_51DBHOH_PET66361_1_A458322/1e6c981d1f978e7e8fac593cae7ba567f092764e (accessed 6 September 2023).
120  Alan Merry, Foreword, PMMRC, *Twelfth Annual Report*, p. 1; 'Executive summary', p. 8.

## CHAPTER 12: Research into maternity outcomes during the 2010s

1  Beverley A. Lawton, Leona F. Wilson, Richard A. Dinsdale, Sally B. Rose, Selina A. Brown, John Tait et al., 'Audit of Severe Acute Maternal Morbidity Describing Reasons for Transfer and Potential Preventability of Admissions to ICU', *Australian and New Zealand Journal of Obstetrics and Gynaecology*, vol. 50, 4, 2010, pp. 346–51, doi: https://doi-org.ezproxy.auckland.ac.nz/10.1111/j.1479-828X.2010.01200.x
2  Beverley A. Lawton, Abby Koch, James Stanley and Stacie E. Geller, 'The Effect of Midwifery Care on Rates of Cesarean Delivery', *International Journal of Gynecology & Obstetrics*, vol. 123, 3, December 2013, pp. 213–16; doi: 10.1016/j.ijgo.2013.06.033
3  Beverley Lawton, Evelyn J. MacDonald, Selina A. Brown, Leona Wilson, James Stanley et al., 'Preventability of Severe Acute Maternal Morbidity', *American Journal of Obstetrics & Gynecology*, vol. 210, 6, June 2014, 557, pp. e1–6, doi: 10.1016/j.ajog.2013.12.032
4  Evelyn J. MacDonald, Stacie E. Geller and Beverley A. Lawton, 'Establishment of a National Severe Maternal Morbidity Preventability Review in New Zealand', *International Journal of Gynecology & Obstetrics*, vol. 135, 1, 2016, pp. 120–23, doi: https://doi.org/10.1016/j.ijgo.2016.03.034
5  Cliff Taylor, 'GP's maternity study reignites issue of supervision for new midwives', *New Zealand Doctor* (*NZD*), 11 November 2015, p. 16.
6  Beverley Lawton, Sara Filoche, Stacie E. Geller, Sue Garrett and James Stanley, 'A Retrospective Cohort Study of the Association Between Midwifery Experience and Perinatal Mortality', *International Journal of Gynecology & Obstetrics*, vol. 132, 1, January 2016, pp. 94–99, doi: https://doi.org/10.1016/j.ijgo.2015.07.003
7  'Midwives hit back at birth danger study', *Stuff*, 21 October 2015, https://www.stuff.co.nz/national/health/73232583/midwives-hit-back-at-birth-danger-study?rm=m
8  Ibid.
9  'Researcher faces backlash from midwives', Radio New Zealand (RNZ), 11 November 2015, https://www.radionz.co.nz/news/national/289438/researcher-faces-backlash-from-midwives

10 'Midwives are in denial, says lobby group', RNZ, 22 October 2015, https://www.rnz.co.nz/news/national/287684/midwives-are-in-denial,-says-lobby-group
11 'Researcher faces backlash from midwives'.
12 Ibid.
13 Amanda Cameron, 'Internship plan posed for midwives', *NZD*, 25 August 2010, p. 19.
14 'Minister u-turned on midwife training', RNZ, 12 November 2015, https://www.radionz.co.nz/news/national/289385/minister-u-turned-on-midwife-training; see also Lawton et al., 'A Retrospective Cohort Study', p. 96.
15 'Midwives hit back at birth danger study'; Cliff Taylor, 'GP's maternity study reignites issue of supervision for new midwives', *NZD*, 11 November 2015, p. 16.
16 'Researcher faces backlash from midwives'; Rachel Wattie, 'Hate mail, formal complaint as study suggests risk to babies', *NZD*, 25 November 2015, p. 5.
17 Rachel Wattie, 'Medical Council won't hound GP over midwives' outcome study', *NZD*, 3 February 2016, p. 15; K. Guilliland, L. Dixon and C. MacDonald, 'A Midwifery Critical Analysis of: A Retrospective Cohort Study of the Association Between Midwifery Experience and Perinatal Mortality (Lawton et al., 2015)', *New Zealand College of Midwives Journal (NZCOMJ)*, vol. 51, 2015, pp. 59–62; Karen Guilliland, Lesley Dixon and Claire MacDonald, 'Correspondence: The Association between Midwifery Experience and Perinatal Mortality', *International Journal of Gynecology & Obstetrics*, vol. 133, 2, May 2016, p. 251, doi: https://doi-org.ezproxy.auckland.ac.nz/10.1016/j.ijgo.2016.02.007; Beverley Lawton, Sara Filoche, Stacie E. Geller and James Stanley, 'Authors' Reply', ibid., vol. 133, 2, May 2016, pp. 252–53, doi: https://obgyn-onlinelibrary-wiley-com.ezproxy.auckland.ac.nz/doi/full/10.1016/j.ijgo.2016.02.008
18 Guilliland, Dixon et al., 'A Midwifery Critical Analysis', p. 62.
19 Ruth Brown, 'Ministry repeats, updates Otago midwifery birth outcomes study', *NZD*, 26 October 2016, p. 5.
20 Fuseworks Media, 'Doubts raised about Lawton's study on graduate midwives', 20 October 2016, http://www.voxy.co.nz/health/5/266128 (accessed 15 October 2022).
21 Brown, 'Ministry repeats'.
22 Lynn C. Sadler, Judith McAra-Couper, Deborah Pittam, Michelle R. Wise and John M. D. Thompson, 'Risk of Perinatal Mortality in the First Year of Midwifery Practice in New Zealand: Analysis of a Retrospective National Cohort', *British Medical Journal Open*, vol. 8, 4, April 2018, doi:10.1136/bmjopen-2017-019026
23 Ibid., p. 5.
24 Ibid., pp. 7, 13.
25 Media release from NZ College of Midwives, 'Research confirms midwifery care by graduates in New Zealand is excellent', *NZD*, 11 April 2018.
26 Bev Lawton, Sibanda Nokuthaba, Stacie Geller et al., 'Submission to Select Health Committee Re: Perinatal mortality safety data associated with pregnancies looked after by first year Midwives', 4 October 2019, p. 1,

https://www.parliament.nz/resource/en-NZ/51SCHE_EVI_66361_HE6357/ f93490c4b0cd512154689226430b7592e75cc143 (accessed 8 March 2023).

27   National Health Committee, *Review of Maternity Services in New Zealand*, National Health Committee, Wellington, September 1999, p. 45, see also p. 7, https://www.moh.govt.nz/notebook/nbbooks. nsf/0/9B3D7BB224CAEC6C4C25681B006EE921/$file/mands2.pdf (accessed 8 March 2023); also reported in *News & Issues: Newsletter from the National Advisory Committee on Health and Disability*, 15, December 1999, p. 4.

28   Don Simmers, 'The Few: New Zealand's Diminishing Number of Rural GPs Providing Maternity Services', *New Zealand Medical Journal*, vol. 119, 1241, 8 September 2006, U2151.

29   Karen Bartholomew, 'The Realities of Choice and Access in the Lead Maternity Carer System: Operationalising Choice Policy in the New Zealand Maternity Reforms', Master of Public Health, University of Auckland, 2010; Karen Bartholomew, Susan M. B. Morton, Polly E. Atatoa Carr, Dinusha K. Bandarai and Cameron C. Grant, 'Provider Engagement and Choice in the Lead Maternity Carer System: Evidence from *Growing Up in New Zealand*', *Australian and New Zealand Journal of Obstetrics and Gynaecology*, vol. 55, 4, 2015, pp. 323–330, doi: 10.1111/ajo.12319; National Health Committee, *Review of Maternity Services*, p. 48.

30   Morton et al, 'Provider Engagement'; National Health Committee, *Review of Maternity Services*, p. 33.

31   Perinatal and Maternal Mortality Review Committee (PMMRC), *Twelfth Annual Report*, Wellington, 2018, p. 26.

32   Guilliland, Dixon et al., 'A Midwifery Critical Analysis', p. 61.

33   AIM: Action to Improve Maternity Consumer Network, Submissions to the Health Select Committee, Consumer concerns with the recently strengthened Midwifery First Year of Practice for new graduate midwives, 24 November 2015, pp. 9–10, 22, https://www.parliament. nz/resource/en-NZ/51SCHE_EVI_51DBHOH_PET66361_1_ A458322/1e6c981d1f978e7e8fac593cae7ba567f092764e (accessed 8 March 2023); Ministry comment to Point 11, in AIM, Comments on the Ministry of Health Response to AIM's 2014/30 Submission to the Health Select Committee on the Midwifery First Year of Practice (MFYP), 18 June 2019, https://www.parliament.nz/resource/en-NZ/51SCHE_EVI_66361_ HE6042/66047345323b7bc8086f62af6c47037924a6a4da (accessed 8 March 2023).

34   AIM submission, 18 June 2019, Points 4, 8.

35   New Zealand College of Midwives, Health Select Committee Response, June 2019, p. 2, https://www.parliament.nz/resource/en-NZ/51SCHE_EVI_66361_ HE6044/975bd026804f29068351416c495cc9e3eaba2e5c (accessed 8 March 2023).

36   Cherry Ngan, 'Should Midwives Be Held to a Different Standard of Care, Given New Zealand's Unique Autonomous Midwife-led Framework?', *Auckland University Law Review*, vol. 23, 2017, pp.119–46, pp. 139– 40; on the Postgraduate Diploma in Obstetrics, see Dawn Miller, Helen Roberts and Don Wilson, 'Future Practice of Graduates of the New Zealand Diploma of

Obstetrics and Gynaecology or Certificate in Women's Health', *New Zealand Medical Journal*, vol. 121, 1282, 19 September 2008, pp. 29–30.
37   Ngan, 'Should Midwives Be Held to a Different Standard of Care', p. 145.
38   Bev Lawton, Sibanda Nokuthaba, Stacie Geller et al., 'Submission to Select Health Committee Re: Perinatal mortality safety data associated with pregnancies looked after by first year Midwives', 4 October 2019, pp. 3–4.
39   Stacie E. Geller, Abigail R. Koch, Caitlin E. Garland, E. Jane MacDonald, Francesca Storey and Beverley Lawton, 'A Global View of Severe Maternal Morbidity: Moving Beyond Maternal Mortality', *Reproductive Health*, vol. 15 (Suppl. 1), 98, 2018, pp. 32–43, doi: https://doi.org/10.1186/s12978-018-0527-2
40   Ellie Wernham, Jason Gurney, James Stanley, Lis Ellison-Loschmann and Diana Sarfati, 'A Comparison of Midwife-Led and Medical-Led Models of Care and Their Relationship to Adverse Fetal and Neonatal Outcomes: A Retrospective Cohort Study in New Zealand', *PLoS Medicine*, vol. 13, 9, 2016:e1002134, doi: 10.1371/journal.pmed.1002134, https://pubmed.ncbi.nlm.nih.gov/27676611/
41   Annemieke C. C. Evers, Hens A. A. Brouwers, Chantal. W. Hukkelhoven et al., 'Perinatal Mortality and Severe Morbidity in Low and High Risk Term Pregnancies in the Netherlands: Prospective Cohort Study', *British Medical Journal*, vol. 341, c5639, 2010, doi: https://doi.org/10.1136/bmj.c5639; Amanda Cameron, 'Tiered Maternity Care questioned', *NZD*, 15 December 2010.
42   Hans Pols, 'Trouble in Paradise', Special issue on Homebirth, *O&G Magazine* vol. 13, 4, Summer 2011, https://www.ogmagazine.org.au/13/4-13/trouble-in-paradise-netherlands-homebirth/
43   M. M. J. Wiegerinck, B. Y. van der Goes, A. C. Ravelli, et al., 'Intrapartum and Neonatal Mortality in Primary Midwife-led and Secondary Obstetrician-led Care in the Amsterdam Region of the Netherlands: A Retrospective Cohort Study', *Midwifery*, vol. 31, 12, 2015, pp. 1168–76, doi: 10.1016/j.midw.2015.08.007
44   Katy Sutcliffe, Jenny Caird, Josephine Kavanagh, Rebecca Rees, Kathryn Oliver et al., 'Comparing Midwife-led and Doctor-led Maternity Care: A Systematic Review of Reviews', *Journal of Advanced Nursing*, vol. 68, 11, 2012, pp. 2376–86, doi: 10.1111/j.1365-2648.2012.05998.x
45   Section: 'Recommendations and Further Research', in Wernham et al., 'A Comparison of Midwife-Led and Medical-Led Models'.
46   Donna Chisholm, 'Birth control', *New Zealand Listener*, 8 October 2016, p. 25; at the time of the interview Wernham was in her second year of a medical degree.
47   The Apgar score is a measure of infant wellbeing immediately post-delivery, with a low score being indicative of an unwell baby.
48   Section: 'Recommendations and Further Research', in Wernham et al., 'A Comparison of Midwife-Led and Medical-Led Models'.
49   Section: 'Strengths and Weaknesses', in ibid.
50   Section: 'Conclusions', in ibid.
51   Jane Sandall, Hora Soltani, Simon Gates, Andrew Shennan and Declan Devane, 'Midwife-led Continuity Models Versus Other Models of Care for Childbearing

52  Women', *Cochrane Database of Systematic Reviews*, vol. 28, 4, 4, April 2016, doi: 10.1002/14651858.CD004667.pub5
52  See Chisholm, 'Birth control', p. 24.
53  Section: 'Strengths and Weaknesses', in Wernham et al., 'A Comparison of Midwife-Led and Medical-Led Models'.
54  Anne-Marie Boxall and Kathy Flitcroft, 'Debate: Open Access: From Little Things, Big Things Grow: A Local Approach to System-wide Maternity Services Reform in the Absence of Definitive Evidence', *Australia and New Zealand Health Policy*, vol. 4, 18, 2007, doi:10.1186/1743-8462-4-18
55  Chisholm, 'Birth control', p. 25.
56  Michelle Duff, 'The maternity study health officials and the College of Midwives fought to undermine', *Stuff*, 22 February 2019, https://www.stuff.co.nz/life-style/parenting/pregnancy/birth/110638963/the-maternity-study-health-officials-and-the-college-of-midwives-fought-to-undermine
57  Natalie Akoorie, 'Higher birth damage rates in midwifery-led care concerns ministry', *New Zealand Herald*, 28 September 2016.
58  Sally Abel, 'Midwifery and Maternity Services in Transition: An Examination of Change Following the Nurses Amendment Act 1990', PhD thesis, University of Auckland, 1997, p. 134.
59  Eileen Goodwin, 'Midwives challenge findings', *Otago Daily Times*, 28 September 2016, https://www.odt.co.nz/news/dunedin/health/midwives-challenge-findings
60  Akoorie, 'Higher birth damage rates in midwifery-led care concerns ministry'.
61  Duff, 'The maternity study health officials and the College of Midwives fought to undermine'.
62  Chisholm, 'Birth control', p. 18.
63  Ibid., p. 23.
64  Ibid., p. 20.
65  Ibid., p. 22.
66  Ibid., p. 23.
67  Media Council, New Zealand College of Midwives against New Zealand Listener, 2557, January 2017, https://www.mediacouncil.org.nz/rulings/new-zealand-college-of-midwives-against-new-zealand-listener, Point 16 (accessed 8 March 2023).
68  Chisholm, 'Birth control', p. 22.
69  Media Council, Points 31, 32.
70  Ibid., Points 41, 51.
71  Ibid., Point 20.
72  Ibid., Point 35.
73  Debb Pittam, Letter to the editor, *New Zealand Listener*, 22 October 2016, p. 4.
74  Ross Howie, Letter to the editor, ibid., 15 October 2016, p. 4.
75  Editor's response, ibid., 22 October 2016, p. 4. The case referred to was presumably 'Provision of care to pregnant woman with high risk factors', in which the Commissioner found the midwife to have 'failed to provide services with reasonable care and skill' breaching Code 4(1),

30 June 2016, 15HDC00540, https://www.hdc.org.nz/decisions/search-decisions/2016/15hdc00540/.
76 Duff, 'The maternity study health officials and the College of Midwives fought to undermine'.
77 New Zealand College of Midwives, Health Select Committee Response, 2019, pp. 2, 10.
78 Frank A. Chervenak, Laurence B. McCullough, Robert L. Brent, Malcolm I. Levene and Birgit Arabin, 'Planned Home Birth: The Professional Responsibility Response', *American Journal of Obstetrics & Gynecology*, vol. 208, 1, 2013, pp. 31–38, 36, doi: 10.1016/j.ajog.2012.10.002
79 Health Quality & Safety Commission New Zealand, Information about deaths of babies and mothers in Aotearoa New Zealand, 2021, https://www.hqsc.govt.nz/our-programmes/mrc/pmmrc/information-about-deaths-of-babies-and-mothers/; PMMRC, *Fourteenth Annual Report*, 2021, Chair's introduction, p. 9, https://www.hqsc.govt.nz/assets/Our-work/Mortality-review-committee/PMMRC/Publications-resources/report-pmmrc-14th-v2.pdf (accessed 8 March 2023).
80 PMMRC, *Twelfth Annual Report*, p. 4.
81 PMMRC, *Fourteenth Annual Report*, p. 16. Commenting on outcomes for Indian women, the report noted that, 'within Aotearoa/New Zealand and internationally, we have an incomplete understanding of what puts women and babies of Indian ethnicity at increased risk.', ibid., p. 140.
82 PMMRC, *Fifteenth Annual Report*, 2022, p. 1.
83 PMMRC, *Fourteenth Annual Report*, pp. 22, 47.
84 Maryanne Twentyman, 'Babies' deaths may be avoidable', *Waikato Times*, 16 October 2010, http://www.stuff.co.nz/national/4240111/Babies-deaths-may-be-avoidable; PMMRC, *Fifteenth Annual Report*, p. 13
85 PMMRC, *Eleventh Annual Report*, 2017, pp. 10, 14, 15, 17, 26.
86 PMMRC, *Fifteenth Annual Report*, Key findings.
87 PMMRC, *Fourteenth Annual Report*, pp. 14, 16, 74.
88 Ibid., p. 17.
89 PMMRC, *Twelfth Annual Report*, p. 6.
90 Adele M. Robertson, 'Rural Women and Maternity Services', in Jean Ross (ed.), *Rural Nursing: Aspects of Practice*, Rural Health Opportunities, Ministry of Health, Dunedin, 2008, p. 180, https://www.health.govt.nz/system/files/documents/publications/rural-nursing-aspects-of-practice-mar08.pdf (accessed 8 March 2023).
91 PMMRC, *Twelfth Annual Report*, p. 26, 44.
92 PMMRC, *Eleventh Annual Report*, p. 9.
93 PMMRC, *Fourteenth Annual Report*, p. 111.
94 Ibid., pp. 16, 111.
95 Ibid., p. 112.
96 Michelle Duff, 'Call for action over maternal suicides', *Dominion Post*, 13 June 2012, http://www.stuff.co.nz/national/health/7097689/Call-for-action-over-maternal-suicides

97   PMMRC, *Fourteenth Annual Report*, pp. 111, 139; Helen Clark Foundation media release, 'Helen Clark Foundation Calls for maternal mental health to be a policy priority in new report', 1 May 2022, https://www.scoop.co.nz/stories/GE2205/S00001/helen-clark-foundation-calls-for-maternal-mental-health-to-be-a-policy-priority-in-new-report.htm
98   PMMRC, *Fifteenth Annual Report*, p. 14.
99   PMMRC, *Fourteenth Annual Report*, p. 18.
100  Ibid., p. 133.
101  Ibid., pp. 136, 138.
102  PMMRC, *Fifteenth Annual Report*, pp. 187, 191, 192, 193, 195, 198, 199.
103  National Maternity Monitoring Group, *Fifth Annual Report*, 2017, pp. 11, 39, 40.
104  Sian Hannagan, 'Reflections on Conference', September 2015, *Home Birth Aotearoa*, https://homebirth.org.nz/magazine/article/reflections-on-conference (accessed 8 March 2023).
105  Lesley Dixon, Karen Guilliland, Julie Pallant, Mary Sidebotham, Jennifer Fenwick, Judith McAra-Couper and Andrea Gilkison, 'The Emotional Wellbeing of New Zealand Midwives: Comparing Responses for Midwives in Caseloading and Shift Work Settings', *NZCOMJ*, vol. 53, December 2017, pp. 5–14.
106  Judith McAra-Couper, 'What Is Shaping the Practice of Health Professionals and the Understanding of the Public in Relation to Increasing Intervention in Childbirth?', PhD thesis, Auckland University of Technology, 2007; Judith McAra-Couper, Marion Jones and Elizabeth Smythe, 'Rising Rates of Intervention in Childbirth', *British Journal of Midwifery*, vol. 18, 3, March 2010, pp. 160–69.
107  Karen Guilliland, webinar: 'Emancipating Midwifery – Reflecting on 30 years of midwifery autonomy', 3 September 2020 (time: 18.22.05), hosted by Alison Eddy, Chief Executive, New Zealand College of Midwives, https://www.midwife.org.nz/news/webinar-emancipating-midwifery-reflecting-on-30-years-of-midwifery-autonomy/
108  PMMRC, *Fifteenth Annual Report*, p. 201.
109  Bill Kirkup, 'The Report of the Morecambe Bay Investigation March 2015', https://assets.publishing.service.gov.uk/government/uploads/system/uploads/attachment_data/file/408480/47487_MBI_Accessible_v0.1.pdf (accessed 8 March 2023).
110  Ibid., p. 6.
111  Ibid., pp. 14, 183.
112  Royal College of Midwives, https://www.rcm.org.uk/promoting/professional-practice/maternity-transformation/ (accessed 8 March 2023).
113  Donna Ockenden (chair), Independent Report: Ockenden Review: Summary of Findings, Conclusions and Essential Actions, 20 March 2022, https://www.gov.uk/government/publications/final-report-of-the-ockenden-review/ockenden-review-summary-of-findings-conclusions-and-essential-actions (accessed 8 March 2023).
114  Donna Ockenden (chair), 'Emerging Findings and Recommendations from the Independent Review of Maternity Services at the Shrewsbury

and Telford Hospital NHS Trust, Our First Report following 250 Clinical Reviews, 10 December 2020', https://www.ockendenmaternityreview.org.uk/wp-content/uploads/2020/12/ockenden-report.pdf (accessed 8 March 2023).
115 Ockenden Review, Report 2022: Executive Summary.
116 Ockenden Review, Report 2020, p. 13; Report 2022: Patterns of repeated poor care.
117 Ockenden Review, Report 2022: Failure in governance and leadership.
118 Ibid.: Local actions for learning, and immediate and essential actions.
119 'NHS trust used "quack" therapy on new mothers', *The Times*, 20 August 2022, p. 16.
120 Ibid.; 'The quack remedies being peddled by NHS midwives that prove the obsession with natural births really HAS gone too far', *Mail on Sunday*, 28 August 2022, p. 53.
121 Dr Bill Kirkup CBE (chair), 'Reading the Signals: Maternity and Neonatal Services in East Kent – the Report of the Independent Investigation, October 2022', https://assets.publishing.service.gov.uk/government/uploads/system/uploads/attachment_data/file/1111993/reading-the-signals-maternity-and-neonatal-services-in-east-kent_the-report-of-the-independent-investigation_web-accessible.pdf (accessed 8 March 2023).
122 Ibid., pp. 22, 163.
123 *Sunday Times*, 26 March 2022.
124 Royal College of Midwives, *News*, 22 September 2022, https://www.rcm.org.uk/news-views/news/2022/new-independent-maternity-working-group-to-oversee-maternity-transformation-programme-in-england/
125 Sally Pairman, panellist, webinar: 'Emancipating Midwifery – Reflecting on 30 years of midwifery autonomy', 3 September 2020 (time: 18.41.43), hosted by Alison Eddy, Chief Executive, New Zealand College of Midwives, https://www.midwife.org.nz/news/webinar-emancipating-midwifery-reflecting-on-30-years-of-midwifery-autonomy/
126 Sarah Catherall, 'Professor Bev Lawton fighting for change in New Zealand's "flawed" maternity care system', *Stuff*, 10 November 2020, https://www.stuff.co.nz/life-style/well-good/123336039/professor-bev-lawton-fighting-for-change-in-new-zealands-flawed-maternity-care-system

## CONCLUSION: 'NZ – the best place to give birth?'

1 Sally Blundell, 'NZ – the best place to give birth?', *Newsroom*, 4 June 2021, https://www.newsroom.co.nz/nz-the-best-place-to-give-birth
2 Malatest International Consulting and Advisory Services, 'Report: Comparative Study of Maternity Systems, Prepared for the Ministry of Health', November 2012, Wellington, p. 98, https://www.health.govt.nz/system/files/documents/publications/comparative-study-of-maternity-systems-nov13.pdf (accessed 9 March 2023).

3   Karen Guilliland, panellist, webinar: 'Emancipating Midwifery – Reflecting on 30 years of midwifery autonomy', 3 September 2020 (time: 18.24.46), hosted by Alison Eddy, Chief Executive, New Zealand College of Midwives, https://www.midwife.org.nz/news/webinar-emancipating-midwifery-reflecting-on-30-years-of-midwifery-autonomy/
4   Celia P. Grigg and Sally K. Tracy, 'New Zealand's Unique Maternity System', *Women and Birth*, vol. 26, 1, March 2013, p. e64, doi: https://doi.org/10.1016/j.wombi.2012.09.006
5   'Inquiry finds midwife's inadequate care led to baby's death', RNZ, 16 August 2021, https://www.rnz.co.nz/news/national/449281/inquiry-finds-midwife-s-inadequate-care-led-to-baby-s-death
6   'Midwife Failed to Monitor Young Woman for Pre-eclampsia', Report by Deputy Health and Disability Commissioner, Case 19HDC01789, Decision, 25 June 2021, pp. 3, 18, https://www.hdc.org.nz/decisions/search-decisions/2021/19hdc01789/
7   Ibid, p. 12.
8   Blundell, 'NZ – the best place to give birth?.'
9   Case 19HDC01789, Decision, 25 June 2021, pp. 11–12.
10  Ibid., p. 11.
11  'Use of Saline as Placebo Pain Relief During Labour', Report by the Health and Disability Commissioner, Case 18HDC01578, Decision, 13 May 2019, pp. 2, 10, https://www.hdc.org.nz/decisions/search-decisions/2019/18hdc01578/
12  'Midwife censured', *New Zealand Herald*, 1 February 2022, p. A8; Case 18HDC01578, Decision, 13 May 2019, pp. 2, 10.
13  Case 19HDC01789, Decision, 25 June 2021, p. 3.
14  Ibid., pp. 4, 5.
15  Ibid., pp. 1, 18, 20.
16  'Midwife fails to recognise high-risk pregnancy from ultrasound scan', Decision 18HDC01959, Executive summary, https://www.hdc.org.nz/decisions/search-decisions/2021/18hdc01959/
17  Case 19HDC01789, Decision, 25 June 2021, pp. 1, 20.
18  Ibid.
19  Ibid., p. 12.
20  Ollie Neas, 'Risky business', *North & South*, May 2022, pp. 53–55.
21  Case 19HDC01789, Decision, 25 June 2021, p. 11.
22  Ibid., p. 12.
23  Table 4.5, Perinatal and Maternal Mortality Review Committee, *Fifteenth Annual Report*, 2022, p. 81.
24  'Minister u-turned on midwife training', RNZ, 12 November 2015, https://www.radionz.co.nz/news/national/289385/minister-u-turned-on-midwife-training; 'Sharron's Story', in Karen Guilliland and Sally Pairman, *Women's Business: The Story of the New Zealand College of Midwives, 1986–2010*, New Zealand College of Midwives, Christchurch, 2010, p. 195.

# BIBLIOGRAPHY

Archives New Zealand Te Rua Mahara o te Kāwanatanga, Wellington

Department of Health Series 632 (1890–1998); Health Department Workforce Development Series 6804 (c. 1986–1992); Political papers series 7838 (1981–1998), personal and political files created by the Hon. Katherine O'Regan.

University of Auckland Library Manuscripts and Archives Waipapa Taumata Rau Te Tumu Herenda

Joan Donley Papers, MSS & Archives 2007/15 (JDP)

New Zealand College of Midwives, Auckland Region records, MSS & Archives-2007/2 (NZCOM ARP)

## Websites

AIM: Action to Improve Maternity, http://aim.org.nz/

Decisions: Health and Disability Commissioner, https://www.hdc.org.nz/decisions/

Hansard (Debates) New Zealand Parliament, https://www.parliament.nz/en/pb/hansard-debates/historical-hansard/

Perinatal and Maternal Mortality Review Committee, *Annual Reports*, https://www.hqsc.govt.nz/our-programmes/mrc/pmmrc/

Te Tatau o te Whare Kahu Midwifery Council, *Annual Reports*, https://www.midwiferycouncil.health.nz/Public/03.-Publications/Publications-Type-A/Annual-Reports.aspx?hkey=ad216505-605a-44cd-93c8-922bebc33f67

Wise Woman Archives Trust (Inc.), (WWAT), includes Home Birth Association Newsletters – National (1980–1990) and Auckland (1978–1997); Domiciliary Midwives Society Newsletters (1984–1989), Save the Midwives Newsletters (1984–1994), New Zealand College of Midwives Newsletters, and other sources, http://wwat.nz/

## Official reports (by date)

Committee of Inquiry into Maternity Services, Report of, *New Zealand Parliamentary Papers, Appendix to the Journals of the House of Representatives*, H31A, 1938.

New Zealand Department of Health, *A Review of Hospital and Related Services in New Zealand*, Department of Health, Wellington, 1969.

Helen Carpenter, *An Improved System of Nursing Education in New Zealand: Report for Department of Health*, Department of Health, Wellington, 1971.

Ohu Advisory Committee, *Ohu: Alternative Life Style Communities*, Department of Lands and Survey, Wellington, 1975.

Maternity Services Committee, *Maternity Services in New Zealand: A Report*, Board of Health Report Series 26, Government Printer, Wellington, 1976.

Maternity Services Committee, *Obstetrics and the Winds of Change*, Board of Health, Wellington, 1979.

House of Commons (UK), *Second Report from the Social Services Committee, Session 1979–80: Perinatal and Neonatal Mortality, Together with the Proceedings of the Committee and the Minutes of Evidence (including evidence taken by the Social Services and Employment Sub-Committee of the Expenditure Committee in Session 1978–79) and Appendices*, vol. 1 (chair Mrs Renee Short), HMSO, London, 1980.

Maternity Services Committee, *Special Care Services for the Newborn in New Zealand: A Report*, Board of Health Report Series 29, Government Printer, Wellington, 1982.

Maternity Services Committee, *Mother and Baby at Home: The early days: A Report*, Board of Health Report Series 30, Government Printer, Wellington, 1982.

New Zealand Planning Council, *First Report of the Social Monitoring Group: From Birth to Death* (chair Peggy Koopman-Boyden), New Zealand Planning Council, Wellington, 1985.

Health Benefits Review, *Choices for Health Care: Report of the Health Benefits Review* (chair Claudia Scott), Health Benefits Review, Wellington, 1986.

New Zealand Planning Council, *Care and Control: The Role of Institutions in New Zealand, Second Report of the Social Monitoring Group Report* (chair Peggy Koopman-Boyden), New Zealand Planning Council, Wellington, 1987.

Julie Leibrich, Janet Hickling and George Pitt, *In Search of Well-being: Exploratory Research into Complementary Therapies*, Health Services Research and Development Unit, Department of Health, Wellington, 1987.

Jennie Nicol, *A Choice of Birthing: Part 1: Homebirth and Domiciliary Midwifery*, Department of Health, Wellington, 1987.

Women's Health Committee, *Women's Health in New Zealand 1985–1988, Report to the Board of Health*, Health Services Research and Development Unit, Department of Health, 1988.

*Bibliography*

*The Report of the Committee of Inquiry into Allegations Concerning the Treatment of Cervical Cancer at National Women's Hospital and into Other Related Matters* (chair Silvia Cartwright), Government Printing Office, Auckland, 1988.

Women's Health Committee, *Report to the Board of Health 1985–1988*, Wellington, 1988.

Maternity Benefits Tribunal, *Report and Recommendations of the Maternity Benefits Tribunal*, Ministry of Health, Wellington, 1993.

Health Funding Authority, *New Zealand Mothers and Babies: An Analysis of National Maternity Data*, Health Funding Authority, Wellington, 1999.

National Health Committee, *Review of Maternity Services in New Zealand*, National Health Committee, Wellington, 1999.

Health Funding Authority, *Maternity Services: A Reference Document*, Health Funding Authority, Wellington, 2000.

Maternity Services, 'Notice pursuant to Section 88 of the NZ Public Health and Disability Act 2000', 13 April 2007, *New Zealand Gazette*, vol. 41, 13 April 2007, Department of Internal Affairs, Wellington, pp. 1026–1111.

*Review of the Quality, Safety and Management of Maternity Services in the Wellington Region* (chair Barbara Crawford), Ministry of Health, Wellington, October 2008.

*National Women's Annual Clinical Report 2009*, Auckland District Health Board, 2009.

*Petition 2008/23 of Jennifer Maree Hooper, Report of Health Committee, Forty-ninth Parliament* (chair Paul Hutchison), 2010.

*Inquiry Into How to Improve Completion Rates of Childhood Immunisation, 1.6E, Report of the Health Committee, Forty-ninth Parliament* (chair Paul Hutchison), 2011.

Malatest International Consulting and Advisory Services, *Report: Comparative Study of Maternity Systems*, prepared for the Ministry of Health, Wellington, 2012.

Auckland District Health Board and Waitemata District Health Board, *Collaboration Maternity Plan: Working Together to Plan Future Maternity Services to 2025*, Auckland District Health Board and Waitemata District Health Board, Auckland, 2015.

*The Report of the Morecambe Bay Investigation: An Independent Investigation into the Management, Delivery and Outcomes of Care Provided by the Maternity and Neonatal Services at the University Hospitals of Morecambe Bay NHS Foundation Trust from January 2004 to June 2013* (chair Bill Kirkup), HMSO, London, 2015.

*Ockenden Report: Emerging Findings and Recommendations from the Independent Review of Maternity Services at the Shrewsbury and Telford Hospital NHS Trust, Our First Report Following 250 Clinical Reviews* (chair Donna Ockenden), HMSO, London, 2020.

*Independent report: Ockenden review: Summary of Findings, Conclusions and Essential Actions*, Department of Health & Social Care, HMSO, London, 2022.

*Reading the Signals: Maternity and Neonatal Services in East Kent – the Report of the Independent Investigation* (chair Bill Kirkup), HMSO, London, 2022.

## Other online sources (by date)

Department of Health, *Your Pregnancy: To Haputanga me to Whakawhanautanga*, Department of Health, Wellington, 1985, Code 4146, https://www.moh.govt.nz/notebook/nbbooks.nsf/0/50BA5494E2C12B5F4C2565D70018BC95/$file/your-pregnancy.pdf

Department of Health, 'Part 1: What Everyone Should Know', *Nurses Amendment Act 1990: Information for Health Providers, Department of Health, 1990*, Wellington, October 1990, https://www.moh.govt.nz/notebook/nbbooks.nsf/0/7e9811383ed959b34c2565d7000de831/$FILE/Nurses%20Amendment%20Act%201990%20-%20information%20for%20health%20providers.pdf

Perinatal and Maternal Mortality Review Committee, 'Report on Recommendation One by the Wellington Coroner Resulting from Two Cases of Perinatal Death', 21 December 2005, to Hon. Pete Hodgson, AD20-82-2-1, https://www.hqsc.govt.nz/assets/PMMRC/Publications/pmmrchealthreport.pdf

Te Tatau o te Whare Kahu Midwifery Council, 'Competencies for Entry to the Register of Midwives', 2007, https://www.midwiferycouncil.health.nz/common/Uploaded%20files/Midwifery%20Leaders/Competencies%20for%20Entry%20to%20the%20register%20of%20Midwives%202007.pdf

Barnes, Helen Moewaka, Angela Moewaka Barnes, Joanne Baxter, Sue Crengle, Leonie Pihama, Mihi Ratima and Bridget Robson, 'Hapū Ora: Wellbeing in the Early Stages of Life', Whāriki Research Group, Massey University, 2013, https://www.massey.ac.nz/massey/fms/Colleges/College%20of%20Humanities%20and%20Social%20Sciences/Shore/reports/Hapu%20Ora%208%20Nov%202013.pdf

AIM: Action to Improve Maternity Consumer Support Network, 'Submissions to the Health Select Committee: Consumer Concerns with the Recently Strengthened Midwifery First Year of Practice for New Graduate Midwives', 24 November 2015, https://www.parliament.nz/resource/enNZ/51SCHE_EVI_51DBHOH_PET66361_1_A458322/1e6c981d1f978e7e8fac593cae7ba567f092764e

Hannigan, Sian, 'Reflections on Conference', *Home Birth Aotearoa*, September 2015, https://homebirth.org.nz/magazine/article/reflections-on-conference/

Media Council, 'New Zealand College of Midwives against New Zealand Listener', 2557, January 2017, https://www.mediacouncil.org.nz/rulings/new-zealand-college-of-midwives-against-new-zealand-listener

AIM: Action to Improve Maternity Consumer Network, 'Comments on the Ministry of Health Response to AIM's 2014/30 Submission to the Health Select Committee on the Midwifery First Year of Practice (MFYP)', 18 June 2019, https://www.parliament.nz/resource/en-NZ/51SCHE_EVI_66361_HE6042/66047345323b7bc8086f62af6c47037924a6a4da

New Zealand College of Midwives, 'Health Select Committee Response', June 2019, https://www.parliament.nz/resource/en-NZ/51SCHE_EVI_66361_HE6044/975bd026804f29068351416c495cc9e3eaba2e5c

Lawton, Bev, Nokuthaba Sibanda, Stacie Geller et al., 'Submission to Select Health Committee Re: Perinatal Mortality Safety Data Associated with Pregnancies Looked After by First Year Midwives', 4 October 2019, https://www.parliament.nz/resource/en-NZ/51SCHE_EVI_66361_HE6357/f93490c4b0cd512154689226430b7592e75cc143

## Journals, magazines and newsletters

*Broadsheet*; *Centrepoint Magazine*; *Consumer*; *Education Effects: Magazine of Childbirth Educators NZ*; *Health* (Department of Health); *HQ Magazine*; *Maternity Services Consumer Council Newsletter*; *More*; *New Zealand College of Midwives National Newsletter*; *News & Issues: Newsletter from the National Advisory Committee on Health and Disability*; *New Zealand Nursing Journal: Kai Tiaki* (and *Kai Tiaki: Nursing New Zealand*); *New Zealand College of Midwives Journal*; *New Zealand Doctor*; *New Zealand Woman's Weekly*; *Next*; *O&G Magazine*; *Parents Centre Bulletin*; *Time*; *Woman's Day*.

## Books and articles

Abel, Sally and R. A. Kearns, 'Birth Places: A Geographical Perspective on Planned Home Birth in New Zealand', *Social Science & Medicine*, vol. 33, 7, 1991, pp. 825–37.

Ansley, Bruce, 'Babes at risk', *New Zealand Listener*, 5 April 1997, pp. 20–23.

——, 'Another unfortunate experiment?', *New Zealand Listener*, 14 August 1999, pp. 18–21.

Balaskas, Janet, *The Water Birth Book*, Unwin Hyman, London, 2004.

Banks, Maggie, *Breech Birth Woman-Wise*, Birthspirit Books, Hamilton, 1998.

——, *Home Birth Bound: Mending the Broken Weave*, Birthspirit Books, Hamilton, 2000.

Bartholomew, Karen, Susan M. B. Morton, Polly E. Atatoa Carr, Dinusha K. Bandara and Cameron C. Grant, 'Provider Engagement and Choice in the Lead Maternity Carer System: Evidence from Growing Up in New Zealand', *Australian and New Zealand Journal of Obstetrics and Gynaecology*, vol. 55, 4, 2015, pp. 323–30.

Bastian, Hilda, Marc J. N. C. Keirse and Paul A. Lancaster, 'Perinatal Death Associated with Planned Home Birth in Australia: Population Based Study', *British Medical Journal*, vol. 317, 7155, 8 August 1998, pp. 384–88.

Bickley, Joy, 'Watchdogs or Wimps? Nurses' Response to the Cartwright Report', in Sandra Coney (ed.), *Unfinished Business, What Happened to the Cartwright Report*, Women's Health Action, Auckland, 1993, pp. 125–36.

Blanchette, Glenn, 'The Changing Landscape of Maternity Services', in Robin Gauld (ed.), *Continuity and Chaos: Health Care Management and Delivery in New Zealand*, University of Otago Press, Dunedin, 2003, pp. 137–49.

Bonham, Dennis G., 'Maternal and Child Health', in Douglas P. Kennedy (ed.), *Health in the 1970s: A Collection of Informed Opinions*, N. M. Peryer, Christchurch, 1970, pp. 28–29.

Boxall, Anne-Marie and Kathy Flitcroft, 'Debate: Open Access: From Little Things, Big Things Grow: A Local Approach to System-wide Maternity Services Reform in the Absence of Definitive Evidence', *Australia and New Zealand Health Policy*, vol. 4, 18, 2007.

Bryder, Linda, *A Voice for Mothers: The Plunket Society and Infant Welfare 1907–2000*, Auckland University Press, Auckland, 2003.

——, *A History of the 'Unfortunate Experiment' at National Women's Hospital*, Auckland University Press, Auckland, 2009; reprinted as: Linda Bryder, *Women's Bodies and Medical Science: An Inquiry into Cervical Cancer*, Palgrave Macmillan, London, 2010.

——, *The Rise and Fall of National Women's Hospital*, Auckland University Press, Auckland, 2014.

——, '"An area peculiarly our own": Women and Childbirth in Early to Mid-twentieth Century New Zealand', *New Zealand Journal of History*, vol. 51, 1, 2017, pp. 92–112.

——, 'Donley, Joan Elsa', *Dictionary of New Zealand Biography, Te Ara – the Encyclopedia of New Zealand*, https://teara.govt.nz/en/biographies/6d2/donley-joan-elsa

Bunkle, Phillida, *Second Opinion: The Politics of Women's Health in New Zealand*, Oxford University Press, Auckland, 1988.

Burgess, Marie E., *A Guide to the Law for Nurses and Midwives*, Pearson Education New Zealand, Auckland, 4th edn, 2008.

Burgess, Rhonda, Shawn Walker and Alison Barrett, 'Informed Consent to Breech Birth in New Zealand', *New Zealand Medical Journal*, vol. 128, 1418, 24 July 2015, pp. 85–92.

Calvert, Irene, *Birth in Focus: Midwifery in Aotearoa*, Dunmore Press, Palmerston North, 1998.

Carstairs, Catherine, 'The Granola High: Eating Differently in the Late 1960s and 1970s', in Franca Iacovetta, Valerie J. Korinek and Marlene Epp (eds), *Edible Histories, Cultural Politics: Towards a Canadian Food History*, University of Toronto Press, Toronto, 2012, pp. 305–25.

Chalmers, Iain, Murray Enkin and Marc J. N. C. Keirse (eds), *Effective Care in Pregnancy and Childbirth, vol. 1, Pregnancy*, and *vol. 2, Childbirth*, Oxford University Press, Oxford, 1989.

Chalmers, Iain, 'Commentary: The "Unfortunate Experiment" That Was Not, and the Indebtedness of Women and Children to Herbert ("Herb") Green (1916–2001)', *Journal of Clinical Epidemiology*, vol. 122, June 2020, pp. A13–A19.

Chervenak, Frank A., Laurence B. McCullough, Robert L. Brent, Malcolm I. Levene and Birgit Arabin, 'Planned Home Birth: The Professional Responsibility Response', *American Journal of Obstetrics & Gynecology*, vol. 208, 1, January 2013, pp. 31–38.

Cheyne, Christine, Mike O'Brien and Michael Belgrave, *Social Policy in Aotearoa New Zealand: A Critical Introduction*, Oxford University Press, Auckland, 1997.

Chisholm, Donna, 'Failure to deliver', *North & South*, August 2011, pp. 38–50.

——, 'Stand and deliver', *New Zealand Listener*, 14 February 2015, pp. 18–23.

——, 'Birth control', *New Zealand Listener*, 8 October 2016, pp. 18–25.

Clay, John, *R. D. Laing: A Divided Self*, Hodder & Stoughton, London, 1996.

Coney, Sandra, *The Unfortunate Experiment: The Full Story Behind the Inquiry into Cervical Cancer Treatment*, Penguin Books, Auckland, 1988.

Corbett, Jan, 'Second thoughts on the unfortunate experiment at National Women's', *Metro*, July 1990, pp. 54–73.

Crotty, Maria, Andrew T. Ramsay, Rosemary Smart and Annabelle Chan, 'Planned Homebirths in South Australia 1976–1987', *Medical Journal of Australia*, vol. 153, 1990, pp. 664–71.

Davis, Deborah, Sally Baddock, Sally Pairman, Marion Hunter, Cheryl Benn, Don Wilson, Lesley Dixon and Peter Herbison, 'Planned Place of Birth in New Zealand: Does It Affect Mode of Birth and Intervention Rates Among Low-Risk Women?', *Birth*, vol. 38, 2, 2011, pp. 111–19.

de Costa, Caroline, *The Women's Doc: True Stories from My Five Decades Delivering Babies and Making History*, Allen & Unwin, Sydney, 2021.

Dobbie, Mary, *The Trouble with Women: The Story of Parents Centre New Zealand*, Cape Catley, Whatamongo Bay, 1990.

Donley, Joan, *Save the Midwife*, New Women's Press, Auckland, 1986.

——, *Herstory of N.Z. Home Birth Association*, New Zealand Home Birth Association, Auckland, 1992.

——, 'Independent Midwifery in New Zealand', in Tricia Murphy-Black (ed.), *Issues in Midwifery*, Churchill Livingstone, Edinburgh, 1995, pp. 63–80.

——, *Birthrites: Natural vs Unnatural Childbirth in New Zealand*, Full Court Press in association with the New Zealand College of Midwives, Auckland, 1998.

Donley, Joan and Brenda Hinton (first published in 1993, updated in 2019 by Elizabeth Cox), 'Home Birth Associations, 1978–', https://nzhistory.govt.nz/women-together/home-birth-associations

Edwards, Brian, *Helen: Portrait of a Prime Minister*, Exisle Publishers, Auckland, 2001.

Evers, Annemieke C. C., Hens A. A. Brouwers, Chantal W. P. M. Hukkelhoven et al., 'Perinatal Mortality and Severe Morbidity in Low and High Risk Term Pregnancies in the Netherlands: Prospective Cohort Study', *British Medical Journal*, vol. 341, c5639, 2010.

Exton, Lynda, *The Baby Business: What's Happened to Maternity Care in New Zealand?*, Craig Potton Publishing, Nelson, 2008.

Eyley, Claudia Pond and Dan Salmon, *Helen Clark: Inside Stories*, Auckland University Press, Auckland, 2015.

Field, Peggy Anne, 'Impressions of Women's Health in New Zealand', *Midwifery*, vol. 6, 4, 1990, pp. 185–192.

Fleming, Valerie E. M., 'Midwifery in New Zealand: Responding to Changing Times', *Health Care for Women International*, vol. 17, 4, 1996, pp. 343–59.

Flint, Caroline, Polly Poulengeris and Adrian Grant, "The 'Know Your Midwife" Scheme – A Randomised Trial of Continuity of Care by a Team of Midwives', *Midwifery*, vol. 5, 1, March 1989, pp. 11–16.

Gaskin, Ina May, *Spiritual Midwifery*, The Book Publishing Co., The Farm, Summertown, Tennessee, rev. ed., 1978.

Geller Stacie E., Abigail R. Koch, Caitlin E. Garland, E. Jane MacDonald, Francesca Storey and Beverley Lawton, 'A Global View of Severe Maternal Morbidity: Moving Beyond Maternal Mortality', *Reproductive Health*, vol. 15 (Supp 1), 98, 2018.

Gibson Smith, Margaret and Yvonne T. Shadbolt (eds), *Objects and Outcomes: New Zealand Nurses' Association 1909–1983*, New Zealand Nurses' Association, Wellington, 1984.

Glasgow, Kathy, 'Maternity "Shambles"', *New Zealand Health Review*, vol. 1, 1, Autumn 1998, pp. 9–12.

Gordon, Doris, *Backblocks Baby-Doctor: An Autobiography*, Faber & Faber, London, 1955.

Greenlees, Janet and Linda Bryder (eds), *Western Maternity and Medicine, 1880–1990*, Pickering & Chatto, London, 2013.

Grigg, Celia P. and Sally K. Tracy, 'New Zealand's Unique Maternity System', *Women and Birth*, vol. 26, 1, March 2013, pp. e59–e64.

Grigg, Celia P., Sally K. Tracy, Virginia Schmied, Amy Monk and Mark B. Tracy, 'Women's Experiences of Transfer from Primary Maternity Unit to Tertiary Hospital in New Zealand: Part of the Prospective Cohort Evaluating Maternity Units Study', *BMC Pregnancy Childbirth*, vol. 15, 339, 2015.

Guilliland, Karen and Sally Pairman, *The Midwifery Partnership – A Model for Practice*, Department of Nursing and Midwifery, Victoria University of Wellington, Wellington, 1995.

——, *Women's Business: The Story of the New Zealand College of Midwives, 1986–2010*, New Zealand College of Midwives, Christchurch, 2010.

Gulbransen, Graham, John Hilton, Linda McKay and Andrew Cox, 'Home Birth in New Zealand 1973–93: Incidence and Mortality', *New Zealand Medical Journal*, vol. 110, 1040, 28 March 1997, pp. 87–89.

Haines, Leah, 'Another unfortunate experiment', *New Zealand Listener*, 31 January 2009, pp. 14–19.

Hamilton, Bruce, 'Williams, Ulric Gaster', *Dictionary of New Zealand Biography Te Ara – the Encyclopedia of New Zealand*, https://teara.govt.nz/en/biographies/4w19/williams-ulric-gaster

Hedwig, Judy and Valerie Fleming, 'Midwifery Practice in New Zealand: A Dynamic Discipline', in Tricia Murphy-Black (ed.), *Issues in Midwifery*, Churchill Livingstone, Edinburgh, 1995, pp. 207–20.

Henaghan, Mark, *Health Professionals and Trust: The Cure for Healthcare Law and Policy*, Routledge-Cavendish, London, 2011.

Howie, Leonie and Adele Robertson, *Island Nurses: Stories of Birth, Life and Death on Remote Great Barrier Island*, Allen & Unwin, Auckland, 2017.

Illich, Ivan, *Medical Nemesis: The Expropriation of Health*, Calder & Boyars, London, 1975.

Jaye, Chrystal, Zara Mason and Dawn Miller, '"Tossing Out the Baby with the Bath Water": New Zealand General Practitioners on Maternity Care', *Medical Anthropology*, vol. 32, 5, 2013, pp. 448–66.

Kennare, Robyn M., Marc J. N. C. Keirse, Graeme R. Tucker and Annabelle C. Chan, 'Planned Home and Hospital Births in South Australia, 1991–2006: Differences in Outcomes', *Medical Journal of Australia*, vol. 192, 2, 18 January 2010, pp. 76–80.

Kline, Wendy, 'Communicating a New Consciousness: Countercultural Print and the Home Birth Movement in the 1970s', *Bulletin of the History of Medicine*, vol. 89, 3, 2015, pp. 527–56.

——, *Coming Home: How Midwives Changed Birth*, Oxford University Press, New York, 2019.

Laing, Adrian Charles, *R. D. Laing: A Biography*, Chester Springs, Pennsylvania, and Peter Owen, London, 1994.

Lawton, Beverley A., Leona F. Wilson, Richard A. Dinsdale et al., 'Audit of Severe Acute Maternal Morbidity Describing Reasons for Transfer and Potential Preventability of Admissions to ICU', *Australian and New Zealand Journal of Obstetrics and Gynaecology*, vol. 50, 4, 2010, pp. 346–51.

Lawton, Beverley A., Abby Koch, James Stanley and Stacie E. Geller, 'The Effect of Midwifery Care on Rates of Caesarean Delivery', *International Journal of Gynecology & Obstetrics*, vol. 123, 3, 2013, pp. 213–16.

Lawton, Beverley, Evelyn J. MacDonald, Selina A. Brown et al., 'Preventability of Severe Acute Maternal Morbidity', *American Journal of Obstetrics & Gynecology*, vol. 210, 2014, 557, pp. e1–6.

Lawton, Beverley, Sara Filoche, Stacie E. Geller, Sue Garrett and James Stanley, 'A Retrospective Cohort Study of the Association Between Midwifery Experience and Perinatal Mortality', *International Journal of Gynecology & Obstetrics*, vol. 132, 1, 2016, pp. 94–99.

Leap, Nicky and Billie Hunter, *The Midwife's Tale: An Oral History from Handywoman to Professional Midwife*, Scarlet Press, London, 1993.

Lecky-Thompson, Maggie, 'Independent Midwifery in Australia', in Tricia Murphy-Black (ed.), *Issues in Midwifery*, Churchill Livingstone, Edinburgh, 1995, pp. 41–62.

Legat, Nicola, 'Measles on Elm Street: The argument against immunisation', *Metro*, December 1991, pp. 93–103.

Loudon, Irvine, *Death in Childbirth: An International Study of Maternal Care and Maternal Mortality, 1800–1950*, Oxford University Press, Oxford, 1992.

——, 'Childbirth', in Irvine Loudon (ed.), *Western Medicine: An Illustrated History*, Oxford University Press, Oxford, 1997, pp. 206–20.

McAra-Couper, Judith, Marion Jones and Elizabeth Smythe, 'Rising Rates of Intervention in Childbirth', *British Journal of Midwifery*, vol. 18, 3, March 2010, pp. 160–69.

MacDonald, Evelyn J., Stacie E. Geller and Beverley A. Lawton, 'Establishment of a National Severe Maternal Morbidity Preventability Review in New Zealand', *International Journal of Gynecology & Obstetrics*, vol. 135, 1, October 2016, pp. 120–23.

McLoughlin, David, 'The politics of childbirth: Midwives versus doctors', *North & South*, August 1993, pp. 55–69.

Malcolm, Laurence and Nicholas Mays, 'New Zealand's Independent Practitioner Associations: A Working Model of Clinical Governance in Primary Care?', *British Medical Journal*, vol. 319, 7221, 20 November 1999, pp. 1340–42.

Mein Smith, Philippa, *Maternity in Dispute: New Zealand, 1920–1939*, Historical Publications Branch, Department of Internal Affairs, Government Printer, Wellington, 1986.

——, 'Midwifery Re-innovation in New Zealand', in Jennifer Stanton (ed.), *Innovations in Health and Medicine: Diffusion and Resistance in the Twentieth Century*, Routledge, New York, 2002, pp. 169–87.

Michaels, Paula A., *Lamaze: An International History*, Oxford University Press, Oxford, 2014.

Miller, Dawn, Helen Roberts and Don Wilson, 'Future Practice of Graduates of the New Zealand Diploma of Obstetrics and Gynaecology or Certificate in Women's Health', *New Zealand Medical Journal*, vol. 121, 1282, 19 September 2008, pp. 29–38.

Myles, Margaret F., *Textbook for Midwives*, Churchill Livingstone, New York, 9th edn, 1981; 10th edn, 1985.

Neas, Ollie, 'Risky business', *North & South*, May 2022, pp. 53–55.

Ngan, Cherry, 'Should Midwives be Held to a Different Standard of Care, Given New Zealand's Unique Autonomous Midwife-led Framework?', *Auckland University Law Review*, vol. 23, 2017, pp. 119–46.

Nicolson, Malcolm and John E. E. Fleming, *Imaging and Imagining the Fetus: The Development of Obstetric Ultrasound*, Johns Hopkins University Press, Baltimore, 2013.

Nuttall, Alison, '"Taking Advantage of the Facilities and Comforts . . . Offered": Women's Choice of Hospital Delivery in Interwar Edinburgh', in Janet Greenlees and

Linda Bryder (eds), *Western Maternity and Medicine, 1880–1990*, Pickering & Chatto, London, 2013, pp. 65–80.

Oakley, Ann, 'The Sociology of Childbirth: An Autobiographical Journey Through Four Decades of Research', *Sociology of Health & Illness*, vol. 38, 5, June 2016, pp. 689–705.

Ogonowska-Coates, Halina, *Born: Midwives and Women Celebrate 100 Years*, New Zealand College of Midwives, Christchurch, 2004.

Page, Lesley and Rona McCandlish (eds), *The New Midwifery: Science and Sensitivity in Practice*, Churchill Livingstone, Edinburgh, 2006.

Pairman, Sally, Jan Pincombe, Carol Thorogood and Sally Tracy (eds), *Midwifery: Preparation for Practice*, Churchill Livingstone Elsevier, Marrickville, New South Wales, 2006.

Palmer, Geoffrey, *Unbridled Power?: An Interpretation of New Zealand's Constitution and Government*, Victoria University of Wellington, Wellington, 1979.

Papps, Elaine and Irihapeti Ramsden, 'Cultural Safety in Nursing: The New Zealand Experience', *International Journal for Quality in Health Care*, vol. 8, 5, October 1996, pp. 491–97.

Pattison, Neil and R. Teele, 'A Plea for a Comprehensive Perinatal Database', *New Zealand Medical Journal*, vol. 114, 1141, 12 October 2001, pp. 439–40.

Pesce, Andrew F., 'Editorial: Planned Home Birth in Australia: Politics or Science?', *Medical Journal of Australia*, vol. 192, 2, 18 January 2010, pp. 60–61.

Powell, Rhonda, Shawn Walker and Alison Barrett, 'Informed Consent to Breech Birth in New Zealand', *New Zealand Medical Journal*, vol. 128, 1418, 24 July 2015, pp. 85–92.

Raffle, Angela E., Anne Mackie and J. A. Muir Gray, *Screening: Evidence and Practice*, Oxford University Press, Oxford, 2nd edn, 2019.

Raffle, Angela E. and J. A. Muir Gray, 'Review: The 1960s Cervical Screening Incident at National Women's Hospital, Auckland, New Zealand: Insights for Screening Research, Policy Making and Practice', *Journal of Clinical Epidemiology*, vol. 122, June 2020, pp. A8–A13.

Rain, Lynn, *Community: The Story of Riverside 1941–1991*, Riverside Community, Lower Moutere, 1991.

Ray, Pauline, 'Whose body is it? Whose baby is it?', *New Zealand Listener*, 15 March 1980, pp. 20–22.

——, 'Birth: Back to basics', *New Zealand Listener*, 30 April 1983, pp. 20–21.

——, 'Midwives tales', *New Zealand Listener*, 5 November 1983, pp. 16–17.

Reid, Rosemary, 'Obstetric Perspectives: Quality Within Choice', *New Zealand Medical Journal*, vol. 117, 1206, 26 November 2004, U1169.

Reiger, Kereen, 'The Politics of Midwifery in Australia: Tensions, Debates and Opportunities', *Annual Review of Health Social Sciences*, vol. 10, 1, 2000, pp. 53–64.

Revington, Mark, 'Born free', *New Zealand Listener*, 14 August 1999, pp. 18–21.

Robertson, Adele M., 'Rural Women and Maternity Services', in Jean Ross (ed.), *Rural Nursing: Aspects of Practice*, Rural Health Opportunities, Ministry of Health, Dunedin, 2008, pp. 179–200.

Robie, Penelope and David, 'A warm and loving welcome', *New Zealand Listener*, 15 January 1977, pp. 18–19.

Rodenburg, Helen, 'Right Place, Right Time', in Rosy Fenwicke (ed.), *In Practice: The Lives of New Zealand Women Doctors in the 21st Century*, Random House, Auckland, 2004, reprint 2017, pp. 111–24.

Rosenblatt, Roger A., Judith Reinken and Phil Shoemack, 'Is Obstetrics Safe in Small Hospitals? Evidence from New Zealand's Regionalised Perinatal System', *The Lancet*, vol. 326, 8452, 1985, pp. 429–32.

Rothman, Barbara Katz, *In Labor: Women and Power in the Birthplace*, W. W. Norton, New York, 1982.

——, *Recreating Motherhood: Ideology and Technology in a Patriarchal Society*, W. W. Norton, New York, 1989.

Sadler, Lynn C., Judith McAra-Couper, Deborah Pittam, Michelle R. Wise and John M. D. Thompson, 'Risk of Perinatal Mortality in the First Year of Midwifery Practice in New Zealand: Analysis of a Retrospective National Cohort', *British Medical Journal Open*, vol. 8, 4, 7 April 2018.

Sandall Jane, Hora Soltani, Simon Gates, Andrew Shennan and Declan Devane, 'Midwife-led Continuity Models versus Other Models of Care for Childbearing Women', *Cochrane Database of Systematic Reviews*, vol. 4, 4, 28 April 2016, pp. 1–63.

Sargison, Patricia A., *Notable Women in New Zealand Health: Te Auora ki Aotearoa Ona Wahine Rongonui*, Longman Paul, Auckland, 1993.

Savage, Wendy, *A Savage Enquiry: Who Controls Childbirth?*, Virago, London, 1986.

Schrader, Ben, 'Magazines and periodicals – Specialist and lifestyle magazines: 1890s to 2010s', *Te Ara – the Encyclopedia of New Zealand*, http://www.TeAra.govt.nz/en/magazines-and-periodicals/page-5

Scott, E. J. C., 'Myles, Margaret Fraser (1892–1988)', *Oxford Dictionary of National Biography*, Oxford University Press, Oxford, 2013.

Simkin, Penny, 'Tribute: Sheila Kitzinger (1929–2015)', *Birth*, vol. 42, 3, September 2015, pp. 199–201.

Simmers, Don, 'The Few: New Zealand's Diminishing Number of Rural GPs Providing Maternity Services', *New Zealand Medical Journal*, vol. 119, 1241, 2006, U2151.

Skegg, Peter D. G., 'English Medical Law and "Informed Consent": An Antipodean Assessment and Alternative', *Medical Law Review*, vol. 7, 2, Summer 1999, pp. 135–65.

Stewart, Sarah, 'Midwifery in New Zealand: A Cause for Celebration', *MIDIRS [Midwives' Information and Resource Service] Midwifery Digest*, vol. 11, 3, September 2001, pp. 319–22.

Stirling, Pamela, 'Hard labour', *New Zealand Listener*, 12 March 1990, pp. 10–15.

Suarez, Suzanne Hope, 'Midwifery Is Not the Practice of Medicine', *Yale Journal of Law and Feminism*, vol. 5, 1993, pp. 315–64.

Sutcliffe, Katy, Jenny Caird and Josephine Kavanagh, 'Comparing Midwife-led and Doctor-led Maternity Care: A Systematic Review of Reviews', *Journal of Advanced Nursing*, vol. 68, 11, 2012, pp. 2376–86.

Te Huia, Jean, 'Nga Maia Maori Midwives Aotearoa 1993–', *Women Together: A History of Women's Organisations in New Zealand*, 2019, https://nzhistory.govt.nz/women-together/nga-maia-maori-midwives-aotearoa

Tew, Marjorie, 'Place of Birth and Perinatal Mortality', *Journal of the Royal College of General Practitioners*, vol. 35, 277, 1985, pp. 390–94.

——, *A Safer Childbirth? A Critical History of Maternity Care*, Springer, New York, 1990.

Visser, Gerard H. A., 'Obstetric Care in the Netherlands: Relic or Example?', *Journal of Obstetrics and Gynaecology Canada*, vol. 34, 10, October 2012, pp. 971–75.

Wassner, Adelheid, *A Labour of Love: Childbirth at Dunedin Hospital, 1862–1972*, self-published, Dunedin, 1999.

Wernham, Ellie, Jason Gurney, James Stanley, Lis Ellison-Loschmann and Diana Sarfati, 'A Comparison of Midwife-Led and Medical-Led Models of Care and Their Relationship to Adverse Fetal and Neonatal Outcomes: A Retrospective Cohort Study in New Zealand', *PLoS Medicine*, vol. 13, 9, 27 September 2016, e1002134.

Wiegerinck, M. M. J., B. Y. van der Goes, A. C. Ravelli et al., 'Intrapartum and Neonatal Mortality in Primary Midwife-led and Secondary Obstetrician-led Care in the Amsterdam Region of the Netherlands: A Retrospective Cohort Study', *Midwifery*, vol. 31, 12, 31 December 2015, pp. 1168–76.

Wolf, Jacqueline, *Deliver Me from Pain: Anaesthesia and Birth in America*, Johns Hopkins University Press, Baltimore, 2009.

Young, Diony, 'The Midwifery Revolution in New Zealand: What We Can Learn', *Birth*, vol. 23, 3, 1996, pp. 125–27.

Zielinski, Ruth, Kelly Ackerson and Lisa K. Low, 'Planned Home Birth: Benefits, Risks and Opportunities', *International Journal of Women's Health*, vol. 7, 2015, pp. 361–77.

## Theses and dissertations

Abel, Sally, 'Midwifery and Maternity Services in Transition: An Examination of Change following the Nurses Amendment Act 1990', PhD thesis, University of Auckland, 1997.

Ashcroft, Shelley, 'Modern Women or Tree-hugging Hippies? A Foucauldian Discourse Analysis of the New Zealand Media's Representation of Waterbirth', Master of Health Science thesis, Auckland University of Technology, 2007.

Banks, Maggie, 'Out on a Limb: The Personal Mandate to Practise Midwifery by Midwives of the Domiciliary Midwives Society of New Zealand (Incorporated), 1974–1986', PhD thesis, Victoria University of Wellington, 2007.

Bartholomew, Karen, 'The Realities of Choice and Access in the Lead Maternity Carer System: Operationalising Choice Policy in the New Zealand Maternity Reforms', Master of Public Health thesis, University of Auckland, 2010.

Bourke, Gabrielle, 'Illuminating the Dark Hour: Auckland's St Helen's Hospital, 1906–1990', MA thesis, University of Auckland, 2006.

Calvert, Irene, 'Trauma, Relational Trust and the Effects on the Midwife', PhD thesis, Massey University, 2011.

Daellenbach, Rea, 'The Paradox of Success and the Challenge of Change: Home Birth Associations of Aotearoa/New Zealand', PhD thesis, University of Canterbury, 1999.

Dixon, Lesley, 'The Integrated Neurophysiology of Emotions During Labour and Birth: A Feminist Standpoint Exploration of the Women's Perspectives of Labour Progress', PhD thesis, Victoria University of Wellington, 2011.

Fleming, Valerie, 'Partnership, Power and Politics, Feminist Perceptions of Midwifery Practice', PhD thesis, Massey University, 1994.

Grehan, Madonna May, 'Professional Aspirations and Consumer Expectations: Nurses, Midwives, and Women's Health', PhD thesis, University of Melbourne, 2009.

Hendry, Christine Elizabeth O'Rourke, 'Midwifery in New Zealand 1990–2003: The Complexities of Service Provision', Doctor of Midwifery thesis, University of Technology, Sydney, 2003.

Hewson, Alan, 'The History of Obstetrics and Gynaecology in Australia from 1950 to 2010', PhD thesis, University of Newcastle, 2016.

Jeffery, Christina A., 'Whanautanga: The Experiences of Māori Women Who Gave Birth at National Women's Hospital 1958–2004', MA thesis, University of Auckland, 2005.

McAra-Couper, Judith, 'What is Shaping the Practice of Health Professionals and the Understanding of the Public in Relation to Increasing Intervention in Childbirth?', PhD thesis, Auckland University of Technology, 2007.

Maude, Robyn Mary, 'Intelligent Structured Intermittent Auscultation (ISIA): A Mixed Methods Evaluation of an Informed Decision-making Framework for Fetal Heart Rate Monitoring', PhD thesis, Victoria University of Wellington, 2012.

Pairman, Sally, 'Workforce to Profession: An Exploration of New Zealand Midwifery's Professionalising Strategies from 1986 to 2005', Doctor of Midwifery thesis, University of Technology, Sydney, 2005.

Ramsden, Irihapeti Merenia, 'Cultural Safety and Nursing Education in Aotearoa and Te Waipounamu', PhD thesis, Victoria University of Wellington, 2002.

Schmidt, Rachel, 'A Voyage to Motherhood: Pacific Mothers' Lived Experiences of Pregnancy, Childbirth, Postnatal Care and Early Motherhood, 1950–1995', MA thesis, University of Auckland, 2020.

Shaw, Alastair, 'Telling the Truth about People's China', PhD thesis, Victoria University of Wellington, 2010.

Skiff, Samantha, 'Machine-minders and Handmaidens? Hospital Midwives and Childbirth in New Zealand, 1950–1990', MA thesis, University of Auckland, 2014.

Stojanovic, Jane Ellen Esther, 'Placental Birth: A History', PhD thesis, Massey University, 2012.

Surtees, Ruth Joy, 'Midwifery as Feminist Praxis in Aotearoa/New Zealand', PhD thesis, University of Canterbury, 2003.

Sweetman, Claire, 'Safe Deliveries? A Review of New Zealand's Midwifery Regulation through the lens of the Health and Disability Commissioner', Laws 513 – Law and Medicine Research Paper, Faculty of Law, Victoria University of Wellington, 2013.

Wittmer, Jillian, 'Place of Birth: A Longitudinal Study Comparing Delivery Outcome, Maternal Attitudes and Coping', MA thesis, University of Auckland, 1981.

# INDEX

## A

Abel, Sally 144; on 1990 Act 134; and direct-entry midwifery training 194; on doctor–midwife disagreements 184; and Joan Donley 89, 103; on shared care 160, 162
ACC (Accident Compensation Corporation) 148–49, 177, 220, 227, 243, 282
active birth 25, 42, 45
active management of childbirth 41, 252
acupuncture 19–20, 22–24, 198, 245, 292n114
Advanced Diploma 75–76
adverse outcomes 3–4; AIM's research on 217, 268; coroners on 208; Lawton's research on 252; preparing graduates for 280; responsibility for 147; Wernham's research on 262, 265
AIDS 28–29, 201, 203
AIM (Action to Improve Maternity) 214, 217, 242–43, 282–83; evidence accumulated by 246; on hospital interventions 264; and Lawton's research 253; submissions by 215, 258, 268
AIMS (Action to Improve Maternity Services) 166–67
AIMS (Association for Improvement to Maternity Services), UK 44
Albany Maternity and Gynaecology 171–73, 177
Alber, Erwin 203–5
alternative and complementary therapies 21, 25, 32, 198–99, 274

alternative lifestyles 13–16, 117–18, 283
ambulance services 53, 211–12, 227, 245
amniotic fluid embolism 270
anaesthesia 7–8
Anderson, Jacqui 95
Ansley, Bruce 159, 162
antenatal care 8, 12, 152, 169, 220–21, 279
antenatal classes 42, 200, 222, 248–49
antibiotics 8, 53, 191
anti-establishment values 13, 29
anti-vaccination movement 28, 203; see also immunisation
Apgar scores 220, 262, 346n70, 359n47
apprenticeship model 243–44
area health boards 161; and 1990 Act 119; and alternatives to homebirth 85; and midwifery standards 83–84; and midwifery training 130; midwives under contract to 124; see also District Health Boards
Area Health Boards Act 1983 106
Arms, Suzanne 46
aromatherapy 274
asphyxia: birth-related 231, 262; intrapartum 213–14
Association of Radical Midwives, Britain 41, 87
Association of Wellington Midwives 171
asthma 29, 191, 203
Auckland Childbirth Education Association 42
Auckland District Health Board 233, 246, 256

# Index

Auckland Home Birth Association 90; and 1983 Act 74; in 1990s 143; and doctors 64, 161; foundation of 13, 30, 37; and immunisation 27; and MSC 39, 52, 62; and NZNA 73–75; political activism of 92–93
Auckland Hospital Board 107
Auckland Hospital Research Ethical Committee 107
Auckland Maternity Services Consumer Council 149, 166, 199
Auckland Obstetric Standards Review Committee 83
Auckland University of Technology (AUT) 139, 191–92, 218
Auckland Women's Health Council 107
Auckland Women's Liberation Group 19
Australia: homebirth research in 246; Maternity Services Review 2009 237
Australian College of Midwives 87, 237–38
Australian Society of Independent Midwives 87
autism 203
*Avenues* (magazine) 175

## B

*The Baby Business* (Exton) 235–36
back-up services 50, 57, 84, 120–21, 211, 280
Baines, Sue 249
Baird, Tony 36, 40, 55, 65, 83, 184–85, 200, 215
Baker, Karine 172
Balaskas, Janet 25, 44–46, 77, 108
Banks, Maggie: on breech births 186–87, 210; on counterculture 14, 18; on CTG 223, 337n30; on medical model 144, 146; on MSC review 52, 65; on nurses against midwives 71; on partnership model 279
Barlow, Anne 196–97, 234
Barlow, Linda and Adam 212–14, 218, 227, 229, 286n1
Barnett, Feliz 85
Barry, Maggie 168
Bartholomew, Karen 257
base hospitals 16, 50, 81, 244

Bassett, Michael 90, 99, 101, 210
Bastian, Hilda 85, 185
Batchelor, Mary 98
Begg, Evan 190
best practice 239–40, 273
Bethlehem Birthing Centre, Tauranga 244–46
Bevan-Brown, Maurice 33
Beynon, Shannon 238
Bickley, Joy 86, 118
biculturalism 96–97, 153–54
bioscience 194
Birch, Bill 159
Birch, Tony 78
Bird, Christine 39
birth experience 17, 25; benefits for mother 33–35, 165; control over 107; and feminism 38; in hospital 143; overemphasis on 217, 239
birth process: decision-making in 279; fear of 45; recording discussions relating to 219, 280; trusting in 222; whānau involvement in 198
*Birth with R D Laing* (film) 18–19
*Birth Without Violence* (Leboyer) 24, 32
Birthcare, Auckland 84
birthing plans 245
Black, Denise 145
Black, Janet 211
blackstrap molasses 19–21
Blanchette, Glen 171–73, 177–78
blood clotting 270
blood pressure, high 19, 23, 273, 277
blood transfusion 8, 53
Blundell, Sally 276, 278
Board of Health Maternity Services Committee *see* MSC
Bonham, Dennis 11, 27, 51, 84, 231
Bourke, Gabrielle 61, 71, 76
Boyd, Bob 126
Boyd, Elaine 205
brain injuries 105, 188; culpability of midwife for 224, 226–27; lobby groups against 147–48; medical technology blamed for 199, 203; rates of 180; treatment cost of 243
Bramley, Dale 269

breastfeeding 180, 196–97, 248
Bree, Sue 217
breech births 16, 22; deaths following 209–10, 227, 233; in hospital 51; lay midwives and 80; and transfer to hospital 185–87
Brett, Cate 143
Brew, Helen 16, 18–19
Bridgman, Geoff 13, 32, 39, 52, 74, 105
*British Medical Journal* 44, 260–61
*British Medical Journal Open* 256
*Broadsheet* Collective 21
'Broken Dolls' (article) 175
Brown, Margaret 76
Browne, Barbara 170, 173
Buchwald, Gerhard 203
Bunkle, Phillida 38
Burgess, Marie 208
Burgess, Sian 12, 43–46, 141; and GPs 160, 164; on immunisation 248; and Maggie Banks 187, 223, 337n30
burnout 180, 277–78
Butler, Hilary 27–28, 201

## C

Cable, Graeme 83
caesarean section 47, 65, 115, 152; and breech births 210; elective 242–43; emergency 242, 353n69; increased rates of 237; rising rates of 252; and transfer to hospital 183–86
Callaghan, Kerry 33
Calvert, Sarah 37
Cameron, Amanda 249
Cameron, Danielle 111
Campbell, Jennifer *see* Rowan, Jennifer
Canada 41, 139
Canterbury Hospital Board 53
Carlaw, Liz 158, 160
Carll, Joan 236
Carpenter, Helen 75–76
Carpenter Report 74
Cartwright Inquiry 90, 103, 107–10, 185, 231, 237–38
Caygill, David 84, 88, 102, 106, 132
Centre for Women's Health Research 260

Centrepoint Community 14, 18, 24, 42, 44, 55
cerebral haemorrhage 220
cerebral palsy 141, 239, 243
Charkovsky, Igor 25, 292n130
Childbirth Education Association of Otago 42
childbirth educators 19, 42–43, 108, 248–49
Chin, Colin 181
Chinese Cultural Revolution 37
Chisholm, Donna 209, 216–17, 226, 240–41, 244, 264–65
*Choices for Health Care* (report) 100
Christchurch HBA 99, 106, 108
Christchurch Polytechnic 76, 192, 195
Christchurch Women's Hospital 15, 148, 231, 238
Churcher, Barbara 151
civil rights 163
Claridge, Sue 248
Clark, Helen 2, 63; and area health boards 106; and Cartwright Inquiry 109–10; and GP obstetricians 166; and homebirth movement 92, 97–98, 143; on midwife autonomy 70, 103–5, 107, 112, 138; and midwifery training 76, 121, 131–33, 280; and Nurses Amendment Act 1990 110, 113–16, 119–21, 123–30, 133–35; as patron of midwives 162, 174
Clark, Ken 265
Clark, Patricia 55
Clendon, Simon 248
Clentworth, Howard 188–89
clinical supervision 209, 253, 273
Clotworthy, Barbara 151
Coco, Jo 160
Code of Health and Disability Services Consumers' Rights 149–50, 218–20, 222, 224–25, 248, 281
Cole, Sharron 108, 118; 208, 213
Coleman, Jonathan 255
Coleman, Lynn 167, 330n42
College of Natural Medicine, Christchurch 28
College of Obstetricians and Gynaecologists (New Zealand/Australia)

319n35; and 1990 Act 120, 123–24; and Barlow case 229; criticism of 1990s reforms 237–38; on CTG monitoring 223; on hospital transfers 184; merger of Australian and New Zealand colleges 189; on midwife autonomy 130; on primary units 245; and Wernham's research 265
Collins, Anne 115
Collins, Simon 123
colonial oppression 196
communes 13–17, 24, 30, 53, 117–18
Communist Party of New Zealand 36
co-morbidities 275
comprehensive nurses 75
Coney, Sandra 37–38, 166, 168, 237
consumer advocates 3; and 1990 Act 116–17; in College of Midwives 107–8; criticising midwifery model 242–43; and health policy 105–7; in homebirth movement 39, 42, 74, 92–93; lack of Māori as 96
continuity of care 84–85, 134, 144, 165, 193, 274
Cooper, Derryn 13, 32, 37
Cooper, Lorraine 175
Cooper, Warren 175
Copland, Alison 330n42
Corbett, Jan 109
coroners 1, 3; on CTG 223; deaths reported to 234, 238; and Health and Disability Commissioner 218; on homebirth deaths 140–41, 148, 187; on midwife competency 188, 208; reports 2005–2015 208–17, 228
Coroners Act 1988 140
corticosteroids 8
cost-effectiveness 105–6, 114–15, 125, 158
Council for Civil Liberties 93
counterculture 13–15, 30, 153
Coyle, Alice 138
Crampton, Peter 254, 266–68
Crawford, Barbara 233
Crawford, Caroline 202–3
Crawshaw, Jennifer 227
Creech, Wyatt 168
Crombie, Rachel 175
crown health enterprises 161–62

CTG (cardiotocography) 184, 189–90, 214, 220, 222–23
Cullen, Michael 99
cultural safety 169, 195–98, 228
Cunliffe, David 233

D

Daellenbach, Rea 96, 106, 108, 122, 134
Daloz, Laurent 195
Dalton, Tracy 78
Daly-Peoples, Linda 37–38, 56
Davidson, Flora 20
Davies, Valerie 39
Davis, Adelle 19–20, 290n86
de Bock, Cecile 211
de Costa, Caroline 200, 242–43
Denyer, Alison 161, 330n42
Department of Health: 1987 report 64; and 1990 Act 125–27, 134; Advisory Committee on Women's Health 61, 67; on complementary therapies 21, 25, 32; and consumer advocacy 107; and direct-entry training 131–32; educational magazine 40; and Fourth Labour Government 102–3; and HBA 28; and homebirth midwives 10, 50, 61, 66, 74, 83, 85, 158; and lay midwives 79; lobbying 94; on maternity units 84; on nutrition 20; on prescriptions 123; review of 1983 Act 60; Safe Maternity Campaign 8; on ultrasound 26; Working Group on Safe Options for Low-Risk Pregnancy 35, 45, 79, 126; *see also* Ministry of Health
de-skilling 215
Desmond, Natalie 247
diabetes 84, 126, 144, 152, 256, 273
diagnostic skills 280
Dick-Read, Grantly 30, 33
Dillon, Leone 142
direct-entry midwifery training 1, 81–82, 90, 192–95, 280; in 1990 Act 129–32; in Canada 139; lobbying for 103; Māori and Pasifika women and 154, 195–98; and rural areas 179–80; Save the Midwives Association on 75–76

direct-entry midwives 192, 195, 253
District Health Boards (DHBs) 179;
  and maternal morbidity 252; and
  Maternity Services Notice 233;
  midwives contracting with 282
Dixon, Lesley 254
doctors: disagreements with midwives
  142, 183, 189, 220, 226–28; gatekeeper
  role of 102, 128, 160–61; male *see*
  medical profession, male; reintegration
  into maternity services 209; *see also* GPs;
  obstetricians
documentation: by midwives 219–20,
  280; by specialists 189
domiciliary midwives *see* homebirth
  midwives
Domiciliary Midwives Society 66–67,
  118; and 1990 Act 117; advising
  Health Department 107; and College
  of Midwives 142; on cost-effectiveness
  114; and Helen Clark 104; and
  homeopathy 22; lack of Māori
  members 96; and lay midwives 78–79;
  and NZNA 85–86; standards review
  committee 82–83, 119
*Domiciliary Midwives Society Newsletter* 23,
  25, 43, 66, 71, 107
Domino services 84–85
Donley, Joan: on 1971 Act 60–62; and
  1990 Act 89, 112, 114, 117–18;
  awarded OBE 110; and biculturalism
  97; on Bronwen Pelvin 67; and
  Cartwright Inquiry 109–10; celebration
  of 138–40; and College of Midwives
  88, 205–6; criticism of independent
  midwives 142–44; on Direct Entry
  Midwifery Task Force 75; and DMC
  Standards Review Committee 82–83;
  on doctor–midwife relationship 183;
  on GP and midwife payments 159; and
  HBA 90–92; on Health and Disability
  Commission 149, 282; and Helen Clark
  103–5, 280; on homebirth movement
  13; and homebirth package 19–23; and
  hospital medicine 84–85; on hospital
  midwives 152; and international
  movement 41–43, 46; on Māori
  midwives 198; on medical technology
  26, 199–203; on midwife autonomy 71,
  79, 82, 286n3; and midwifery training
  76–77, 81, 192, 215; and MSC survey
  54, 56; and Nga Maia 155; and NZNA
  55, 73, 86; political activism of 93–94,
  100, 102; and politics of homebirth
  36–37, 39–40; and psychology 31;
  at Social Services Select Committee
  123; on water birth 25; on witch hunt
  against homebirths 141; on women's
  empowerment 33–35, 147; on Working
  Group for Safe Options 79, 107
Donnison, Jean 41
Drew, Jenny 42
drugs: midwife opposition to 12, 22, 27;
  prescribing rights 22, 122–24, 126, 128,
  190–91
Duff, Michelle 263, 267, 271–72
Dunkley, Penelope 52
Durham, Gillian 201–3
Durie, Mason 169, 198
duty of care 190

E

Earl, Deborah 189–90
East Kent Maternity Services 274
ecbolics 8, 200
Eddy, Alison 282, 286n3
*Education Effects* (magazine) 248
Edwards, Brian 133
Edwards, Diana 120, 141, 319n36
Elliot, Cameron 209–10
Elliott, Bob 97
Ellison-Loschmann, Lis 196, 261
empirical midwifery 77
English, Bill 168
epidurals 8, 47, 144, 150, 242
episiotomies 21, 38, 150
ergometrine 8, 26–27
Evans, Garry 208–11, 214–17, 232
Evans (Jackson), Rhonda 14, 18, 24,
  42, 55
Exton, Lynda 3, 173–74, 235–36, 238,
  241, 244, 264

## F

The Farm, Tennessee 17–18, 22, 63
Farquhar, Cynthia (Cindy) 209–10, 231, 240–41, 270
Farry, Annabel 193
fathers, in homebirth movement 12
Federation of Women's Health Councils 178, 190
female principle 205
feminism: contemporary forms of 242, 284; and homebirth movement 36–42, 45–46, 94–95; and midwifery 77, 108, 145–46, 156; second-wave 33, 37, 41; Western notions of 153
Ferguson, William 160–61, 167, 172–73, 176, 180, 236, 329n17, 330n42
fetal abnormalities 126
fetal distress 141, 148, 184–85, 222
fetal hypoxia 184
fetal movements 26, 220, 223
fetal surveillance education 270, 281
Field, Peggy Anne 101
Fitchett, Tony 164, 173
Fitzpatrick, Val 71
Fleming, Valerie 75, 144
Flint, Caroline 76, 87, 194
flying squads 53–54, 120, 122, 124, 245
forceps 16, 32, 115, 150, 184
Fountain, Barbara 170, 172
freedom of choice 42, 55, 91, 140, 158
*Frontline* (TV programme) 140–41
Furness General Hospital, UK 272

## G

Gadsby, Jon 175
Gane, Adrian 329n17
Gaskin, Ina May 16–19, 46, 63, 187
Gaskin, Stephen 16–17, 46
Geller, Stacie 254
general practice, maternity care in 167, 172, 176–77; *see also* GPs
Gibson, Gillian 238
Gilbertson, Tina 63, 86
Gillanders, Stan 11–12, 21
Gloriavale Christian Community 14
Gluckman, Peter 241

Godbold, Rosemary 218–20, 280
*The Good Fight* 238–39, 242
Gordon, Doris 95
GP obstetricians 3, 57; and acupuncture 23; collaboration with 157; exodus of 156, 158, 165–68, 170, 173, 175–78, 235–37, 259; and homebirth midwives 62, 64, 68, 160; on homebirth movement 13; and homeopathy 46; and LMC scheme 164–65, 181; and natural childbirth 142; in rural areas 179; use of term 328n2; *see also* homebirth doctors
GPs (general practitioners) 1, 3; collaboration with midwives 41, 158–61, 170, 178; instruction in obstetrics 57; and LMC scheme 162–64; midwives equivalent to 259; Pasifika women and 97; supervision of midwives 60–66
Graf, Friedrich 46
Graham Downs Community 118
Grant, Jeff 129
Gray, Robin 100
Great Barrier Island primary healthcare service 179
Green, Herb 109
Grehan, Madonna 72
Grey, Sandy 138, 161
Grieve, John 13, 63
'Growing up in New Zealand' study 257
Guilliland, Karen: and 1990 Act 118, 127–28, 130–31, 134, 272, 280; and Bev Lawton 253, 255; on biculturalism 153; and Cartwright Report 108–9; on consumer support for midwives 166; and criticism of midwifery model 241–42, 244; and Department of Health 107; on Direct Entry Midwifery Task Force 75; on doctor–midwife relationship 183–85, 258; and feminism 145; on fetal-centrism 217; and Garry Evans 209; on GPs and shared care 157, 170, 172–73, 175; and Health and Disability Commissioner 226; on immunisation 279; on lay midwives 79; on LMC scheme 163, 188–89; lobbying by 95–96, 101–3; and Lynda Exton 236; on Māori midwives 154–55, 339n77;

Guilliland, Karen (*cont.*) on medical technology 105, 202, 204; and midwife autonomy 139, 152; and midwifery training 192; on Nurses Act 1971 60; on Nursing Council 282; and NZNA 77, 86; on partnership model 146, 151, 154, 237, 276; as president of College of Midwives 40, 111; and Save the Midwives 92; on shortage of midwives 277; at Social Services Select Committee 123–24; and Wernham's research 263; and women's empowerment 34–35

Gulbransen, Graham 329n17, 330n42

Gunn, Jackie 192

Gurney, Jason 261

Guthrie, Margaret 217, 243

# H

Hahnemann, Samuel 21

Hammond, Mary 118

Handiside, Teenah 127

Hardie Boys, Bryan 63, 115

Harison, Christopher 16, 18, 53

Harrington, Chris 126–28, 136

Harrower, Micky 43, 45, 75, 78, 92

Harte, Helen Mountain 197–98

Hasslacher, Barbara 24, 64, 78

HBA (Home Birth Association) 10–13; and 1983 Act 59; and 1990 Act 116–17; bicultural conference 96–97; and College of Midwives 108, 154; and Department of Health 107; disbanding of national organisation 73, 93; doctors at conferences 36, 55, 63; foundation of 90; on homebirth package 20–21; and immunisation 27–29; and midwife pay 158; and midwifery standards review committees 83; on MSC 51; national lobbying by 94; promoting homebirth 30–34, 39, 47–48; and psychology 31; on 'real' midwives 71; on ultrasound 199; *see also* Home Birth Aotearoa

*HBA Auckland Newsletter* 94, 104, 160, 164

*HBA Newsletter* 90–92, 311n9; and 1983 Act 99–100; Donley and Baird in 40; editors of 43; GPs mentioned in 330n42; on homeopathy 21–22; on international movement 41, 43; taken over by Auckland 93; on technology 26–28; on vitamin K 200; on water births 25

The Health Alternatives for Women 39

Health and Disability Commissioner (HDC) 3, 137, 218–28, 267, 282–83, 361n75; and Jean O'Neil 188; and Jennifer Rowan 213; on partnership 279

Health and Disability Commissioner Act 1994 149

Health and Disability Services Act 1993 149, 161

Health Benefits Review 1986 100, 126

health foods 12

Health Funding Authority (HFA) 170, 180

health policy, consumer involvement in 105–6

Health Practitioners Competence Assurance Act 2003 207–8, 250

Health Practitioners Disciplinary Tribunal 218, 222, 282

health promotion 74, 208

Health Quality & Safety Commission New Zealand 232, 240, 246, 269

Health Select Committee 230; on immunisation 249; Lawton's submission to 260; and The Good Fight petition 239

heart monitoring, fetal 9, 184, 214, 220–23, 238, 273, 337n30; *see also* CTG

Helem, Ursula 14, 92

Helen Clark Foundation 270

Henaghan, Mark 184, 226

Henderson, Graeme 53

Hendry, Chris 174, 177

hepatitis B 28

Hercus, Ann 98–99, 101, 131

Herrick, R. 54

high-risk birth 39, 152, 188, 209, 260, 275

Te Hiiri Hauora 155

Hill, Anthony 218, 221, 225–26, 279

Hillary, Edmund 34

Hilton, John 23, 160–61, 329n17

Hinton, Brenda 143; on 1990 Act

112; and Direct Entry Midwifery Task Force 75; and DMS standards review committee 82; on doctor–midwife disagreements 185; and *HBA Newsletter* 19, 26, 43, 91, 97; on immunisation 201; and Save the Midwives 92
hippies 13–15; *see also* counterculture
Hodgson, Pete 232–33
Hogg, Vanya 38
Hokianga 22, 78–79
Hokianga Health Trust 171, 174
Holden, Helen 165
holistic approach 132, 179, 198–99
holistic/social model 182, 280
Holland, Dawn 194
Home Birth Aotearoa 216–17
homebirth: alternatives to 84–85; GPs involved with 160; midwives as persuaders for 279; negative outcomes of 140–41, 148, 183, 211, 219; numbers after 1990 Act 137, 142–43, 145, 226, 348n113; and perinatal mortality 261; studies on New Zealand outcomes 246; submitting information on 232; in Sweetman's analysis 220–21; vetting of women for 65, 183; *see also* hospital transfers; neonatal deaths
Homebirth Australia 43, 85
homebirth conferences 2, 43
homebirth doctors 13, 23, 63–64, 160, 164, 278, 329n17, 330n42
homebirth midwives 2; and 1983 Act 58; and 1990 Act 116; and counterculture 14–15, 18, 20–22; demands for autonomy *see* midwifery autonomy; Helen Clark and 104; independence prior to 1990 84; international situation of 42–43, 46; MSC report on 50, 52–54, 56; names for 10; nursing training for 74; practising alone 65–69; quality of 102; rates of pay 54, 63, 93, 101, 142; 158; relationship with doctors 60–62; training for 73; in UK 46; using medicalised framework 143–45; and women's empowerment 39
homebirth movement 1–2, 7; in 1970s and 1980s 10–13; and autonomy 70; and Cartwright Inquiry 109–10; celebrating Donley 139; and College of Midwives 137, 156, 205, 278, 284; and consumer advocacy 106; and the counterculture 13–18; criticism of midwives 142–45; and Fourth Labour Government 100–1; international 41–47; medical professionals and 49, 53; Pākehā domination of 153; persuading wider society 30–48; political activism of 90–96; rejecting modern technology 26–29; representativeness of 112
homebirth package 19–25, 206
homeopathy 12, 21–22, 24, 221, 293n150; lay midwives and 80; in midwifery model 198, 200; visiting experts on 28, 46
Hooper, Jenn: and AIM 242–45; on childbirth philosophy 278–79; Chisholm interviewing 241, 264; and The Good Fight 239; and Lawton's research 253–54, 258; on midwife accountability 282; and Nathan case 214, 217
Horowitz, L. 204
hospital births: early discharge after 55–56; growth in twentieth century 7–9; ideological opposition to 14, 18–19, 38; improved experience of 143; medical professionals on 49; midwives in charge during 188; and psychology 31–32; safety of 44; and women's empowerment 34–36
Hospital Boards' Association 53
hospital internships: coroners recommending 215–16; and direct-entry midwifery training 194; Hooper calling for 258; Lawton recommending 253–54, 281; public pressure for 240–41; Wellington Area Review on 234–35
hospital medicine, homebirth midwives and 3, 70, 82, 85, 88
hospital midwives: conducting homebirths 78; as de-skilled 215; homebirth midwives on 71–73; and independent midwives 189; and midwifery model 206; and partnership

hospital midwives (cont.) model 150–53, 156; petition by 240; relationship with doctors 60–61
hospital transfers 52, 244–46; delayed or refused by midwives 148, 211, 238, 265, 273; flying squads for 54; from homebirth 56; homebirth movement and 107; protocols on 182–87, 206, 221, 250
Howie, Ross 9, 217, 266
Hudson, Erin 248
Hugill, Colleen 212
humanism 51
Hunt, Jonathan 113, 124–25
Hunter, Dale 140–41, 211
Huntly Birthcare 214, 216
Hutchison, Paul 239, 249
Hutt Hospital, Lower Hutt 180, 188
Hutt Valley 18, 50
hypertension 126, 191, 256
HypnoBirthing 245
hypoxic ischaemic encephalopathy 220, 346n72

I

IAS (Immunisation Awareness Society) 27, 201–3, 247–49
ICEA (International Childbirth Education Association) 42, 138
Illich, Ivan 19, 290n82
immunisation 27–29, 182; adherence to directives 230; in early 21st century 247–50; in midwifery model 199, 201–3, 206, 279
Immunisation Advisory Centre 205, 247–48
incubators 8
indemnity insurance 83, 148–49
independent midwives 3, 46, 182; accountability of 237; capabilities of 188–89, 280–81, 284; coroner criticisms of 209–10; and indemnity insurance 149; relationship with doctors 183; scarcity in rural areas 277; supervision of 253; using medical framework 142–45
independent practitioner associations 172, 332n93

Indian women 256–57, 269, 361n81
induced labour 23, 32, 186, 188
infant mortality rates 72, 197, 232, 236
influenza 249–50
informed choice 187, 193, 203–4, 210, 219–20, 248–49
informed consent: to immunisation 201, 205, 247; as legal defence 227; in midwifery practice 219–20, 267, 279
Inquiry into Maternity Services (1938) 8
Insull, Tim 167
intensive-care units 211, 214, 252, 269
International Confederation of Midwives 46, 51
International Home Birth Movement 45
International Homebirth Conference, London 1987 2, 43–44, 78, 297n84
*International Journal of Gynecology and Obstetrics* 253, 255
International Medical Council on Vaccination 28
International Midwives Day 138
international systematic reviews 262
intracranial haemorrhage 200
ipecac 22

J

Jackson, Rhonda *see* Evans, Rhonda
Jennings, Peter 188
Jerusalem (commune) 15
Joan Donley Midwifery Research Collaboration 139
Johnson, Lannes 161, 238
Judd, Carly 22, 78–79

K

Kaa, Emere 198
Kainamu, Reena 198
Kaitāia 25, 43, 78–79
Karetai, Margaret 330n42
Keall, Judy 121, 125, 130–31
Keirse, Marc 185
Kemp, Henriette 25, 74, 93, 98, 100
Key, John 244
King, Annette 99, 166, 171, 173–76, 278

# Index

Kirk, Jenny 102, 113, 115, 122, 128, 131
Kirk, Norman 13
Kirkup, Bill 272, 274
Kitzinger, Sheila 34, 44–47
Kline, Wendy 17, 41, 78
Koopman-Boyden, Peggy 48, 115

## L

laboratory services 125, 161
labour, prolonged 214, 238
Labour Party: and 1983 Act 58–59, 90; first government 8; fourth government 74, 100–6; homebirth movement and 93–94, 98–100; third government 13
Laing, R. D. 16, 18, 31–32
Lamaze 17, 19
Lancaster, Paul 185
Larkin, Judy 39, 74, 92
Lauder, Erica 330n42
Lawton, Beverley (Bev) 232, 252–56, 260–61, 263–66, 268, 275, 281
Lawton, Maureen 119, 124, 132–33
lay midwives 16, 22; autonomy of 77–80; international 41–42; and water birth 25
Leachy, Roger 25
Leap, Nicky 146–47
Leboyer, Frederick 24, 32
Lecky-Thompson, Maggie 78, 86–87, 152, 245, 307n55
Leggat, Alistair 329n17
lesbian separatism 38
Let Mothers Choose 175
life experience 192, 239
Ligtermoet, Henny 43
*Little Treasures* (magazine) 168
LMC (Lead Maternity Carer) system 161–63, 182; auditing and accountability in 250; bonuses under 239; choice of providers under 257; contracts outside 170–74, 181; and GP exodus 176–77, 277–78; Guilliland on 276; and hospital staff 228, 234; and immunisation data 205, 247, 249; informed consent in 219; midwives in charge under 188–91, 255; and National Health Committee review 169; and neonatal deaths 211, 214–15, 253; in practice 164–67; referral to specialists under 252; responsibility for outcome under 263; and rural areas 179; and vitamin K prophylaxis 220
Loudon, Irvine 9
Loveridge, Graham 67, 204
Lovett, Lisa 203
low-risk pregnancies 45, 102, 121, 126–27, 133–34, 161, 280
Lydall, Wendy 203

## M

MacGregor, Duncan 9
MacKay, Pippa 170, 173, 177, 180, 243
Mackintosh, Andrew 55
Malatest Report 177, 180
Malcolm, Aussie 59, 93, 98
male doctors *see* medical profession, male
Malloy, Tim 180
Mandela, Nelson 163
Mannion, Lisa 148
Mantell, Colin 38, 197–98
Manu, Upali 167
Māori midwives 137, 339n77; and direct-entry training 195–97; and LMC scheme 174; recruitment of 154–56; training 81
Māori population 3
Māori service providers 174
Māori women: birth outcomes for 232, 260, 269; differing choices of 197–98; and homebirth movement 95–98, 153; homebirths 11, 79; hospital births 9; inequality of care for 263; and maternal morbidity 252; in National Health Committee review 168–69; and perinatal mortality 256, 272, 275, 277–79, 281, 283; in primary units 244; and suicide 270
Maori Women's Welfare League 154–55
Margaret Marsh Defence Fund Trust 41
Marr, Heather 117
Martis, Ruth 114, 131
Matenga, Gordon 1, 208, 211–14
maternal morbidity, severe 252, 260

maternal mortality 9, 27; PMMRC on 231, 240, 250, 270; in UK 272–73
Maternal Mortality Review Committee 231
Maternity Action 38, 92, 106–7
Maternity Action Alliance 108, 154
maternity benefit 8, 10, 55, 161; for doctors 119, 158; homebirth midwives claiming 50, 100, 125; and Nurses Amendment Act 1990 159
maternity care: concerns about quality of 250; evidence-based standards for 234; gaps in provision of 226; politicisation of 4
maternity hospitals 9; access agreement for 228; midwives working in 61, 72; reforming 51, 56; small 106, 119
maternity nursing 9, 41, 57, 80
maternity services: 1990s reforms to 161–62, 238; calls for audit of 231–33; consumer lobby in 166–67; HBA involvement in 106–7; and homebirths 49–50; marae-based 154–55; primary 112, 158–59, 177, 208, 284; role of hospitals in 84
Maternity Services Notice 226, 233–34
Maternity Transformation Programme (UK) 273–74
maternity units, small 56, 76, 81, 84
maternity wards 86
Matpro (Maternity Project) 171
Matthews, Maggie 140, 211
McAleer, Dorothy 9
McAra-Couper, Judith 18, 135, 194, 256, 271, 282
McClay, Roger 59
McCoy, Celeste 25, 46, 114
McCully, Murray 122, 129
McElrea, Richard 148
McFarland, Lynley 15, 63, 72, 85
Macfarlane, Barbara 13, 37, 39, 52, 92
McGarry, Sean 329n17
McGeorge, Victor 31McKay, Don 61
McKinnon, Don 102, 115–16, 122, 129, 131
McLean, Lyn 11, 13, 71; and Aussie Malcolm 98; on hospital midwives 73; and MSC 56; on nutrition 20–21; on politics of homebirth 39; and psychology 31
McLoughlin, David 110, 143, 157–59, 184
McNeil, Kathryn 162
McTigue, Maurice 96
meconium 68, 141–42, 147
medical advice 186, 227
Medical Audit Board (Netherlands) 82, 84
medical control 2, 89; arguments about safety as 156; and conflicting advice 147; Domino services as 85; threat of return to 238, 282; and transfer to hospital 206
Medical Council 67, 255
Medical Disciplinary Committee 142
medical intervention: midwives dismissive of 32, 34, 105, 222–23; mothers refusing 227; responsibility to accept 83; support for 40
medical model of childbirth 3, 208; and Cartwright Inquiry 109; homebirth movement opposing 37, 42; and midwife training 215, 264, 280; midwives adhering to 83–84, 144, 147, 151–52, 156; midwives opposing 182, 186–87, 191, 198, 274; use of term 206
Medical Practitioners Disciplinary Committee 183–84
medical profession: and 1990 Act 122, 128; male 34, 48, 108–9; nurses criticised for supporting 152
medical technology 3; College of Midwives and 182, 189; government questioning 89, 105; McAra-Couper on 271; rejection of 19, 26–29, 198–205, 284
Mein Smith, Philippa 110
men's involvement in childbirth 37–38, 41
Mental Health Foundation 31
mentoring 230; in direct-entry midwifery training 194–95, 235, 258; of Jennifer Rowan 212–13; recommended by Health and Disability Commissioner 218
Merry, Alan 246

Metcalfe, Wallace 63–64
*Metro* (magazine) 29, 108
Michaels, Paula 17
middle-class women 13, 29, 37, 45, 156
Middlemore Hospital, Auckland 151–52, 189
midwife autonomy 2, 50; and 1990 Act 67, 69, 115, 117, 120–21, 123–26, 134–36; and accountability 282; campaign for 71; celebration of 138–40; challenges to 140, 237; College of Midwives on 46, 234; and Dutch model 80–85, 88; and Fourth Labour Government 103–4; and lay midwifery 77–80; and LMC system 162; meaning of 70; and medical supervision 62–64; and Midwifery Council 207; NZNA on 86; and patient safety 228; and qualifications 75–77
midwifery: golden age of 72, 114; modern philosophy of 193; *see also* partnership model of midwifery
midwifery care: safe 208; substandard 189, 219–21, 224–25, 227–29, 243
Midwifery Council Competence Review Panel 227
Midwifery Council New Zealand 3, 108, 206, 275; accountability to 282–83; and Bev Lawton 254; competencies established by 207–8, 219, 223–24, 250; and coroner criticisms 215–16; on Crawshaw prosecution 227; first decade of 230; foundation of 207; HDC reports to 218; mentoring programme 258; on new graduates 225; suspending Hugill 212; suspending Matthews 211; Timutimu on 154; Tony Ryall and 241
Midwifery First Year of Practice (MFYP) 212, 235, 258
midwifery knowledge 187, 192–93
midwifery model of childbirth: criticisms of 228, 230, 275, 277; and direct-entry training 192, 194–95, 280; hospital midwives excluded from 151; and independent midwives 145, 182; and modern technology 198–206; opposed to medical model 140, 144, 194, 208

*Midwifery: Preparation for Practice* 185, 188, 207
midwifery qualification 57, 75
midwifery standards review committees 83, 142
midwifery training 3, 9–10, 75–76; academic structure of 81; Chisholm on 241; coroner criticisms of 209, 211, 213, 216; and Health and Disability Commissioner 226; in hospitals 9; Ngan on 259; and nursing training 57; *see also* direct-entry midwifery training
midwifery-led care 3; accessibility issues 276–78; accountability issues 281–83; College of Midwives defence of 251, 284; criticisms of 219, 235, 237, 242, 246–47, 250; and obstetricians 178; philosophical issues 278–79; research on 251–54, 256, 260–63, 265–66; and suicide 270; training issues 280–81
midwives: empowerment of 271; legal status of 1–2; *see also* homebirth midwives; hospital midwives; independent midwives; lay midwives; new graduate midwives; nurse-midwives; self-employed midwives
Midwives Act 1904 197
Midwives Registration Act 1904 9
'Midwives United Song' 91
Miller, Neil 204
Mills, Jackie 166, 330n42
Ministry of Health 3; data on maternity care 234, 246, 253; group schemes contracting with 171–73; on hospital internships 258; and immunisation data 247, 249; lobbying of 101; and Lynda Exton 236; Maternity Advisory Group 178; and midwifery leaders 230; National Maternity Monitoring Group 267, 271; and rural areas 178; and Sadler study 255–56; and Wernham's research 263; *see also* PMMRC
Ministry of Women's Affairs 101, 108
Minnell, Pat 62, 76
MMPO (Midwifery and Maternity Providers Organisation) 174, 179
Moonen, Kiet 16

Moore, Amale 188
*More* (magazine) 27
Morecambe Bay investigation 272–74
Morton, Susan 257
*Mother and Baby at Home – The Early Days* 50, 56, 56–58, 82–83, 99
mothers, partnership with 2
Motueka Women's Electoral Lobby 117
MSC (Maternity Services Committee) 2, 10, 283; 1979 pamphlet 50–51; 1979–80 inquiry into homebirths 16, 18, 39, 52–56, 65, 246; 1982 report *see Mother and Baby at Home – The Early Days*; and 1983 Act 59; activism targeting 93; on homebirth in communes 14; replacement by Women's Health Committee 74
Muir, Terryll 221
Muller, Veronica 22, 160
multidisciplinarity 270–71, 273–74, 277, 284
Munro, Rob 96
Murdoch, Campbell 29
Myers, Estelle 25
Myles, Maggie 72, 305n17

# N

Nacey, Mary 93, 99
Nambassa festivals 16–19
narcotics 105, 127, 191
Nash, Diana 35, 165, 329n17, 330n42
Nathan, Casey Missy Turama and Nathan-Tukiri, Kymani 214, 216–17, 286n1
National Council of Māori Nurses 154
National Council of Women (NCW) 68, 283; on 1983 Act 60; on 1990 Act 114–15, 119, 124–25, 130; on homebirth 52, 54; and shared care 166
National Health Committee, review of maternity services 168–70, 172, 180–81, 205, 257
National Home Birth Publicity Week 91–93
National Homebirth Australia 43
National Immunisation Register 249
National Maternity Services Coordinator 167
National Party 14, 94, 98, 129, 235; and midwives and GPs 157, 159; and Nurses Amendment Act 1990 115
National Women's Hospital, Auckland 9, 11, 103; Bert Potter on 55; closure of 165; courses at 51, 57; and elective caesareans 242, 353n69; flying squad at 53; *see also* Cartwright Inquiry
natural childbirth 2–3, 30; advocates of 108; changing attitudes to 242, 284; and epidurals 47; informed consent to 227; Maggie Myles on 72; midwives' ideology of 117, 147–48, 272–74, 278; psychological arguments for 32–33; right to 121
naturopathy 22, 198, 203
Nealie, John 16
Nelson Area Health Board 117
Nelson HBA 15, 106, 117
neoliberalism 159
neonatal care, high-tech 33, 104–5
neonatal deaths: Bev Lawton on 253; coroner's reports on 140–41, 148, 187, 208–16; Health and Disability Commissioner on 223, 227–28; from intracranial haemorrhage 200; PMMRC data on 250, 269; and uterine rupture 185; and Wellington Area Review 233; *see also* perinatal mortality
neonatal encephalopathy 231, 246, 262, 269
Netherlands 68; homebirth in 57–58, 61, 119; homebirth midwives in 50; midwife autonomy in 80–85, 126; pain relief in 242; perinatal mortality in 260–61; primary units in 245
new graduate midwives: and adverse outcomes 253–57, 267–68, 281; and coroners' reports 211–12, 215–16; petition of concern about 240; substandard care by 224–26, 229; training and supervision of 216–17, 241, 250, 258; and Wellington Area Review 233–34
New Zealand China Friendship Society 23, 36

# Index

New Zealand College of Midwives 1–3, 34; and 1990 Act 46–47, 95, 117–18, 125, 128, 130–31; 1990 conference 110–11; 2010 history 208; and AIM 243–44; on Australian review 237–38; and Barlow case 229; and Bev Lawton 252–54, 258; celebrating autonomy 137–38; code of ethics 217; complaints to Press Council 214, 265; contemporary criticisms of 284; and coroners 209–11, 215; and disciplinary processes 283; foundation of 86–88, 90, 107; and GPs 160–61, 170, 172–73; Helen Clark and 105, 110, 113, 121, 125; and homebirth deaths 141–42; and hospital medicine 70; and hospital midwives 240; on immunisation 247–49; and Irihapeti Ramsden 196; and lay midwives 79–80; and LMC scheme 162; and Lynda Exton 236; on medical technology 199–200, 204–5; and midwifery model 182, 205–6; on midwifery training 133, 194, 258–59, 268, 280; on multidisciplinarity 274–75; and partnership model 145–46, 151, 156, 180, 279; partnership with Māori 153–56, 196; on pay for midwives 159; and prescribing 191; reviews by 225, 234; and rural areas 178; and Sadler's research 256; and shared care schemes 278; on transfers to hospital 183–84; and Wellington Area Review 233, 235; and Wernham's research 263; and women doctors 164; *see also* MMPO

*New Zealand College of Midwives Handbook for Practice* 142, 219, 222–23

*New Zealand College of Midwives Journal*: and Bev Lawton 255; on bioscience 194; on breech births 186, 210; criticism of independent midwives 144–45; Donley in 40, 139, 199; on Health and Disability Commissioner 218–19; on LMC scheme 163; on medical technology 199, 203, 205; myths about the past in 197; on partnership model 111; Wagner in 47

New Zealand College of Obstetricians and Gynaecologists *see* College of Obstetricians and Gynaecologists (New Zealand/Australia)

*New Zealand Doctor* (magazine) 107, 167; on 1990s reforms 238, 266; on Bev Lawton 253; on doctor–midwife disagreements 189; on GP obstetricians and shared care 166–68, 170, 172, 175–76, 236; Guilliland in 154; on immunisation 249; on maternity services audit 232; on petitions 240; reporting on midwives' conferences 144, 162

New Zealand General Practitioners' Association 123, 167

*New Zealand Listener* (magazine): and 1983 Act 73; and 1990 Act 67–68; on Australian review 237–38; on coroners and midwife competency 215–17; on homebirth movement 22, 24, 91, 94; on lay midwives 78; and LMC scheme 166; and MSC survey 54–55; on vaginal examinations 210; and Wernham's research 264–66

New Zealand Medical Association 83, 257; and 1980 MSC inquiry 54; and 1990 Act 120, 123, 128; and LMC scheme 162; on maternity care payments 159; on midwifery training 130; and review of maternity services 167

New Zealand Medical Women's Association 120, 123, 141

New Zealand Planning Council 48, 115

New Zealand Register of Acupuncturists 23

*New Zealand Woman's Weekly* (magazine) 11–12, 27, 31, 39, 168

New Zealand Women's Health Network 37

Ngā Maia Māori Midwives Aotearoa 155–56, 195

Nga Puna Ora Te Atiawa 154

Ngan, Cherry 259

Ngan Kee, Digby 227

Ngati Porou Hauora Board 171

NHI (National Health Index) 232

Nicol, Jennie 101

Nixon, Leon 330n42

Noble-Spruell, Carolyn 46

non-interventionist philosophy 1, 185, 194, 213, 222, 278–79
normal birth 46, 62; equivalency of midwives and GPs for 162; ideological positions on 184, 278–80; midwives' role in 76, 104, 114, 134, 241; and Royal College of Midwives 274; war against 89
normal life event, birth as 195, 207–8, 211, 241, 278–79
*North & South* (magazine) 4, 110, 114, 143, 157, 240, 282
Northland Area Health Board 108
Nottingham University Hospitals NHS Trust 274
nurse-midwives 41, 71, 205, 253
Nurses Act 1971 50, 57, 60, 68
Nurses Act 1977 61, 114
Nurses Amendment Act 1983 58–60, 73–74, 88, 99–100, 105–6
Nurses Amendment Act 1990 1–2, 7, 89, 110–13, 135–36; amendments to 125–29; and autonomy 133–35; and Cartwright Inquiry 109–10; consequences of 137–38, 140–44, 156, 266, 277; debate on 47; direct-entry midwifery training in 129–33; and GPs 157–58; and homebirth 114–16; and Māori 153; precursors to 52; and prescription authority 190; at select committee 121–25; submissions on 116–21; and transfer to hospitals 182–83
Nurses and Midwives Board 73
Nurses and Midwives Registration Act 1925 9
nursing: alignment with midwifery 72–73, 152; and Cartwright Inquiry 108–9; *see also* obstetric nursing
Nursing Council of New Zealand 66, 74, 106; and 1990 Act 128; and homebirth midwives 141, 186–87, 221; and midwifery training 129, 131, 193; professional misconduct charges 148, 282; requirements for midwifery registration 75–76
nursing training: in 1970s 14; general 9, 57, 73–76, 131; impact on midwives

76–77, 192; requirement for midwives 1, 130, 179–80
nutrition 12, 20, 82, 248
NZNA (New Zealand Nurses' Association) 2, 49; and 1990 Act 116, 118; and midwives 73–74
NZNA Midwives' and Obstetric Nurses' Special Interest Section: 1980 policy statement 55, 58, 73; on homebirth 49, 51–52, 68, 85–88; on midwifery training 75, 77

# O

Oakley, Ann 44–46
O'Brien, Gayle 61, 67, 132
obstetric advisory committees 83
obstetric nursing, unsupervised 58, 60–62; *see also* NZNA
Obstetric Regulations 1985 86
Obstetric Review Committee 107
Obstetrical and Gynaecological Society 53, 65, 83
obstetricians: homebirth movement opposing 36–40, 43, 45–47, 49, 89; hospital 126, 189, 223; in LMC scheme 164; poor relationships with midwives 235; specialist 40, 177–78
obstetrics 8; education in 57; Maggie Myles on 72; threats to 40, 45
Ockenden, Donna 273–74
Odent, Michel 24–25, 44–46, 94
Ohu scheme 13
O'Neil, Jean 188–89
O'Regan, Katherine 96, 111, 114, 122, 128–29, 131, 135, 141
Orr, Leonard 32
osteopaths 22, 28, 198
Otago Polytechnic 192–94, 204
*Our Bodies Ourselves* 37, 295n41
oxytocin 8, 144, 199–200

# P

Page, Lesley 138, 157
pain management, without drugs 24–25
pain relief 7–8, 23, 47, 127, 189, 242, 279

Pairman, Sally 3, 18, 25, 63; and 1990 Act 123, 128, 130, 134, 139, 280; on biculturalism 153; and College of Midwives 111; on Donley and Clark 103; and feminism 145; and fetal heart monitoring 223; and historical myths 197; on hospital midwives 152–53; and LMC scheme 163; lobbying by 95–96, 101; on Māori midwives 339n77; on Marilyn Waring 95; on midwife autonomy 134–35, 282, 286n3; on midwifery training 76, 192–93, 195, 240; and Midwives Council 206; on multidisciplinarity 274–75; and NZNA 77, 86; on partnership model 146–47, 150–51, 237, 279; on pay for midwives 159

Pākehā women: and homebirth movement 11, 13, 90, 97, 154; hospital births 9

Palmer, Geoffrey 103, 122, 133

Palmerston North Hospital 15, 18, 53

Paraku, Lisa 268

Parents Centre 18, 33, 42, 93; and 1990 Act 118; and NZ College of Midwives 108, 154; and rural maternity services 178; and shared care 166, 176

Parents for Safe Births 137, 147–48, 150

Parker, Jess 54

partnership model of midwifery 137, 146–53, 156, 193, 276, 279, 282

Pasifika women: birth outcomes for 232, 252, 256, 269, 272; and homebirth movement 96–98, 154; inequality of care for 263; in National Health Committee review 168–69; training as midwives 81, 155

Paterson, Ron 149–50, 218–21, 224, 227–28

patient safety 131, 163, 228, 234

patients' rights, breaches of 218, 221

Patterson, Jean 17

Pattison, Neil 231

Paul, Charlotte 264

Pearce, Joseph Chilton 32

peer review 82, 120, 239

Pelvin, Bronwen 93; and 1990 Act 86, 117–18; and doctors 66–69; and Helen Clark 104; and homebirth deaths 142; and hospital medicine 85; on lay midwives 79–80; and midwife accountability 283; on midwife autonomy 107, 135; in midwifery textbooks 194; on midwifery training 77; at Ministry of Health 267, 271; and NZCOM 87; on partnership model 147–48, 150; and Riverside Community 14–15, 289n53; and *Spiritual Midwifery* 18; on women's empowerment 34–35

perinatal database 168, 231–32, 239

perinatal mortality: in Australia 309n100; for Māori women 275; and midwife experience 253, 256, 260; in the Netherlands 261; New Zealand rates 52, 232, 236, 275; PMMRC on 240; and safety 141; UK inquiry on 56; *see also* neonatal deaths

perineum, inadequate care of 225

pethidine 190, 212, 279

petitions 167, 175, 239–40

Petousis-Harris, Helen 248

petticoat government 95

pharmacists 258–59

pharmacology 126, 190–91

Pittam, Deb 217, 256, 265–66, 271

placenta: burial of 196–98; retained 53

*PLOS Medicine* (journal) 260

Plunket nurses 54, 74, 306n27

Plunket Society 27, 167

PMMRC (Perinatal and Maternal Mortality Review Committee) 3, 209–10, 230–32, 250, 268–72, 284; AIM and 243; deaths reported to 234, 236; and LMC system 257–58; on midwifery training 281; reports 240, 243, 246, 269–70

polio 27–28, 204

polycose tests 144

posterior presentation 22–23, 80, 150, 221, 279

postnatal care 20, 57, 158, 167; National Health Committee review on 169; in rural areas 179

postnatal depression 173

postpartum haemorrhage 200; drugs to treat 8, 22, 27; and homebirths 78; treatment in hospital 11, 53
post-term birth 185
Potter, Bert 14, 24, 55
Poutasi, Karen 132
power inequalities 146, 150
pre-eclampsia 220, 277, 279, 281
Prendergast, Kerry 171
prescribing rights 22, 122–24, 126, 128, 190–91; *see also* drugs
Press Council 214, 265–66
pre-term birth 8, 269
Primal Health Research Centre 44
primary birthing units 3, 151–52, 230, 244–46; ethnicity and deprivation in 269; hospital transfer from 227, 238–39; lack of medical facilities 216; neonatal deaths in 212, 281
professional development 68, 221
professional misconduct 148, 188, 219, 222, 307n55
psychology, and homebirth 31–33
psychosexual experience 34, 47
Public Health and Disability Act 2000 231, 233, 250
Puea O Pua 155
puerperal sepsis 8

## Q

quality assurance 120, 123
Queen Mary Hospital, Dunedin 227

## R

Railton, Phil 329n17, 330n42
Rama, Joanne 155–56
Ramsden, Irihapeti 96, 154, 196
raspberry leaf tea 19, 21
Rau-Kupa, Marjorie 96
Rāwene hospital 78
Ray, Pauline 54
Raymond, Janice 330n42
rebirthing 32
record-keeping *see* documentation, by midwives

referral criteria 85, 184, 186, 213, 217, 244
Register of Midwives 207, 222, 250
Reid, Rosemary 231
resuscitation: attempts at 187, 270; Ockenden review on 273; poor 220, 224, 239, 243
RHAs (regional health authorities) 161–62, 170, 172, 180
Richardson, Ruth 99–100
risk assessments 85, 218, 273
risk factors 65, 84
risk selection 261
Ritchie, David 28, 293n150
River Ridge Birthing Centre, Hamilton 212
Riverside Community 15, 118, 271, 289n53
Robertson, Adele 179–80
Robertson, Lois 124–25
Robertson, Vicki 177
Rodenburg, Helen 162, 171, 175–76
Ronayne, Ian 71–72
Rose, Edna 151
Rosevear, Sylvia 214, 216
Rothman, Barbara Katz 147, 159
Rowan (Campbell), Jennifer 212–14, 241
Royal Australian and New Zealand College of Obstetricians and Gynaecologists *see* College of Obstetricians and Gynaecologists
Royal College of Midwives 87, 148, 251, 274
Royal College of Nursing Australia 179
Royal College of Obstetricians and Gynaecologists 26; New Zealand Council of 52, 54
Royal New Zealand College of General Practitioners 170–71, 176
rural areas, maternity care in 167, 169, 171, 174, 178–80, 244–45, 277–78
Rushmer, Philip 160–61
Ruzek, Sheryl 41
Ryall, Tony 232–33, 235, 239, 241

## S

Sadler, Lynn 256, 260, 267, 281
safe care 207, 267

Safe Maternity Campaign (1920s) 8
safety issues, professionals disagreeing on 147
Sage, Jennifer 56
Salvation Army Women's Organisation 119
SAMCL 170, 172–73
Sarfati, Diana 261, 263–64, 267
Savage, Wendy 44, 46
*Save the Midwife* (Donley) 71, 138, 165
Save the Midwives Association 73–74, 88, 92, 99–100, 108, 117; Direct Entry Midwifery Task Force 43, 75–77, 80–81, 94–95, 131, 154, 192
Scanlan, Margaret 71–72
scaremongering 237, 247, 251, 254, 263
Scheibner, Viera 28, 203
Scott, Claudia 100
secondary care 151, 178, 184
the self, discourses of 193
self-determination, women's 39, 96, 111
self-employed midwives 171, 195, 213; becoming hospital midwives 228; in MMPO 174; in Wellington Area Review 234–35, 238
self-esteem 35–36
self-responsibility 19, 106
*Sensitive Midwifery* (Flint) 87, 194
septicaemia 252
service clubs, women's branches of 95
sexual politics 37
Shanks, Margaret 165, 170
shared care 157–60, 181; group schemes for 169–75, 177, 180, 206, 278; and LMC scheme 164, 166; National Health Committee review and 168–70; pay under 159
Sharplin, Anne 14, 75, 92
Shaw, Sally 131
Shields, Margaret 58–59, 116
Shipley, Jenny 162–63
Shrewsbury and Telford Hospital NHS Trust 273
SIDS (sudden infant death syndrome) 28–29, 203, 232
Simmers, Don 178–79
Singer, Jan 330n42
Sissons, Anne 189

Skiff, Samantha 61, 71, 76
Skinner, Joan 146, 150, 181, 219
Sloan, David 85
Smail, Sheryl 76, 79, 104, 125, 132–33
Smith, Barbara 109
Smith, Ian 211
smoking 11–12, 20, 51, 216, 223, 256, 264
Snead, Eva 203
social birth 17
Social Security Act 1964 159
Social Services Select Committee 121, 129
South Link Health (SLH) 172–73
specialist care: in hospital 97, 127, 151; late referrals to 169, 252
*Spiritual Midwifery* (Gaskin) 16–18
St Andrews Medical Centre, Hamilton 158
St George's Private Hospital, Christchurch 53
St Helen's Hospital, Auckland 61, 71
St Helen's hospitals 9–10, 61–62, 236; midwifery training at 51, 72, 75–76
Stanbridge, Chris 213, 227
Stanley, James 261
Stent, Robyn 186
Stewart, Sarah 138, 153
stillbirths 180, 219, 221, 232, 238, 273
Stimpson, Glenda 52, 61
Stirling, Pamela 63, 67–68, 79–80, 127, 266–67
Stojanovic, Jane 18
Stone, Peter 188, 233
Strid, Judi 39; criticism of independent midwives 144; and Direct Entry Midwifery Task Force 75, 80, 131; and international movement 46–47; on medical technology 200; on political activism 96; on prescription rights 190; and Save the Midwives 92
suicide 270
Supplementary Order Paper 66 116, 121–25, 128
Supplementary Order Paper 67 129–31
Sutherland, Allan 142, 184–85, 259, 278
Sutherland, Nancy 42
Swagerman-Fugle, Saskia Marama 209
Sweetman, Claire 219–22, 224, 226, 280
systemic failure 229

## T

Tait, John 271
Tapsell, Peter 59, 116
Te Tātai Haouroa o Hine Centre for Women's Health 275
technology: obstetrics and 36, 39; rejection of 26–27
Terry, Jayne 274
Tew, Marjorie 44
Thames Hospital Board 83
tikanga Māori 153, 197
Tilyard, Murray 172
Timutimu, Mina 154–55
Tizard, Bob 93
Tohunga Suppression Act 196–97, 339n83
toxaemia 8, 51
Treaty of Waitangi 96–97, 137, 153–54
Tui Community 118
Tukiri, Hayden 214
Tukuitonga, Collin 247–48
Tuohy, Pat 236, 263
Tupara, Hope 195, 197–98
Turner, Nikki 247, 249
Tutukaka Dolphin Centre 25
twin pregnancy 185

## U

UK (United Kingdom): flying squads in 53, 124; GP obstetricians in 177; homebirth midwives in 50, 76, 194; homebirth movement in 56; inquiries in 272–75; maternal mortality in 231, 250; and New Zealand midwifery model 138, 157; suicide in 270
ultrasound scans 9, 72; health board policies on 107; interpreting 281; opposition to 26, 91, 144, 199
umbilical shock 32
'unfortunate experiment': at National Women's Hospital 108–10; New Zealand's maternity reforms as 237–38
Union Health Centres 171
United Nations World Conference for Women 101
United Women's Convention 50, 299n3
University of Auckland, Community Health Project 26, 33
Upton, Simon 190
uterine rupture 185–86, 188

## V

Vaccination Information Network 203
vaginal examinations 209–11
Vague, Stephanie 215
Venkataiah, Rukmini 16
vitamin K 26, 199–200, 220

## W

Waata, Mandy 35, 38, 78
Wagner, Marsden 44–47, 110–11, 140, 199, 202
Waikato Area Health Board 83, 119, 124
Waikato District Health Board 229, 233
Waikato Women's Hospital 186–87
Wall, Carole 51
Wall, Rose 277–81, 283
Wanganui Area Health Board 119
Ware, Maria 18, 22
Waring, Marilyn 94–95, 98, 100, 117
water births 25, 44, 59
Waterford Birthing Centre, Hamilton 214
Watson, Yvette 14
Waugh, Heather 71
Wellington Area Health Board 85, 107
Wellington Area Review 2008 233–35, 238
Wellington HBA 11–12, 46, 93–94, 99, 101
Wellington Hospital 252
Wellington Women's Health Research Centre 252
Wernham, Ellie 260–68, 272–73
West, Dave 12
Te Whatu Ora 269
Wheeler, Kim 151
White, Gillian 210, 343n13
whooping cough 20, 27
Wilcox, Jonathan 68, 226
Wilde, Fran 99

Wiles, Anton 170
Williams, Lynda 26; on 1983 Act 99; on 1990 Act 136; and biculturalism 97; and childbirth education 42; on Direct Entry Midwifery Task Force 75; and DMS standards review committee 82; on *HBA Newsletter* 90; on Health and Disability Commission 149; on immunisation 248; and LMC scheme 166–67; lobbying by 102; and Save the Midwives 92; and women's empowerment 33–34
Williams, Ulric 203
Wishart, Kitty 19–20, 23
Witchalls, Julia M. 54
Witt, Janne 166
Witten, Michelle 141–42, 147–48
Wolf, Jacqueline 242
womanhood, affirmation of 217
women's bodies 37, 39, 183
Women's Division Federated Farmers 118–19, 150
women's empowerment 2, 33–37, 39, 45, 146
women's groups, and 1990 Act 116
Women's Health Committee 74, 94
Women's Health Conference 1982 92
women's health movement 37, 39, 89, 107
women's liberation 36
Wood, Pamela 197
World Health Organization 45, 75, 231; on child mortality 57; definition of midwives 73, 77, 305n20; SHE and HE scenarios 101
Wormald, Muriel 173

## Y

Yates, Anne 233
yeast 19–20
yoga 21, 24
Young, Carolyn 20, 51; on 1990 Act 110; and doctors 62, 65, 160, 164; and *HBA Newsletter* 91; and hospital practice 143
Young, Catherine 76
Young, Diony 42, 138

Younge, Roy 244
Yusak, Monica 330n42

## Z

Zimmer, Coralie 205

**LINDA BRYDER** gained her MA (1st Class Hons) at the University of Auckland in 1980, and her DPhil in the history of science at the University of Oxford in 1985. Her doctoral thesis was published by Oxford University Press as *Below the Magic Mountain: A Social History of Tuberculosis in Twentieth-Century Britain* (1988). Linda held a research fellowship at The Queen's College, Oxford, from 1984 to 1988, and was awarded a British Academy Post-Doctoral Fellowship in 1987.

Since returning to New Zealand in 1988, Linda has taught history at the University of Auckland and in 2008 was appointed professor. She has an extensive publication list in the social history of health and medicine, including over one hundred peer-reviewed journal articles and book chapters, and significant monographs in the history of women and children's health, including *A Voice for Mothers: The Plunket Society and Infant Welfare, 1907–2000* (2003), *A History of the 'Unfortunate Experiment' at National Women's Hospital* (2009) and *The Rise and Fall of National Women's Hospital: A History* (2014), all published by AUP.

In 2014 she was awarded an inaugural University of Auckland Research Excellence Award. From 2007 to 2023 she held an honorary chair at the London School of Hygiene & Tropical Medicine. She is a Fellow of the Royal Society of New Zealand Te Apārangi. A founding editor of the Oxford journal *Social History of Medicine*, Linda has served on the editorial board of several international medical history journals and co-edits the *New Zealand Journal of History*. She is currently President of the Australian and New Zealand Society of the History of Medicine.